PEDIATRIC EMERGENCIES

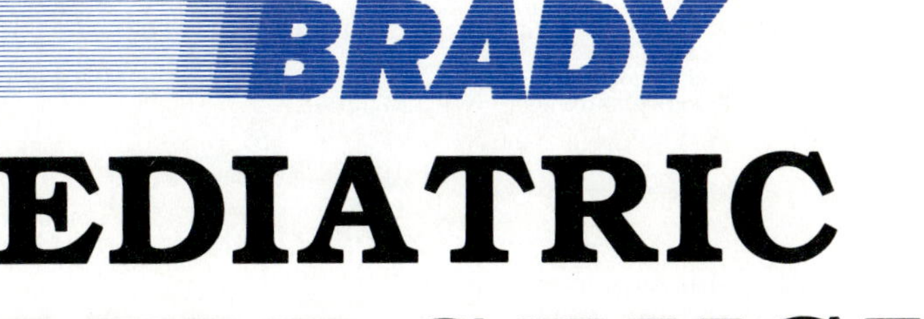

PEDIATRIC EMERGENCIES

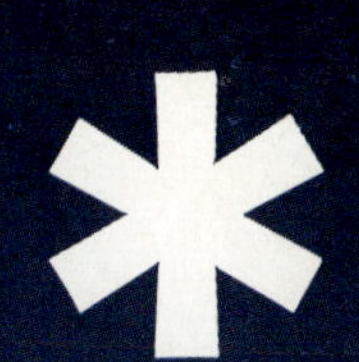

A Manual for Prehospital Care Providers

Martin R. Eichelberger M.D.

Jane W. Ball R.N., DR.P.H.

Geraldine S. Pratsch R.N., M.P.H.

Eliane Runion B.S.W.

BRADY
A Prentice Hall Division
Englewood Cliffs, New Jersey 07632

Library of Congress Cataloging-in-Publication Data

Pediatric emergencies : a manual for prehospital care providers /
    Martin R. Eichelberger . . . [et al.].
        p.   cm.
    Rev. ed. of: Pediatric emergencies manual. c1984.
    Includes bibliographical references and index.
    ISBN 0–89303–803–2
    1. Pediatric emergencies.   I. Eichelberger, Martin.
II. Pediatric emergencies manual.
    [DNLM: 1. Accidents—in infancy & childhood—handbooks.
    2. Emergencies—in infancy & childhood—handbooks.   WS 39 P3706]
RJ370.P4264   1992
618.92′ 0025—dc20
DNLM/DLC
for Library of Congress   91–20573
                                                                        CIP

Acquisitions editor: Natalie Anderson
Editorial/production supervision: Ed Jones
Interior design: Andy Zutis
Cover design: Ben Santora
Cover photo: F.P.G.
Prepress buyer: Mary McCartney & Ilene Levy
Manufacturing buyer: Ed O'Dougherty
Editorial Assistant: Louise Fullam

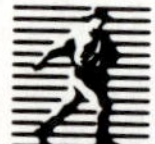

This book was previously published
under the title *Pediatric Emergencies Manual*,
M.R. Eichelberger and G. Stossel-Pratsch, eds.,
Rockville, Md.: Aspen Publishers, 1984.

Chapter 4 was contributed by
Michael McAdams, NREMT-P.

Printed in the United States of America
10 9 8 7 6 5 4 3 2 1

ISBN   0-89303-803-2

Prentice-Hall International (UK) Limited, *London*
Prentice-Hall of Australia Pty. Limited, *Sydney*
Prentice-Hall Canada Inc., *Toronto*
Prentice-Hall Hispanoamericana, S.A., *Mexico*
Prentice-Hall of India Private Limited, *New Delhi*
Prentice-Hall of Japan, Inc., *Tokyo*
Simon & Schuster Asia Pte. Ltd, *Singapore*
Editora Prentice-Hall do Brasil, Ltda, *Rio de Janeiro*

Dedication

This text is dedicated to all Prehospital Care Providers and the children and families in their care.

Prehospital Care Providers have become champions in changing the EMS system to accommodate the child. We salute all of you in your professionalism and dedication!

Contents

3   General Pediatric Assessment

4   Equipment and Procedures for Management of ABC's

Pediatric Cardiopulmonary Resuscitation **5**

77

Respiratory Emergencies **6**

101

12   Burns
183

13   Child Abuse
195

14   Newborn Management
207

Apnea and Sudden Infant Death Syndrome **15**
219

Suicide in Children and Adolescents **16**
227

Crisis and Stress Management **17**
235

Index

Preface

The past decade has seen a rapid expansion in the provision of improved emergency care for children by the Emergency Medical Services community nationwide. This interest was triggered by federal initiatives which provided funding from the Department of Transportation, National Highway Traffic Safety Administration (DOT, NHTSA) and the Department of Health and Human Services, Bureau of Maternal and Child Health (DHHS, BMCH).

In 1983, Children's National Medical Center (CNMC) received funding from the Devore Foundation, Washington, DC, to develop and offer a continuing medical education program for prehospital providers in pediatric emergency care. This experience led to the national Pediatric Emergency Medical Services Training Program (PEMSTP), funded by DOT and DHHS. This four-year project trained 190 EMS instructors from all 50 states, the District of Columbia, and two US territories in pediatric emergency care. These instructors were encouraged to disseminate the pediatric knowledge and skills they learned in their respective states.

The information contained in *Pediatric Emergencies* is the result of valuable experience we obtained while conducting prehospital education programs for EMS providers and instructors. These students shared their insights and suggestions to help shape the organization and content in this text, which is much more extensive than our first text, *Pediatric Emergencies Manual.*

The Emergency Medical Trauma Center at CNMC recognizes the importance of prehospital care within its Continuum of Care philosophy. This continuum is initiated with Prevention activities, and includes organized care in the Prehospital, Emergency Department, Intensive Care Unit, General Care Unit, and Rehabilitation phases of care. The interdisciplinary nature of the pediatric emergency care requires that both the prehospital and hospital team approach to the seriously ill or injured child be standardized and cohesive for an optimal outcome.

Pediatric Emergencies is written to document a standard of prehospital pediatric emergency care for both the basic and advanced levels of prehospital care providers. It is the intent of this text to convey that children are uniquely different from adults in anatomic, physiologic, and emotional characteristics that need special consideration when managing serious illness or injury.

The first chapters address the complex emotional and psychosocial characteristics of the child and family. The text identifies by developmental stage how each child deals with the fear of being in an emergency situation. The parents are equally anxious and may display a range of emotions that prehospital care providers must recognize and manage. Having an understanding of the interdependent relationship between the parent and child enables the prehospital provider to better manage the child's care and to assist the child and family to work through their crisis.

Subsequent chapters of pediatric assessment and procedures for management of the ABCs are the keystones necessary in becoming proficient and confident in managing the pediatric patient. The assessment chapter gives the "how to" guidelines for approaching the child and the rationale. The descriptions of the anatomy and physiology identify the uniqueness of the child and justify the procedures discussed. The procedures chapter is thorough in explaining management strategies tailored to the pediatric patient. For example, because airway management is so important, significant attention is paid to all appropriate methods of basic and advanced life support airway management.

We have made every attempt to be comprehensive in presenting medical and trauma emergencies. Frequently encountered conditions are covered, such as respiratory conditions and blunt trauma, as well as those less frequently encountered, such as diabetic ketoacidosis and penetrating trauma. These chapters are organized with an overview of each condition, the physiologic responses of the child, assessment guidelines, and management. Both basic and advanced care is delineated to guide pediatric management for providers of different skill levels.

Several other chapters highlight the role of the prehospital provider in the emergency management of children. The newborn, small and unresisting, demands solid skill and knowledge to prevent rapid physiologic deterioration. The newborn chapter focuses on the care of the infant after birth and safe transport to the hospital. Management of the newborn in distress is emphasized to ensure optimal care. Emergency care of the child with special care needs due to a chronic health condition or terminal illness have also been addressed. There is a growing number of children with these conditions cared for at home with high technology equipment who may access EMS.

One concern addressed in the educational sessions conducted at CNMC was the feelings triggered in prehospital providers when managing the child and family in emergency situations. Feelings run strong when the prehospital provider sees his or her own child in the patient, confronts the injustice of child abuse or neglect, or relives the tragedy of a child's death. Handling parents who may be unreasonable and demanding adds another dimension to the duties of the prehospital provider which cause stress. For this reason, a chapter on stress recognition and management has been included.

The authors have attempted to provide a knowledge and skill base for the prehospital provider to become confident and competent in delivering care to seriously ill or injured children and their families. We remain impressed with the level of dedication, enthusiasm, and child advocacy prehospital providers express in their quest for more knowledge about emergency care of children. We hope many of your current and future questions will be answered by this text.

MARTIN R. EICHELBERGER, M.D.
JANE W. BALL, RN, DrPH
GERALDINE S. PRATSCH, RN, MPH
ELIANE F. RUNION, BSW

Acknowledgments

The authors are grateful to Prentice Hall for the opportunity to develop and design a pediatric emergency textbook to meet the current needs of prehospital care providers across the United States. The efforts of Natalie Anderson, our editor, and Ed Jones, our production editor, have enabled us to provide you with a high quality text. George Dodson created the strong visual appeal of this text with his sensitive photography of children. We are also grateful to the parents, children, and prehospital care providers who gave their time for long photography sessions, to get the techniques just right.

Development of this book would not have occurred without the continuing requests and encouragement of the EMT instructors who attended the Pediatric Emergency Medical Services Training Program (PEMSTP) at Children's National Medical Center over the past five years. We learned as much from these individuals as we taught. Without them, there would have been little incentive to get the original book rewritten and published.

We must give special recognition to Mike McAdams, NREMT-P, a graduate of PEMSTP, and friend of the Emergency Trauma Services. He not only contributed the Equipment and Procedures chapter for the book; he answered numerous questions and helped organize the photography sessions.

Another individual deserving special recognition is John Clark, NREMT-P, the present coordinator of PEMSTP and other pediatric prehospital educational programs. He willingly provided frequent consultations and suggestions to improve the final manuscript.

Finally, we must acknowledge and thank our families, who willingly gave us the time and support to complete the manuscript.

About the Authors

Martin R. Eichelberger, M.D., F.A.C.S., F.A.A.P., is Professor of Surgery and Pediatrics at the George Washington University School of Medicine, and Director of Emergency Trauma Services, Children's National Medical Center in Washington, DC. A special interest in children led to development of a pediatric emergency curriculum of specialized knowledge, skills, and equipment for the prehospital provider. This commitment presently extends to childhood injury prevention as president of the National SAFE KIDS Campaign. As a member of many local, state, and federal initiatives, he represents the needs of children and their families. He is also the author of many publications and a research investigator on all aspects of care of the seriously ill or injured child from prevention through pediatric trauma systems development and rehabilitation.

Jane W. Ball, R.N., Dr.P.H., is the Program Director of the Pediatric Emergency Education and Research Center for the Emergency Trauma Services of Children's National Medical Center, Washington, DC. She was the coordinator of the Pediatric Emergencies Medical Services Training Program, a nationwide federally funded project for instructors of prehospital care providers. She continues to teach prehospital providers, to advocate improved pediatric emergency education for prehospital care providers, and to develop pediatric emergency education programs for other health care professionals.

Geraldine L. Pratsch, R.N., M.P.H., is the Pediatric Emergency Education Coordinator for the Emergency Trauma Services of the Children's National Medical Center, Washington, D.C. She has been responsible for the development of regional and national prehospital education programs, workshops, and conferences since 1983. She is currently involved in the federal initiative to provide comprehensive health care delivery services for seriously ill and injured children through the Emergency Medical Services for Children Act.

Eliane F. Runion, B.S.W., is the Advocacy Coordinator for Children's National Medical Center, Washington, D.C. She is a graduate of the University of Maryland EMS Degree Program and served as the Assistant Coordinator of the Pediatric Emergency Medical Services Training Program from 1985 through 1988. She volunteered as an EMT-A between 1980 and 1989, and has also been active as a mental health professional on the Critical Incident Stress Debriefing Team for the Maryland Institute for Emergency Medical Services Systems for the past nine years.

PEDIATRIC EMERGENCIES

The Child's Response to Emergencies

OBJECTIVES

When you have completed this chapter you should be able to

* List and describe five stages of child development.
* List two primary concerns of a child at each developmental age group in an emergency situation.
* Identify three responses the emergency medical technician (EMT) can use with a child at each developmental age in an emergency situation.

There is no way of knowing what is really going through a child's mind as he or she is taken away in an ambulance at the time of illness or injury. Seeing children in pain is difficult, especially when we have children of our own. We need to strike a balance among performing our duties in a professional manner, wishing to comfort the child, and identifying with the parents in their moment of helplessness, anxiety, and guilt.

Emergency medical technicians (EMTs) and *paramedics need to be concerned with a child's emotional well-being, even during life-threatening events.* A child that experiences such a frightening situation as being hit by a car and then having strangers touch him, apply equipment, and place him in an ambulance is vulnerable to emotional setbacks. Even under the best of circumstances (when the feelings of the child are taken into consideration and care for the physical illness or injury is successful), a child may experience regression, nightmares, and mistrust of adults.

When approaching the scene remember a child's primary emotion is *fear* (Figure 1.1).

- Fear of being hurt and of having his or her body invaded and disfigured;
- Fear of being separated from the people and places that are familiar and of never returning home again;
- Fear of the unknown.

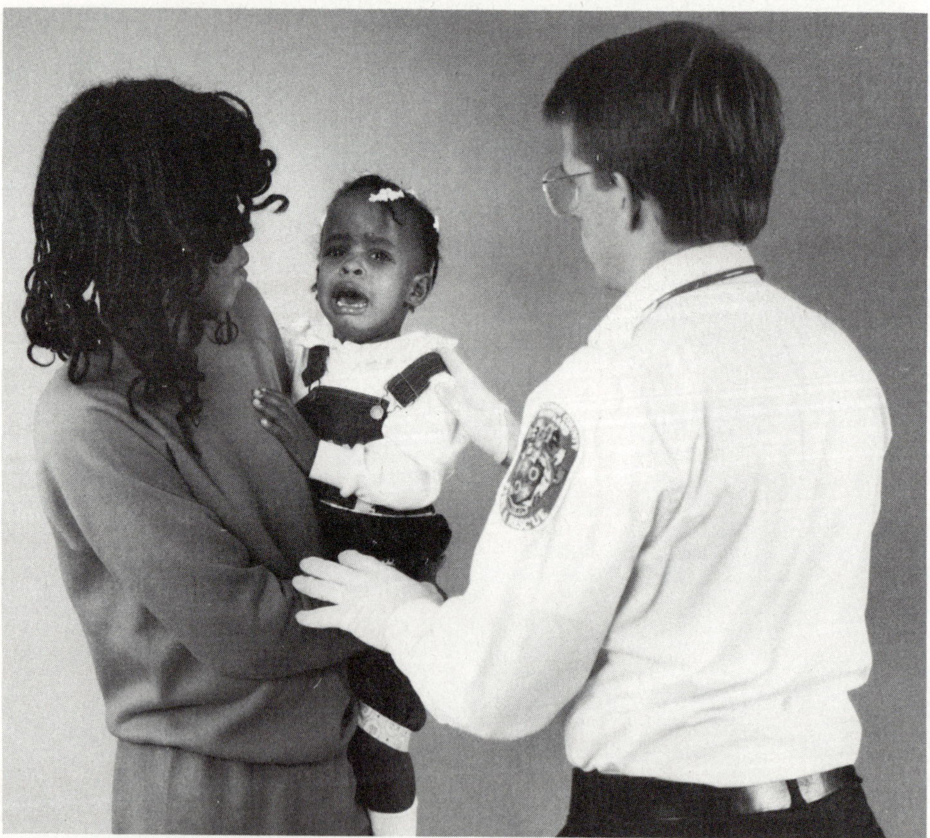

FIGURE 1.1 The child's primary emotion is fear.

The child will be distressed by the general air of panic and confusion that usually surrounds an emergency.

Prehospital treatment must be based on knowledge of the normal emotional and physiologic development of children. Well-intentioned treatment without the sufficient knowledge and skills in caring for a child's emotions places children and their families at unnecessary emotional risk.

The Approach to the Child and Family

Rights of Children and Parents

Children and parents have a right to know what is being done and what to expect will be done to their bodies. For example, if the child is anxious and/or the parent is present, describe the treatment, directing it to the child in age-appropriate language ("I need to put this long board under your leg to keep it from moving"). However, the language used for the child may not be appropriate for the parent. Do not "talk down" to the parents. The parent/child relationship is extremely important to the child at this time, and children will seek consolation from parents. Do all that you can to provide for the child that parental emotional support (Figure 1.2).

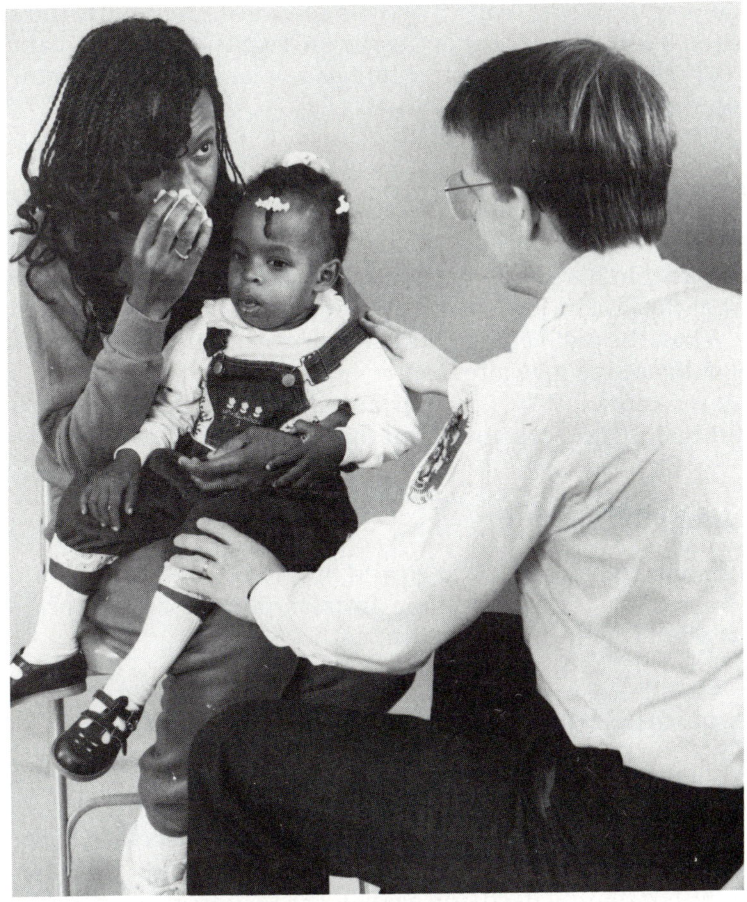

FIGURE 1.2 Providing emotional support to the parent.

Appropriate Language

Identify and use language of body parts that children will understand, such as *leg* and *tummy*. Avoid medical terms such as *femur* or *spleen*. Using unfamiliar terms will make both child and parent more anxious in an already tense situation.

Dealing with Pain

Always warn the child if a procedure or treatment will cause pain. Never say "This won't hurt" if it will. It is difficult to determine a child's level of pain, and thus the slightest movement of an extremity could trigger an outburst. If you know a procedure is going to hurt, have all equipment ready, then tell the child what has to be done, do it, then say "I'm sorry, I know that hurts." Do not let anticipation of pain build by allowing time between preparation for the procedure and doing it.

Pain is very difficult for a preschool-age child to describe or localize. School-age children may be able to describe the intensity of pain on a scale of 1–5 (5 being the worst pain ever felt and 1 being mild discomfort such as a splinter). Ask the child to point to where the pain is to determine the location.

Never minimize the hurt or intimidate the child by saying "That doesn't hurt" or "Big boys don't cry," be a "brave boy" or a "good girl." Sometimes the child seems too old chronologically to be crying and seems to be acting like a "baby." In this instance, deal with the behavior as it occurs. If a 10-year-old is acting like a 4-year-old, then treat that child as a 4-year-old. Remember, the child has no control over events, and crying is a coping mechanism.

Honesty

Be as honest as possible; however, use discretion. It is not necessary to tell the child that his or her mother is in critical condition and may not survive, or that the child's leg is severely damaged and he or she might lose it.

When the child or parents ask you questions you cannot answer do not feel obligated to give a reason or explanation. It is perfectly all right to say "I don't know." When the parent and child cannot be reassured that the child is all right, reassure them that everything possible is being done.

Sense of Hearing

Hearing is the last sense to go and first to return for the child slipping into unconsciousness or emerging from it. Therefore, assume the child can hear what is being said at all times.

Emotional and Behavioral Development

An understanding of the emotional and behavioral development of infants and children is necessary for the EMT and paramedic to appropriately manage the child during prehospital care. As described in this chapter, the age breakdown is the accepted definition of infant, toddler, preschooler, etc., as commonly used and seen in the pediatric and growth-and-development literature.

Infant

The first year of life is one of rapid change. The newborn infant is physically and mentally immature and emotionally reacts at an instinctive level. The 12-month-old walks, talks, and exercises some independence, letting everyone know he or she has "arrived."

Birth to 6 Months

Young infants recognize the faces and voices of their parents and are emotionally tied to them. Infants experiencing pain in any portion of their body are unable to localize it. They have a whole-body response (crying, withdrawal, flexion of extremities) to any painful stimuli. This age group is physically easier to examine because infants are not very strong. On the other hand, because of small anatomic body parts, the infant's physiologic condition will deteriorate rapidly if not properly managed (Figure 1.3).

6 to 12 Months

Older infants have a clear need of a parent or primary-care provider because they are very distressed by separation (Figure 1.4). They are not old enough to understand what is happening to them, and they resist being examined. If held in mother's arms the infant will be more cooperative.

Your Approach at the Scene

Infants express emotional and physical distress through crying. Infants cope by seeking close physical contact with a parent or familiar per-

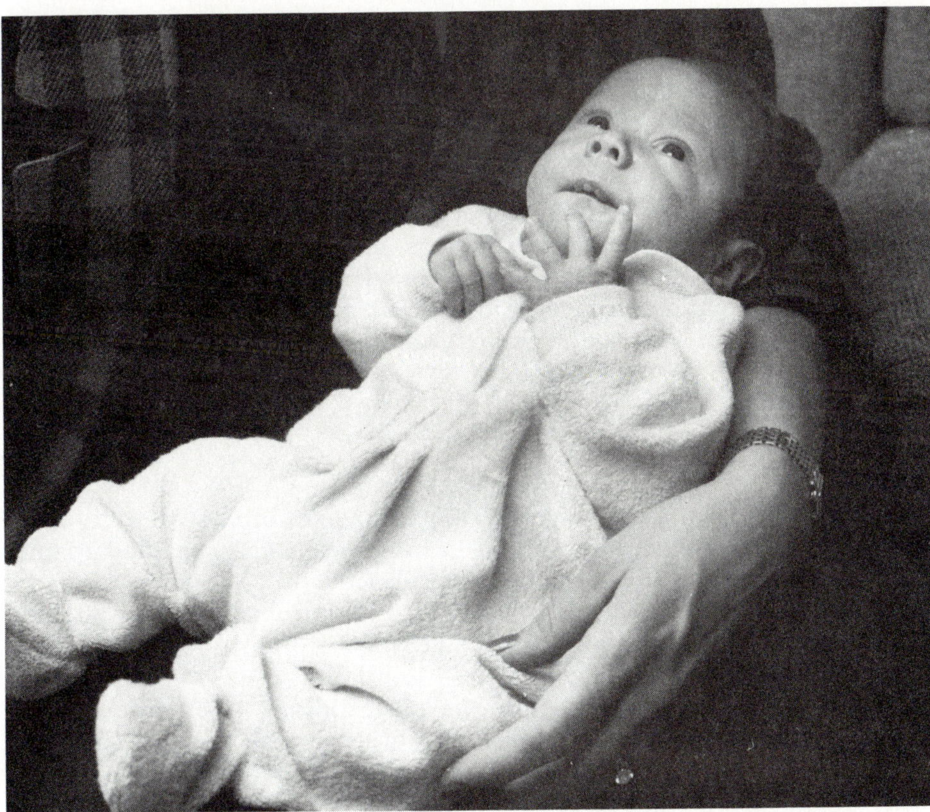

FIGURE 1.3   Infant less than 6 months.

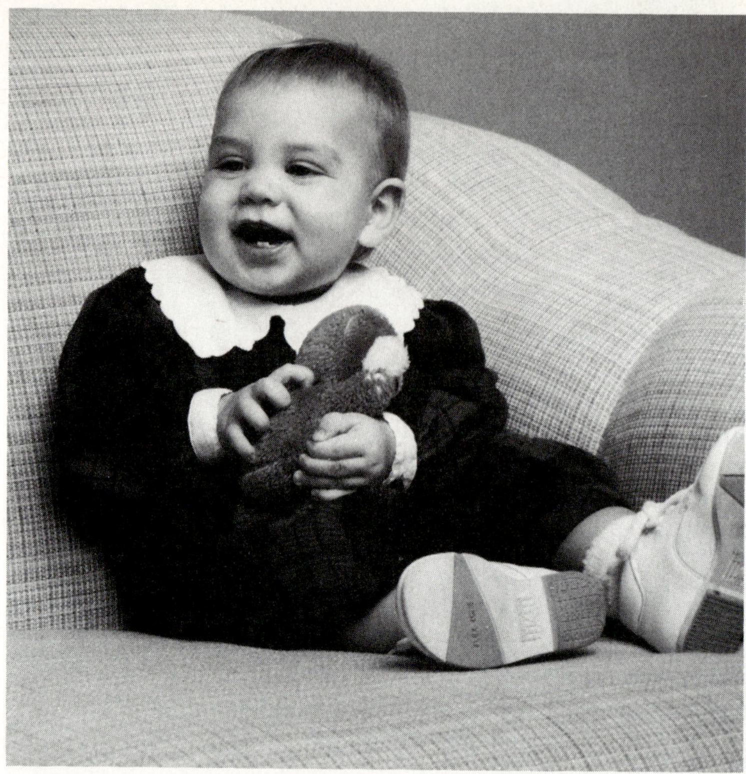

son. If the condition permits, swaddle the younger infant in a blanket to provide a feeling of security. Allow the older infant to suck a thumb, pacifier, or bottle for comfort.

In emergencies, parents will be upset. Be calm and reassure them that everything is going to be all right or that everything possible is being done. If you feel the parent will not interfere with treatment, let one parent ride in the back of the ambulance to provide a history and to comfort the infant. This may relieve some parental distress. Examine the infant in the parent's arms or lap, if there is no suspected cervical spine injury (Figure 1.5). Respect the child's "space." Do not rush to touch and examine the child without first observing the child's condition. (Refer to Chapter 3.)

Toddler

Development

Children between 1 and 3 years enjoy an age of intense activity and discovery. The toddler's philosophy of life is: Holes need to be filled up (including ears, nose, and mouth); everything needs to be touched, tasted, and manipulated; no one except a parent is to be trusted; nothing should be agreed to; and displeasure should be shown often and loudly (See Figure 1.6.).

Children 1 to 3 years of age are the most difficult to examine, even when they are not ill or injured. Problems are magnified by illness or injury. Toddlers will physically push you away, cry, scream, squirm, and do whatever is necessary to prevent you from touching them. Here you need to be flexible and take opportunities to perform the physical exam as the

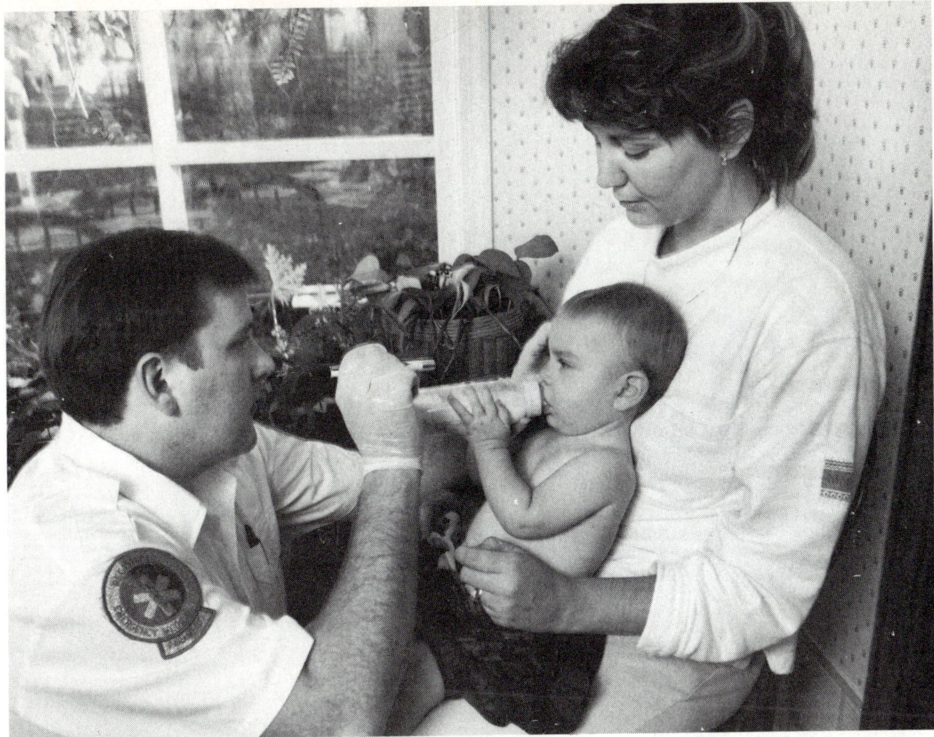

FIGURE 1.5 Examining infant in mother's lap. Allow infant to suck a bottle for comfort during the examination.

opportunity presents itself. This is where the *toe-to-head* assessment is the most beneficial, going from the less threatening parts of the body to the more threatening parts. In cases where the toddler is very uncooperative, concentrate on the component of the physical exam that is most important in obtaining information concerning the chief complaint. For example, if the child is having respiratory problems, concentrate on signs and symptoms of respiratory distress and level of consciousness and forego examination of the abdomen and extremities, etc.

Toddlers are the age group most likely to experience short-term and long-term emotional problems as a result of the emergency. Therefore, handle them with special care. Toddlers are terrified of separation from what is familiar, particularly the parent or primary-care provider. They do not understand that things are being done for their benefit. They have limited language skills and thus have difficulty understanding verbal explanations.

The toddler's biggest fear is the possibility of separation from the parent or that which is familiar, such as a toy or stuffed animal. Fear of strangers is also strongly expressed. The toddler copes by seeking physical contact with the parent. A dependency object such as toy, stuffed animal, or blanket is often used by the toddler for a feeling of security.

Your Approach at the Scene

Talk to the child in a reassuring and quiet tone of voice, repeating a phrase such as "You are going to be all right." Tone of voice conveys reassurance even though the child may not understand your words. If restraining the child is needed, be as gentle as possible. When necessary, human restraints are preferable to mechanical ones. Be sure the child has any de-

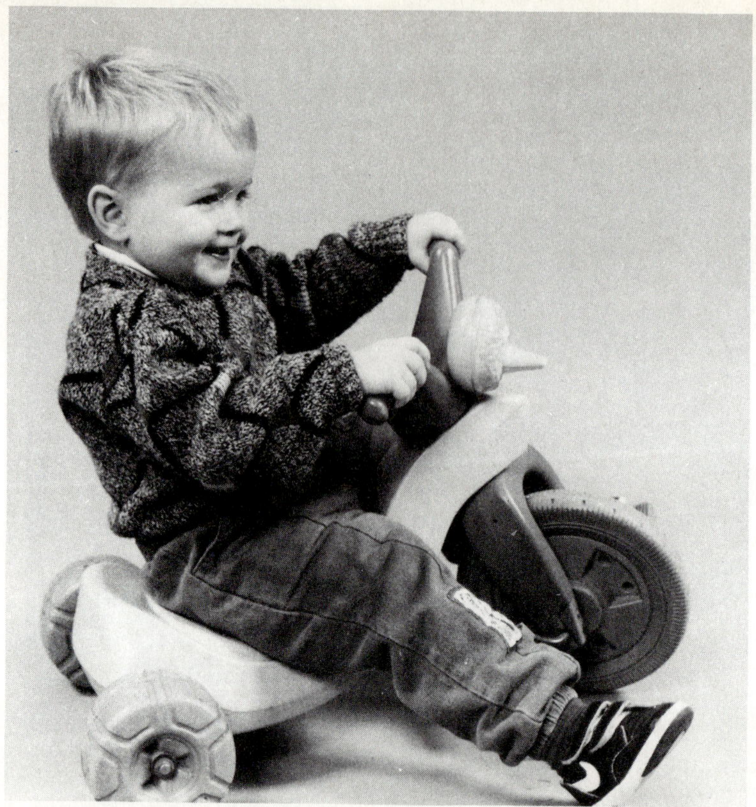

FIGURE 1.6 Toddler.

pendency object alongside while being transported in the ambulance (Figure 1.7). Some rescue units have a stuffed animal onboard to distract the child or use it to help with the examination. If a stuffed animal is given to the child it may be problematic in retrieving it at the end of the run. In this instance, repossessing it seems inappropriate. Keep the parent nearby; allow the parent to touch or hold the child so as to calm him or her and to assist during your examination.

Preschooler

Development

During the preschool period (3 to 5 years of age), basic skills such as walking, running, talking, toilet training, etc., have been accomplished and are being refined. Running, once an enjoyment within itself, is now a means to a bigger and better end. This child has full awareness of the external body and body parts. Concrete thinking and literal interpretation of what is heard is normal. The preschooler has a vivid imagination and can dramatize events (Figure 1.8).

Preschoolers are likely to believe an accident or injury is their fault, regardless of whether or not they had a role in bringing it about. While they have better verbal skills, they do not have complex language skills and can misinterpret common words. They do not understand their internal anatomy. Preschoolers continue to have the fears of younger children, particularly of separation and abandonment. Use of the *toe-to-head* approach for

The Child's Response to Emergencies

FIGURE 1.7 Toddler
with dependency objects.

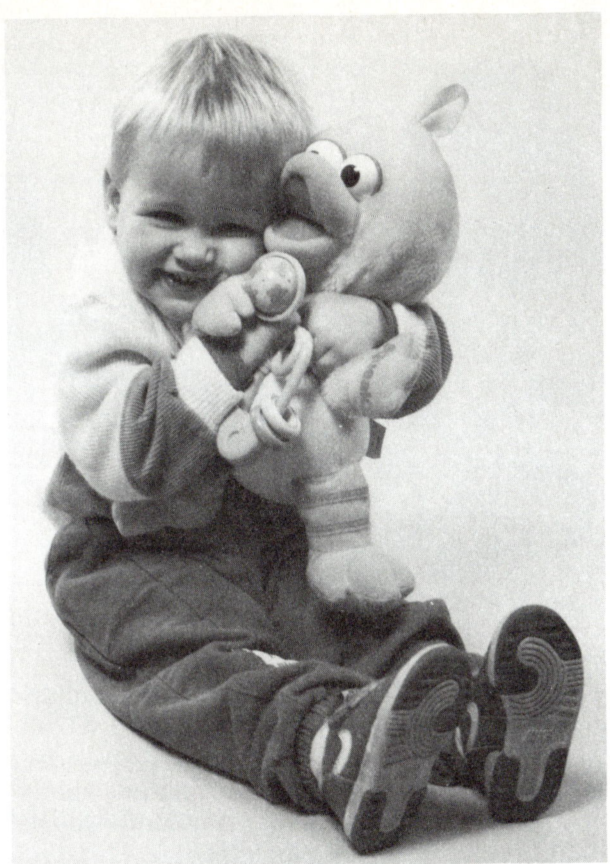

FIGURE 1.8 Preschooler.

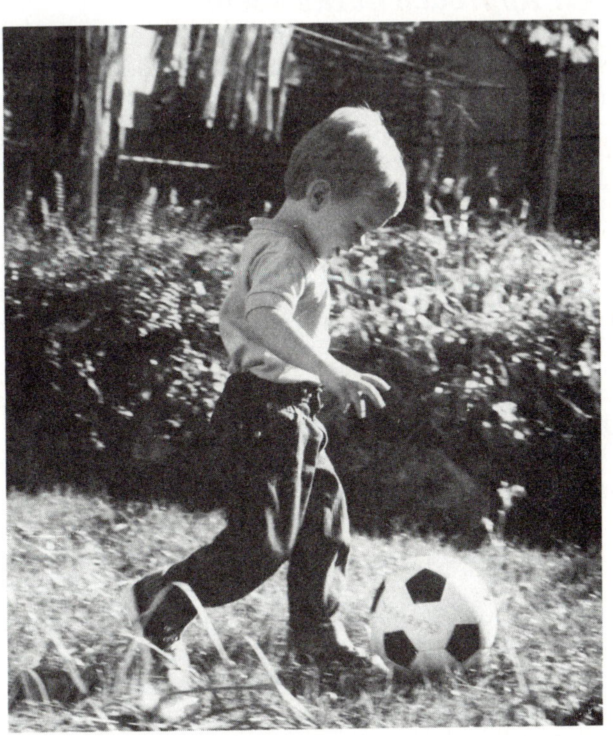

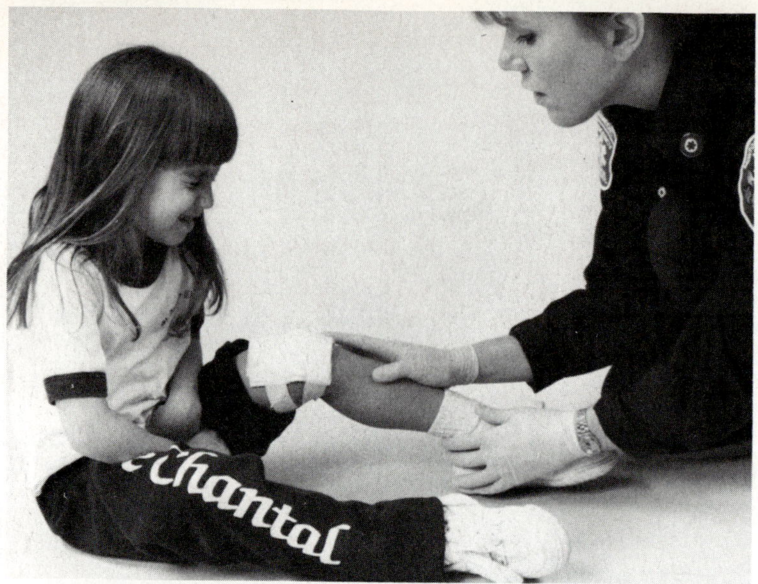

FIGURE 1.9   Cover the injury to reduce the child's anxiety.

the assessment is also appropriate for these children, depending on the circumstances and age of the child.

Preschoolers are very frightened of physical injury and especially the sight of blood on their body. Fears related to body integrity such as mutilation or body intactness are intense. Band-Aids help in covering the wound so that the child can avoid looking at it.

When coping with pain, the preschooler's need for the parent is still great, especially the young preschooler. Oftentimes they regress to a younger stage of behavior, crying or resisting examination and care.

Your Approach at the Scene

Approach the child slowly. These children might appear to understand what is occurring when actually they do not. Be certain that your reassuring and quiet tone of voice gets through to the child, even if nothing else does. Employ the toe-to-head assessment if appropriate.

Use simple words to describe the care to be given; do this for the benefit of both the parent and the child. Let the child know it is okay to cry. If there is a visible injury, particularly a bloody one, clean it and dress it (Figure 1.9). Blood in the eyes from a scalp wound can be far more terrifying to children than the extent of the injury suggests to you.

School Age

Development

The 6-to-12-year age group covers a wide range of differing levels of behavior and development. During these middle childhood years the child learns and develops through games, contacts with peers, relationships with family, and the environment of home, school, and community (Figure 1.10).

School-age children can understand rational explanations and are probably the easiest to examine and manage. However, they are still frightened and may see illness or injury as a punishment. The school-age child fears pain, punishment, and separation from family and friends. While

 School-age children.

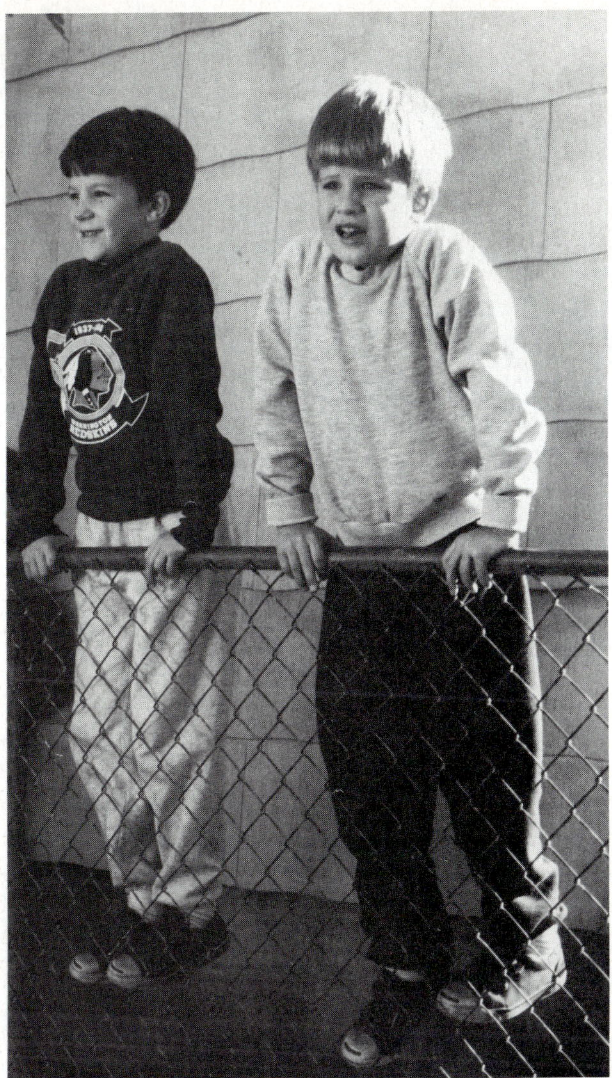

these children do not understand technical words, they have simple understanding of internal anatomy. Issues of modesty are very important, and these children do not like their bodies exposed to strangers. Concerns about death and disability emerge during this stage of development.

Early school-age children may regress under stress of an emergency. Parents are needed to validate the child's reactions to the illness or injury in order to help the child adjust. How the parents cope will influence how the child copes.

Your Approach at the Scene

Include the child in conversation, particularly when obtaining the history. Direct the history questions to the child and explain in simple terms what you are doing during examination and treatment. The head-to-toe assessment is appropriate with these children. The parent will appropriately respond to history questions and appreciate the explanation of care. Do not belittle the child's pain or threaten or cajole the child who protests. This will help reassure both child and parent that everything possible is being done. Make every attempt to cover the child's body so that it is not unduly exposed (Figure 1.11).

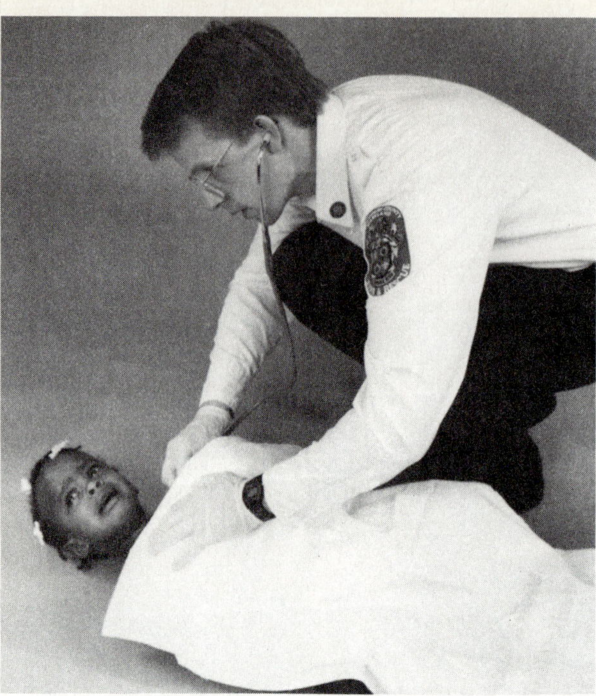

This child will be interested in what is in the ambulance. Explain the function of the equipment and indicate that not all pieces of equipment will be used. To the best of your ability, prepare the child for what is going to be done at the hospital.

Adolescent

Development

The period between 13 and 18 years is an age of many changes and decisions as the adolescent leaves childhood and enters the world of the young adult in search of independence. Because adolescents possess concrete thinking and are developing abstract thinking, they can deal with the present and project into the future. The adolescent has incredible drive and energy and commonly engages in "magical thinking" with feelings of indestructability (Figure 1.12).

Adolescents generally understand what is happening and are often the best historians. On the other hand, adolescents are tremendously preoccupied with their bodies even when not threatened by illness or injury. These concerns are intensified when there is bodily injury. They fear permanent disability or disfigurement and they are aware of the possibility of their own death. Modesty is a very real issue with this group.

Adolescents of both sexes are capable of a "hysterical" reaction to illness or injury, which often impresses outsiders as "overdoing" it. Instances of "mass hysteria" may be observed in adolescents, as when a great number of children seem to suffer food poisoning or are overcome by fumes, etc. Generally, even "hysterical" adolescents respond to quiet reassurance.

Your Approach at the Scene

Try to have the assessment of the adolescent done by someone of the same sex (Figure 1.13). In all cases, respect the teenager's feelings of mod-

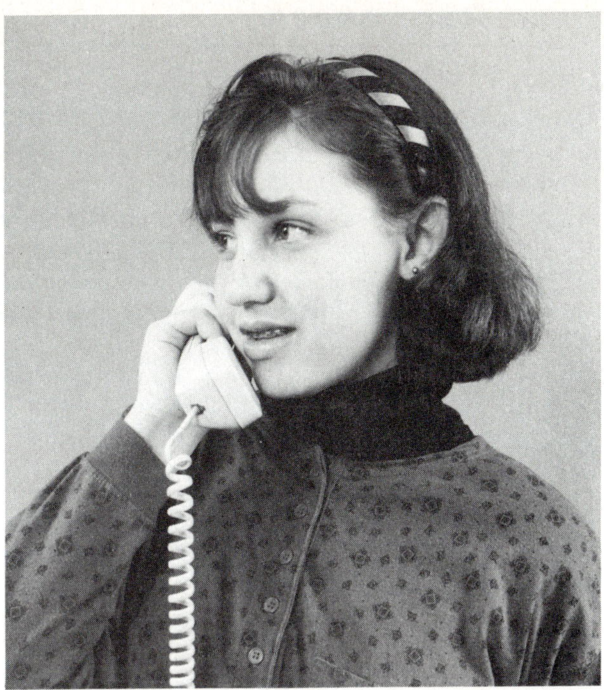

FIGURE 1.12 Adolescent.

esty. Reassure the adolescent that he or she is not going to die (even if you feel that is possible). Instead, say that "We are doing everything we can as fast as possible to get you to the hospital for the care you need." If the adolescent appears "hysterical" and seems to be overreacting, be tolerant of this; do not get caught up in the hysteria or become angry about it. In most cases the parents do not need to accompany the teenager in the ambulance. Explain to the adolescent what is happening and what will probably happen at the hospital.

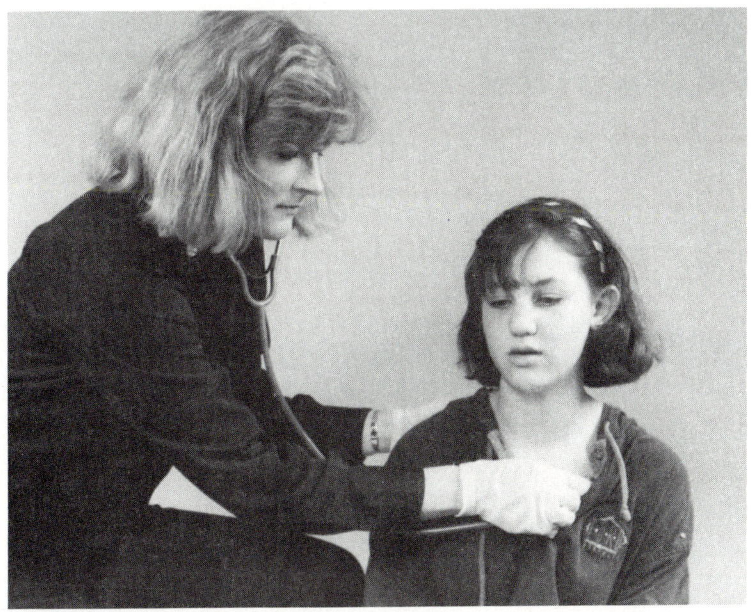

FIGURE 1.13 Try to provide assessment of the adolescent by an EMT of same sex.

GATZ, R. R., "Children's responses to emergency department care," *Annals of Emergency Medicine,* 13, no. 5 (May 1984), pp. 322–333.

KEMP, V., "The relationship of temperament and children's crying behavior during a stressful situation," *Children's Health Care,* 13, no. 2 (1984), pp. 59–63.

PONTIOUS, S. L., "Practical Piaget: Helping children understand," *American Journal of Nursing,* 82, no. 1 (January 1982), pp. 114–117.

RAVENSCROFT, K., "Psychological considerations for the child with acute trauma." In Randolph, J., and others, eds., *The Injured Child.* Chicago: Yearbook Medical Publishers, 1979, pp. 31–42.

REYNOLDS, E. A., and RAMENOFSKY, M. L., "Emotional impact of trauma on toddlers," *Maternal Child Nursing,* 13 (March/April 1988), pp. 106–109.

SHANAGERGER, J., "Children's rights and EMS," *JEMS,* 12, no. 2 (February 1987), pp. 60–61.

Family Members' Response to Their Child's Emergency

OBJECTIVES

When you have completed this chapter you should be able to

* Describe three types of reactions or emotions exhibited by parents in an emergency involving their child.
* Describe three different methods for dealing with the family in a pediatric emergency.

Families in Emergency Situations

Pediatric professionals who care for children realize that treating the child requires treating the family as well. When the child experiences discomfort and pain with illness or injury, the parents suffer almost equally with anxiety and emotional stress.

In an emergency, the parents' reaction to the child's emergency condition is "acute grief." This is a normal reaction to a distressing situation manifested by psychological and somatic symptoms. The range of emotions associated with the grief expressed by parents includes fear, shock, denial, guilt, anger, and loss of control. Whatever behavior the parent is demonstrating when you arrive at the scene is the way that particular parent is managing grief *at that particular time.* Parents' behavior may, however, change dramatically during the time prehospital care is provided (Figure 2.1).

The most common parental reaction noted by EMTs and paramedics is *fear.* Relinquishing their child to your care, not knowing what will happen next, and worrying about the child's eventual outcome leave parents feeling helpless. Because of this, parents may ask questions such as:

- "Is my child going to die?"
- "Is his brain O.K.?"
- "Will he walk again?"

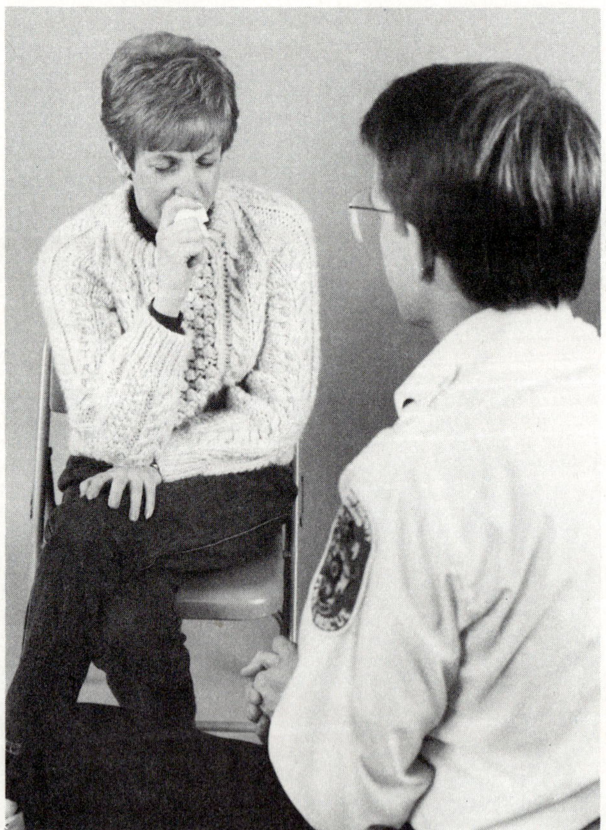

FIGURE 2.1 Parents display a range of emotions in response to their child's emergency condition.

Parents in emotional shock respond differently. They are pale, quiet, and uncommunicative; they are withdrawn, stare into space, and may be unaware of another's presence.

Sometimes parents become very demanding in an attempt to control the situation and help their child. This can be a very uncomfortable situation for the EMT. Sometimes these parents may get in your way, preventing you from doing your job effectively.

When responding to a pediatric emergency, the EMT should respond to the parent in the following ways:

- Acknowledge the feelings of the parent.
- Reassure the parent that "it's okay to feel the way you do."
- Redirect the parents' energies to help you in some way in caring for their child.
- Remain calm and appear in control to help parents deal with their anxiety.
- Project confidence to family members so they trust you and believe that everything possible is being done to stabilize the child's condition and to provide transport as soon as possible to the hospital.

Guidelines for Verbal and Nonverbal Communication with Parents

Set the Tone During the Rescue

- Introduce yourself and identify your job responsibilities.
- Call the child by name; also use the surname of the parent. For example, "Mrs. Blake, we will be taking Jimmy to the trauma center at Children's Hospital."

Remember That Your First Priority Is to the Ill or Injured Child

- Help family members with their crisis without compromising patient care. Patient care is your main objective and responsibility, and it should never be compromised. However, dealing with the parents is a fact of life, and this chapter will assist you in coping with parental reactions to a child in crisis.
- Initiate your assessment in an efficient and rapid manner. Parents are reassured when their child is cared for by professionals who take their work seriously and who project a concerned and caring attitude.

Keep Calm: You Are in a Crisis-Management Situation

- Through all of this, the one positive emotion that you must foster and project to the family is trust.

- Keep calm, even though you may be apprehensive about the situation.

- Project an image that everything possible is being done and the best possible care is being delivered so as to ease anxious family members. Professionalism is important to gain the trust of the parents.

Keep the Parents Informed and Keep the Language Simple

- Anticipate what type of information parents want and need to know (Figure 2.2).

- Explain as you proceed with the examination and treatment or give a short synopsis of the overall condition of the child. For example: "I'm feeling Susie's abdomen for any internal bumps or bruises" or "The blood on Tim's head is from a laceration; it will probably need some stitches. We have a pressure dressing on the wound to stop the bleeding until we get to the emergency room." The responses you get to this type of interaction help you determine how the parent is handling the situation.

Ask for the Parents' Assistance

- The parent and child should not be separated unless the parent is totally out of control and interfering with your care.

- Ask parents who are capable, "Would you hold his [her] hands while I look at his [her] chest and abdomen?" (See Figure 2.3.)

- If the child is seriously injured, ask, "Would you please stand here? I may need your help." Try to make the parents feel they are participating in the care given to their child.

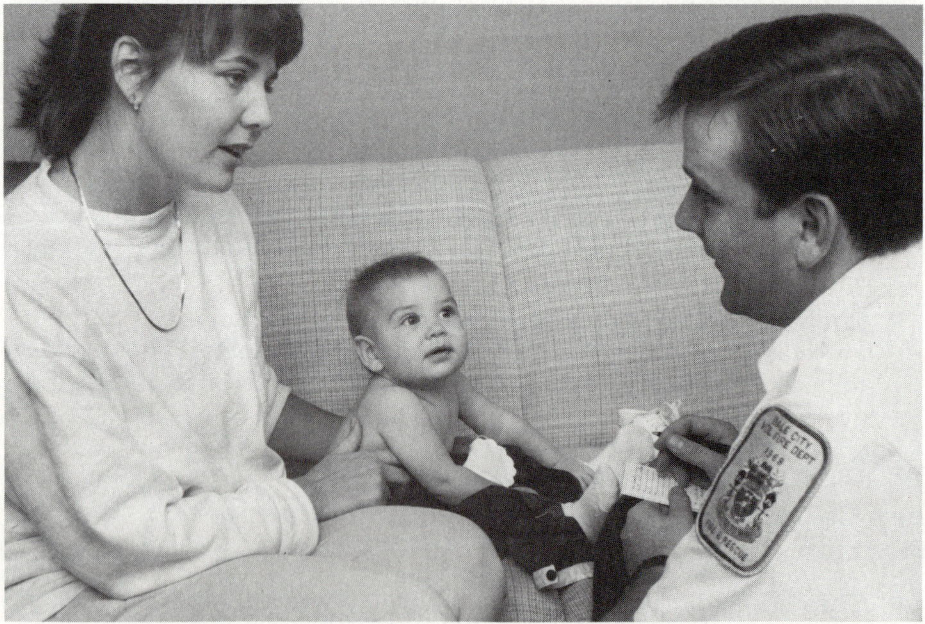

FIGURE 2.2 Provide information to parent.

Family Members' Response to Their Child's Emergency

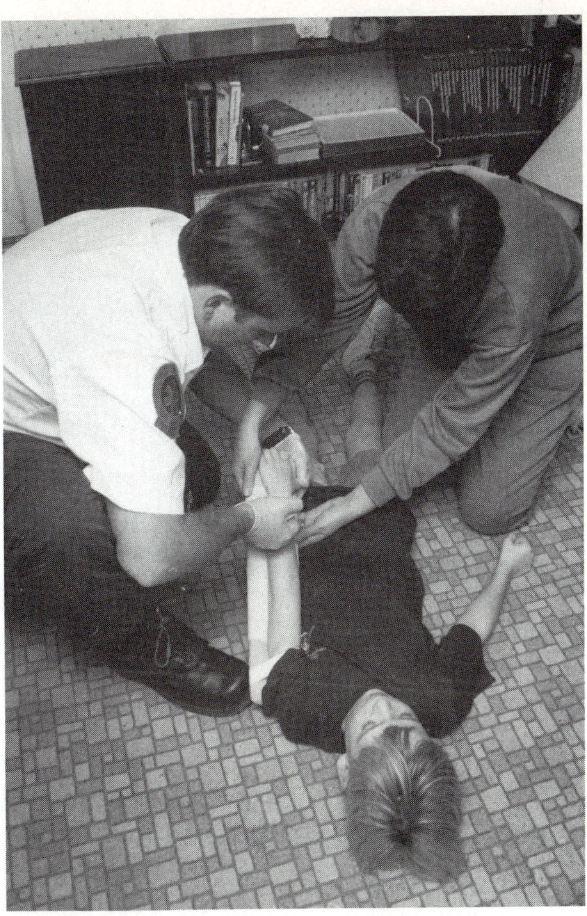

Be Honest with the Parent and Child

- If you must perform a procedure that is particularly painful for the child, explain what needs to be done and the reason. For example: "Billy, I'm going to put your leg in this splint and it's going to hurt for a short time. The splint prevents further injury to your leg until we get to the hospital. While I'm doing that, I want you to squeeze your Dad's hand as hard as you can, and it's okay to cry."

Provide Parents with Some Words of Reassurance About Their Child's Condition

- Emphasize the positive. "Your child is breathing fine. His blood pressure is good. He may have a broken leg, but he has good toe movement and good pulses in the foot."
- Avoid giving the parents *false* reassurances with such phrases as "Sam will be fine" if that is not the case. You may be promising more than the best medical care can deliver.
- If the situation is grave and the parents ask, "Is she going to die?" tell them, "I don't know; we're going to do our best for your daughter." With that statement you are being honest and preparing them for the potential grief (Figure 2.4).
- At the hospital, professionals are available to help parents through the death of their child and to begin the grieving process.

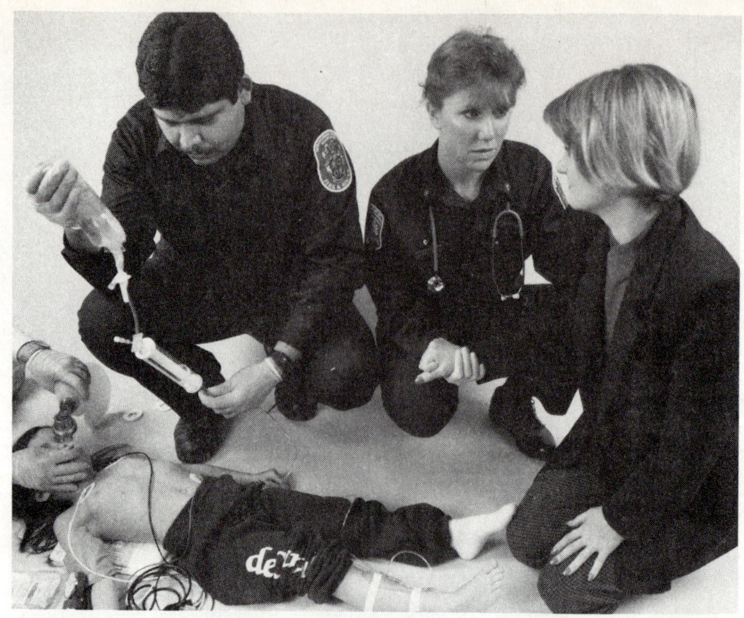

FIGURE 2.4   Showing concern for the parent during treatment of the child.

Do Not Show Family Members or Bystanders Your Personal Negative Feelings Concerning the Circumstances at the Scene

- Your initial reaction sets the tone of how the parents will respond and cooperate with the treatment of their child from the scene through hospital care.

- If you reveal your negative feelings, family members may either panic and try to interfere with treatment or assume additional guilt. Many parents blame themselves for any serious illness or injury of their child. If they feel that you or other professionals blame them for what happened to their child, their psychological adjustments may be more difficult.

- Situations where the gate was left unlocked or the household cleaning agent was left within reach should be evaluated objectively, without verbal or nonverbal judgment. When abuse or neglect is suspected, refer this information to the appropriate hospital personnel or community social service agency.

- Even when abuse is suspected, the parent and child should be transported together. These children have the same fears of separation from parents as do other children. (See Chapter 13, "Child Abuse.")

Show Concern for the Family Members During the Process of Management and Transport

- Remind parents to lock their doors, turn off the stove, and make arrangements with neighbors to look after their other children.

- Assess the parents' ability to drive to the hospital. If possible, find a

friend, neighbor, or police to transport them. If they drive themselves, remind them to drive safely and not to try to keep up with
the ambulance. Tell them to obey all traffic laws, and say you will
meet them at the hospital.

- Be sure the parent knows the name and location of the hospital
where you are taking the child. Make sure someone has directions if
it is distant.

- When at the hospital, show them where to sit, offer tissues, and before you leave say goodbye and offer words of encouragement. Any
act of kindness will be remembered.

Accept the Parents' Reaction to the Situation

- Whether the parents are angry, hysterical, or in shock, they are
doing the best they can in this very trying and unreal situation.
Your acceptance of their behavior affords them permission to start
working through their fears and grief to face reality.

What About the Feelings of the First Responder?

- After you have had a particularly difficult situation involving a
child, talk to someone about it. Talking to a colleague, partner, hospital staff member, or unit supervisor may help you cope with the
very difficult work that you are asked to perform. (See Chapter 17
for additional details.)

Table 2.1 lists some of the common reactions that parents have in an
emergency involving their child and offers examples of EMT interventions.

TABLE 2.1   Common Parental Reactions to Sudden, Life-Threatening Conditions

Parental Behavior During First Impact of Crisis	Reason for the Behavior	Suggested Responses
Shock or Denial		
Parents may be in a daze and seem incapable of absorbing the reality of the illness/injury.	Sometimes it is too difficult to integrate the loss or potential loss of the child into the conscious process of the mind.	Do not force the parent to face reality. Remain calm, use simple but direct explanations, and offer reassurance and support.
The "numb" reaction makes it difficult to understand explanations about the situation.	Numbness enables the parent to *slowly* begin to feel the impact of the seriousness of the situation.	Parents in denial sometimes do not hear the assessment information being told to them. Keep the parent informed concerning the child's condition and the need for transport. You may need to repeat the information to them before they process what is being said.
Parents in a state of denial react by saying, "I don't believe it." "He was fine when I put him to bed." "There must be a mistake," etc.	Denial is a normal mechanism of trying to keep the terrible truth from hitting all at once.	

(continued)

Parental Behavior During First Impact of Crisis	Reason for the Behavior	Suggested Responses

Crying, Screaming, Intense Rage, and Bitterness

Some parents react immediately with an intense emotional display to the potential loss of the child or the potential loss of normal functioning.	The suddeness and severity of the illness or injury may make it impossible for the parent to use denial as a defense.	You may feel uncomfortable with the parents expressing their feelings openly. Don't discourage them. Do listen, give information, and provide reassurance.
Some will lash out at God, the spouse, the sibling, the school, the babysitter, the driver of the other vehicle, the doctor who didn't find anything wrong last week, etc. Some will cry out and remain in one place; others will be agitated and pace the floor, slam their fists into walls, or physically lash out at those rendering care.	Crying openly and intensely is a common way of dealing with tragedy. In some cases parents may be displaying what could be interpreted as overreacting, when in reality the parent may be getting ready for the worst.	Often, parents become embarrased about their open expressions of sorrow, rage, etc. Reassure them that such expressions are normal under the circumstances. Let them know that other parents react this way when their child's life is threatened.

Expressions of Guilt and Self-Blame by the Parent

In the event of sudden illness the parent may blame himself or herself for "not paying enough attention to the sore throat or fever"—"for cancelling last week's checkup"—for not giving enough cough medicine," etc.	Parents look for a "reason" for the catastrophe. It is better to blame something than for it to occur randomly. If one could figure out why something happened, one could keep it from happening again.	Listen to the parents' anguish. Let them verbalize their thoughts. If the parent says, "My teenager said that I should go to work—that he would stay in bed and would be fine," and the mother found him unconscious when she came home, reassure the mother that she made the best decision she could at the time. Generally, teenagers who get sick do fine with some rest. No one can blame the mother for going to work. Most would have done the same thing under the circumstances.
If the child is injured the parent will often blame himself or herself for "letting him ride his bicycle," "for crossing the busy street," "for driving too fast," "for letting him play football," etc. If anger was expressed (or felt) the parent may be feeling very guilty.	Some guilt may have deep roots. Some has to do with recent events in which something unpleasant occurred to strain the parent-child relationship.	

Controlling Hysterical Behavior Toward the EMT

Parents may become so agitated that they interfere with the examination and treatment of their child. They tell the EMTs that they (the EMTs) do not know what they are doing—that the child should not be treated at the scene, that the procedures are worthless, etc.	Parents feel it is their role to protect and nurture their children from all threats. In most instances, it is healthy for parents to try to exert "some" control over events in the life of the child.	In most instances, the parents' need to control may work to the advantage of the EMT. The EMT can have the parent hold the child's hand, comfort the child, accompany the child to the hospital, provide a good medical history, help explain why certain procedures must be carried out, etc.
In some instances, parents may exert physical control over the EMT.	It is an innate response of some parents to physically protect children from a perceived harm.	However, if the parent is out of control and interferes with the care of the child, the EMT must get help from a relative, friend, police, etc., so as to restrain and comfort the parent.

BRAULIN, J. L. D., ROOK, J., and SILLS, G. M., "Families in crisis: The impact of trauma," *Critical Care Quarterly*, 5, no. 3 (1982), pp. 38–46.

KARPEN, M., "Pediatric training for paramedics," *Emergency*, 20, no. 10 (October 1988), pp. 62–63.

LININGER, M., "Cultural diversities of health and nursing care," *Nursing Clinics of North America*, 12, no. 1 (March 1977), pp. 5–18.

General Pediatric Assessment

3

OBJECTIVES

When you have completed this chapter you should be able to

✳ Identify one anatomic or physiologic difference between children and adults for each of the following areas:
  - Skin and body surface area
  - Head
  - Airway, including the nose, mouth, and trachea
  - Chest
  - Abdomen
  - Blood volume

✳ List approaches to improve the child's cooperation during the physical examination.

✳ Identify four areas to consider when taking the child's history.

✳ Identify important observations to make about the child's appearance and condition before touching the child.

✳ Describe important factors in taking and interpreting each of the following vital signs:
  - Pulse
  - Respirations
  - Blood pressure
  - Temperature

Anatomy and Physiology

To interpret the findings from a physical examination of infants and children, it is important to understand the differences in anatomy and physiology between children and adults. Most special features of the child's anatomy and physiology are directly related to their smaller size and the continual growth and development of body systems. See Figure 3.1 for an overview of the unique anatomic and physiologic features of children.

Skin and Body Surface Area

Children's body surface area is proportionately larger for their body mass than an adult's. The head of an infant or young child accounts for approximately 20% of the total body surface area, and is larger and heavier in comparison to the rest of the body, until about 4 years of age. Proportions of body surface area by body part change throughout childhood, assuming adult dimensions by about 10 years of age. (See Figure 12.3, page 188.)

The skin of both infants and young children is thinner and more delicate, containing less subcutaneous fat, than an adult's. The same exposure to burn injury will result in deeper burns than what adults receive.

The large surface area for body mass and thinner layer of subcutaneous fat contribute to problems in maintaining body temperature. For this

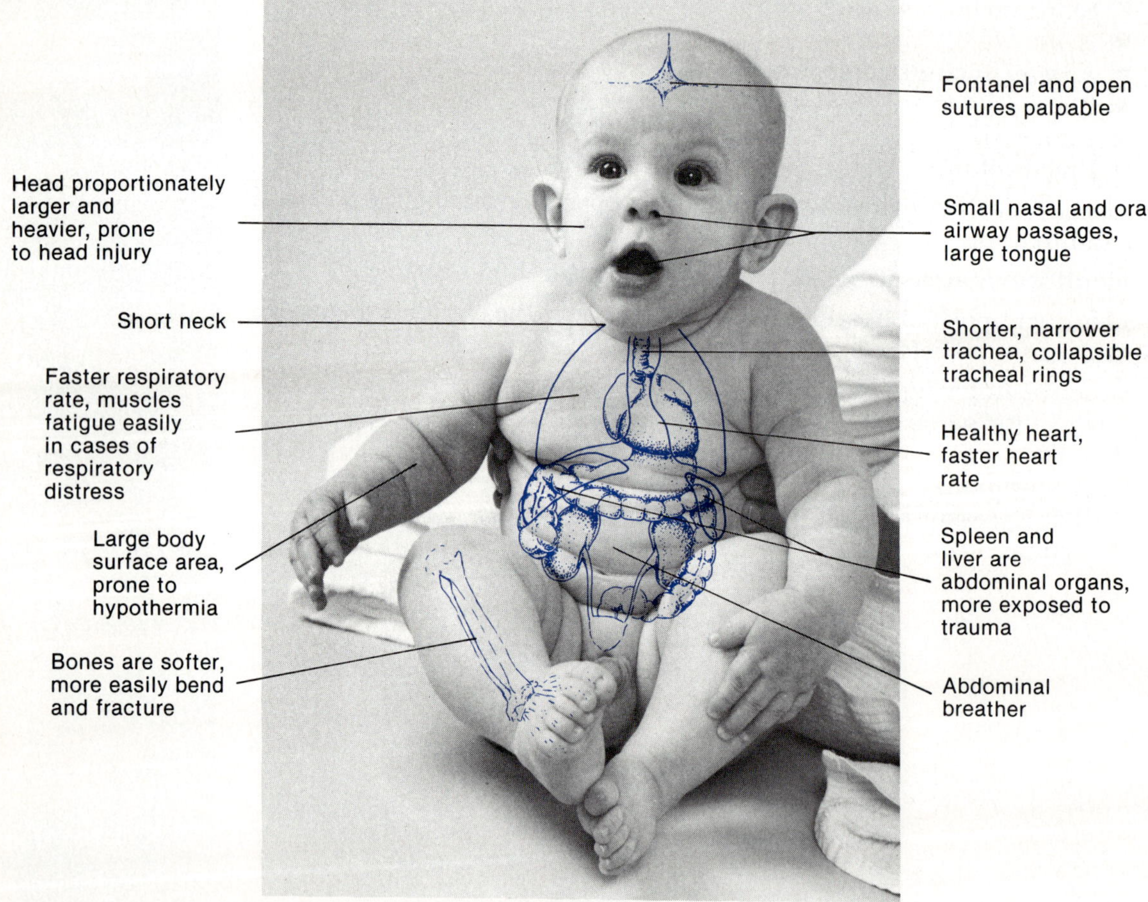

FIGURE 3.1 The unique anatomic and physiologic features of children.

reason, children are more prone to develop *hypothermia.* Newborns are further compromised because their body temperature regulatory mechanisms are not well developed. The child should be kept warm with minimal exposure to the environment. Resuscitation efforts and drug therapies are not as effective in a hypothermic child.

Head

The bones of the skull are soft and separated by cartilage until about 5 years of age. The cartilage suture lines permit growth and expansion of the skull as the brain grows. Because the skull is expandable, the child may be able to survive increased intracranial pressure for a *short* time without major complications.

Fontanelles are diamond-shaped soft spots of fibrous tissue found at the top of the skull where three or four individual bones will eventually fuse together. This fibrous tissue is very strong, and in normal circumstances it adequately protects the brain from injury. The anterior fontanelle closes (is covered by bone) between 12 and 18 months of age, and the posterior fontanelle closes by 2 months of age (Figure 3.2).

All of the brain cells a person will ever have are present at birth; however, they are not fully developed. Neurologic development proceeds over several years as the brain cells grow in size and nerve endings develop and connect. Brain cell development is complete by 5 years of age. Motor development proceeds from the head to the trunk and distally to the extremities as nerve connections develop. For this reason, head control develops before an infant can sit or walk.

The developing brain of an infant or young child is sensitive to poisons, infections, and injury, which may result in major neurologic defects. The brain tissue is thinner, softer, and more flexible than an adult's. The *dura,* the tissue surrounding the brain, is firmly attached to the skull in children

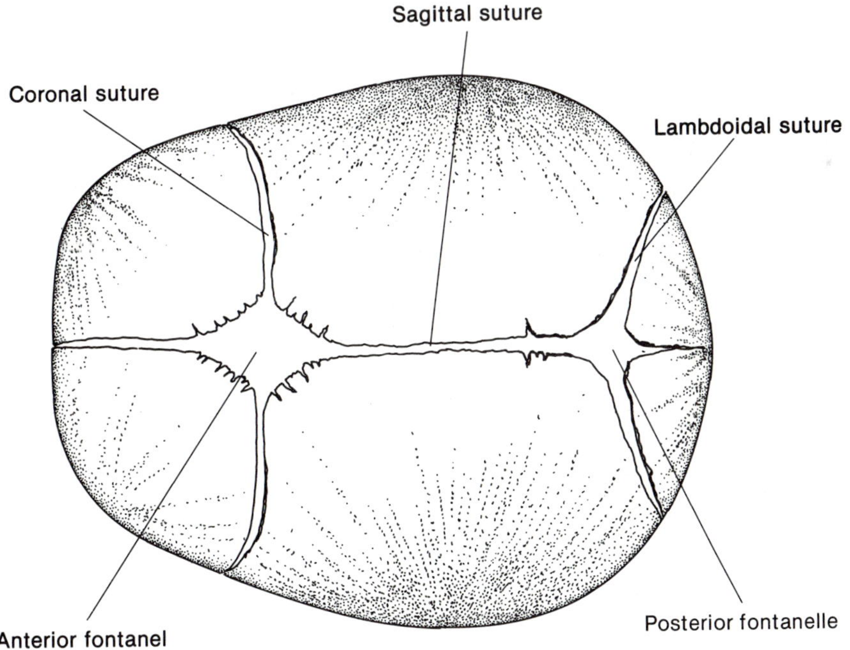

FIGURE 3.2 Location of the anterior and posterior fontanelles on the infant's skull.

and is more likely to be torn away with injury and result in bleeding into the subdural spaces.

Airway

The face of the young child is smaller than an adult's, but not necessarily small in proportion to head size. The nasal bridge is flat and flexible. Nasal passages are small in diameter, becoming easily obstructed with foreign objects or secretions. Newborns and young infants are obligate nose breathers, meaning they do not automatically open the mouth to breathe when the nose becomes obstructed. They will develop respiratory distress if nasal passages become obstructed. See Figure 3.3 for illustration of the airway characteristics.

The child's tongue is large in comparison to the size of the mouth. Pressure on the soft tissues under the chin can easily press the tongue to the roof of the mouth and cause an airway obstruction. The muscles controlling the jaw are immature, permitting the tongue to fall back into the throat and obstructing the airway when the child is supine. For these reasons, the tongue is the major cause of airway obstruction in children.

The size of the trachea is small in comparison to an adult's; thus, any inflammation or swelling in the airway seriously compromises ventilation (Figure 3.4).

- The diameter of the trachea is approximately 4 mm in an infant (about the diameter of a drinking straw) compared to 20 mm in an

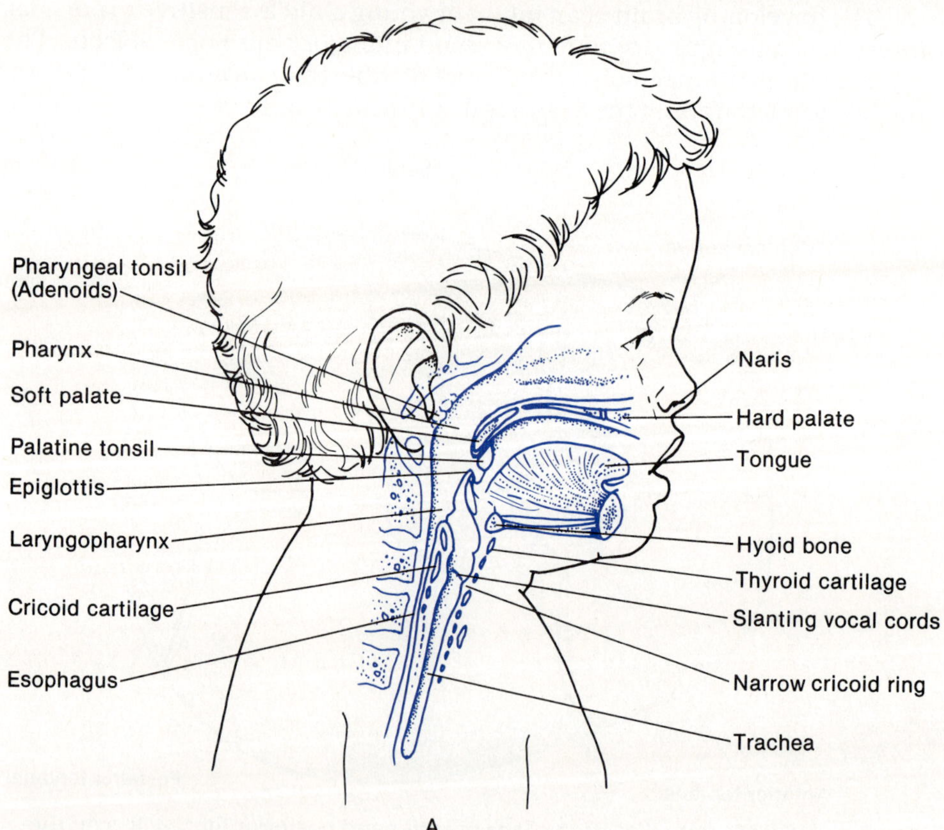

FIGURE 3.3 (a) Anatomic features of the young child's airway, contrasted with that of (b) the adult's airway.

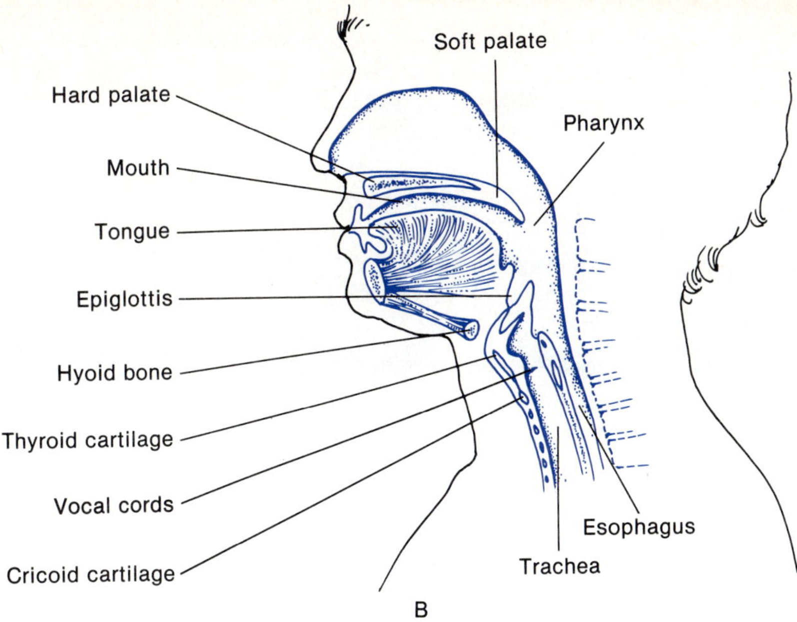

FIGURE 3.3 (Continued)

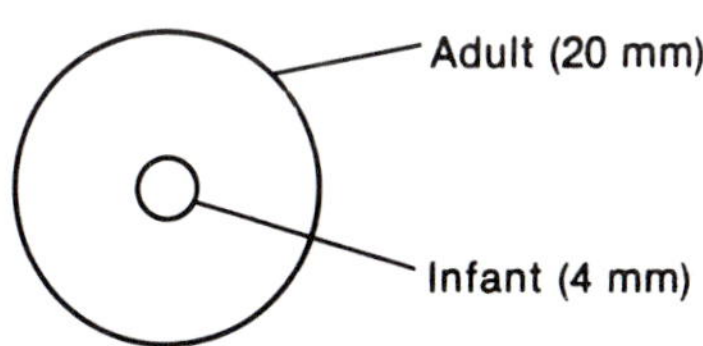

FIGURE 3.4 Comparison of the size (diameter) of the infant's trachea compared to the adult's.

adult. The smallest tracheal diameter is in the subglottic area at the cricoid (until about age 8) rather than at the cords.

- The length of the trachea is 4 to 5 cm in a newborn and 7 cm by 18 months; this compares to 12 cm in an adult.

The tracheal cartilage rings are more elastic in children and collapse easily. Hyperextension or flexion of the child's neck can crimp the trachea, leading to an airway obstruction.

The larynx is higher and more anterior in the child, at the level of the 3rd or 4th cervical vertebrae, compared to the 5th or 6th cervical vertebrae in the adult. This high position contributes to aspiration by the child, especially if the neck is hyperextended. The epiglottic folds are more elastic and interfere with visualization of the vocal cords during intubation. Neutral or "sniffing" position is the best for managing the child's airway.

Chest and Lungs

The rib cage of both infant and young child is more elastic and flexible as it is composed of more cartilage than bone. Rib fractures are less common in children; this is because the force of injury is dissipated over the chest. Lung tissue is fragile, and pulmonary contusion is the most common result of a thoracic injury. In addition, the child has a mobile mediastinum with a greater tendency to develop a tension pneumothorax.

Chest muscles are not well developed in children, and the diaphragm is the primary muscle for ventilatory effort. The healthy child will have minimal chest movement with respirations; however, the abdomen should

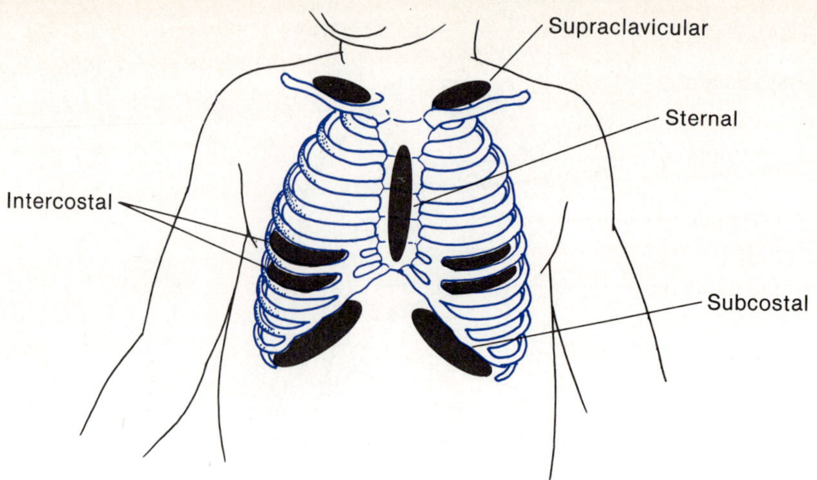

FIGURE 3.5 Retractions associated with respiratory distress: intercostal, suprasternal, subcostal, and sternal.

rise with inspiration and fall with expiration. Chest muscles are accessory respiratory muscles in the young child, used in cases of respiratory distress. Retractions are the result of the flexible rib cage and use of accessory muscles for breathing. Intercostal retractions (between the ribs) are seen with mild respiratory distress. Sternal (sternum sinking on inspiration) and supraclavicular (in the neck above the clavicles) retractions are seen as respiratory distress progresses in severity (Figure 3.5).

Normal respiratory rates vary with age; the younger the child, the faster the rate (see Table 3.1). Stress of any kind (fear, fever, excitement) will stimulate an increase in the child's respiratory rate. This hyperventilation may lead to gastric dilatation. Hypoxia results in a progressively more rapid respiratory rate if not treated with oxygen.

- Breathing becomes ineffective at rates faster than 60 breaths per minute in children. Air moves only in the upper airway, never reaching the lungs, when hyperventilation occurs. This leads to respiratory failure if not managed properly.

- Children have immature chest muscles and cannot sustain an excessively rapid respiratory rate. They will tire and subsequently decrease their respiratory rate, indicating development of ventilatory failure. Hypoxemia progresses and respiratory arrest may result if oxygen and/or ventilatory assistance is not provided.

TABLE 3.1 Normal Vital Signs for Children of Various Age Groups

Age Group	Respiratory Rate	Heart Rate	Systolic Blood Pressure
Newborn	30–50	120–160	50–70
Infant (1–12 months)	20–30	80–140	70–100
Toddler (1–3 years)	20–30	80–130	80–110
Preschooler (3–5 years)	20–30	80–120	80–110
School Age (6–12 years)	20–30	70–110	80–120
Adolescent (13+ years)	12–20	55–105	100–120

General Pediatric Assessment

Infants and children breathe two to three times faster and more shallowly than adults. Both smaller volume and less pressure are needed to ventilate the lungs. Children's tidal volume is proportional to their weight, 5–7 ml/kg, as with adults; therefore, a 12-month-old child weighing 10 kg would have a tidal volume of 70 ml. Only 16–20 cm water pressure (measured by manometer during bag mask ventilation) is usually needed to ventilate a healthy child's lungs. This amount of pressure causes a visible chest rise. Slightly higher pressures will be needed for the initial resuscitation of newborns and for children with diseased lungs (cystic fibrosis).

Children also have a higher metabolic rate than that of adults, leading to a higher oxygen requirement, 6–8 l/kg/minute in children compared to 3–4 l/kg/minute in an adult. (This is a metabolic oxygen requirement rather than oxygen flow rate used in patient management.) Hypoxemia develops more rapidly in children when ventilation is compromised.

Heart and Circulation

The child's heart is strong and healthy, unless a congenital heart defect is present. Newborns must make the transition from fetal to pulmonary circulation, usually completed during the first days after birth. Congenital heart defects, such as narrowed valves or abnormal openings between chambers, may result in hypoxemia, respiratory distress, and congestive heart failure in some children.

The normal heart rate varies by age and often increases in response to fear, exercise, hypoxia, and hypovolemia. Infants increase their cardiac output principally by increasing their heart rate. As with the respiratory rate, there is a normal heart rate range for children in various age groups (see Table 3.1).

- Tachycardia (an excessively high heart rate) is often a response to a demand for more oxygen to the brain. This may result from an increased metabolic rate, such as in a febrile illness, or from hypovolemia.
- Bradycardia (an excessively low heart rate) is a response to hypoxemia when tachycardia fails to adequately correct tissue hypoxia. Bradycardia is the initial response to hypoxemia in neonates. It is usually a sign of impending cardiac arrest.

The normal range for systolic blood pressure is also related to the age of the child (Table 3.1). Children do not become hypotensive with volume loss as rapidly as do adults. They are able to compensate for a while by increasing vascular resistance by constricting their veins and increasing their heart rate. When these compensating mechanisms are surpassed, as in cases of severe shock, *hypotension will suddenly develop*, usually after a 20 percent or greater volume loss has occurred.

The total circulating blood volume of a child is less than that of an adult; however, children will lose the same amount of blood as an adult from a comparable laceration. Because the child's head is proportionately larger, a greater percentage of the child's total blood volume goes to the head. The child's total blood volume (80–90 ml/kg) is proportional to the body weight (see Table 3.2). The newborn, averaging 3.5 kg or 7 lb, thus has approximately 300 ml of blood, slightly more than a cup.

TABLE 3.2 Total Blood Volume by Age Group and Weight

Age	Mean Weight		Approximate Blood Volume
	kg	lb	
Newborn	3–5	6–11	240–400
1 Year	10	22	800
3 Years	15	33	1200
5 Years	20	44	1600
8 Years	25	55	2000
10 Years	30	66	2400
15 Years	50	110	4000

Abdomen

A child's liver and spleen are also proportionately larger and more vascular than that of an adult's. Because the organs are larger, they have less protection by the rib cage and extend into the abdomen. The child's abdominal muscles are also immature and provide these organs less protection from injury.

Extremities

The child's arms and legs grow in length from the growth plates, located on each end of the long bones. Bones start out as cartilage and then harden, or ossify, as minerals are deposited in the cartilage. For this reason, children's bones are softer than those of an adult's; this holds true until puberty. Consequently, children's bones are easily fractured by bending and splintering.

All of the muscle fibers a child develops are present at birth; however, the fibers lengthen and develop throughout childhood as the bones grow.

Nervous System

The child's nervous system develops and matures throughout childhood. The nervous system controls conscious state, communication, motor, coordination, and sensory abilities.

Motor development occurs constantly, proceeding bilaterally in a head-to-toe progression. Motor development occurs in an established pattern, but each child has a personal timetable for achievement of specific functions such as sitting, controlled hand movement, and walking. Coordination is slower to develop and contributes to many falls and injuries.

Sensation is present in all portions of the body at birth. A young infant feels pain but does not have the ability to localize pain and isolate a response to pain to the involved extremity. As nerve connections develop, response to pain becomes much more localized.

Motor and sensory development are most advanced in the cranial nerves at birth because of their life-sustaining function and protective reflexes. These nerves control such functions as blinking, sucking and swallowing, vision, and hearing.

As part of the pediatric assessment, much information about the child's condition will be obtained by observing the scene and environment in which the child is found. Clues in the environment may help the field provider to determine the child's problem. Such clues may include the presence of pill bottles, plants, or household cleaners; position in which the child is found; and a mechanism of injury.

It is equally important to observe the interaction between the child and parent or other care provider. Children generally seek reassurance and comfort from these persons when afraid, ill, or in pain. Passive children who either do not seek or appear to expect such comfort are demonstrating inappropriate behavior. They should be assessed first for an altered level of consciousness. When such a child is alert and conscious, consider the possibility of child abuse or neglect.

The elements of the pediatric history are the same as those collected for adults:

- Reason why EMS was activated.
- Present illness—symptoms and their characteristics; duration; change in symptoms over time; did something precipitate the event? treatment already attempted; has the child seen a doctor for this problem?
- Past medical history—significant health problems; any chronic diseases? prematurity, congenital defects, major injuries or surgery, last time the child was at a doctor?
- Medications—those taken for the present illness (including aspirin, Tylenol, or other over-the-counter preparation); when was last dose given? what medications are used routinely for other illnesses?
- Allergies—to foods, medications, plants; type of response.
- Patient's weight—best estimate, or what it was at last visit to doctor.

The *AMPLE* mnemonic is one method used by prehospital providers to remember key elements of the patient history.

A = Allergies
M = Medications
P = Past history
L = Last meal
E = Events leading up to current problem.

If the patient is an infant, some additional information about the health problems of the mother during the pregnancy should be obtained, such as mother's expected delivery date, presence of high blood pressure or vaginal bleeding, and use of any drugs.

For young children it will be necessary to obtain the history from the parent or care provider. However, once a child is old enough to verbalize, which is about 4 years of age, include the child in the history taking. Ask simple questions the child can understand and answer, such as, "Show me with your finger where it hurts."

Enhancing Cooperation for the Examination

Once the prehospital provider has surveyed the scene and determined that the child has no immediately life-threatening injuries, it is important to gain the child's trust before proceeding with the rest of the examination. The child needs a "transition phase" to become comfortable with the EMT or paramedic and any unfamiliar equipment to be used. *If the child has any life-threatening injuries, intervention begins immediately, without regard for the child's adjustment to the field provider.*

Some units carry teddy bears or dolls to give to small children in their care. If such a toy is not available on your unit, try to use one of the child's favorite toys. A toy like this gives the child something to hold onto for security. It can also be used to obtain a better history from the child, such as pointing out "where it hurts" (Figure 3.6).

To reassure the nonacutely ill child, project a calm and friendly manner. Include the child in the conversation with the parent. Ask questions such as "What happened?" "How do you feel?" "Can you point with one finger to where it hurts?" When speaking to the child, use age-appropriate language and a quiet tone of voice. Whenever possible, speak to the child at the child's eye level.

Certain words may cause more anxiety in a child and should be avoided, if possible, even in discussions with your partner. *Cut* implies pain; *laceration* will not be understood by young children and may cause less anxiety to the child when discussing care with your partner.

Take, as in "take a blood pressure," implies removal of something. Alternate wording to explain this procedure to the child could be "measure how hard your heart is working." *Bleeding* may cause children to think that all their blood will leak out.

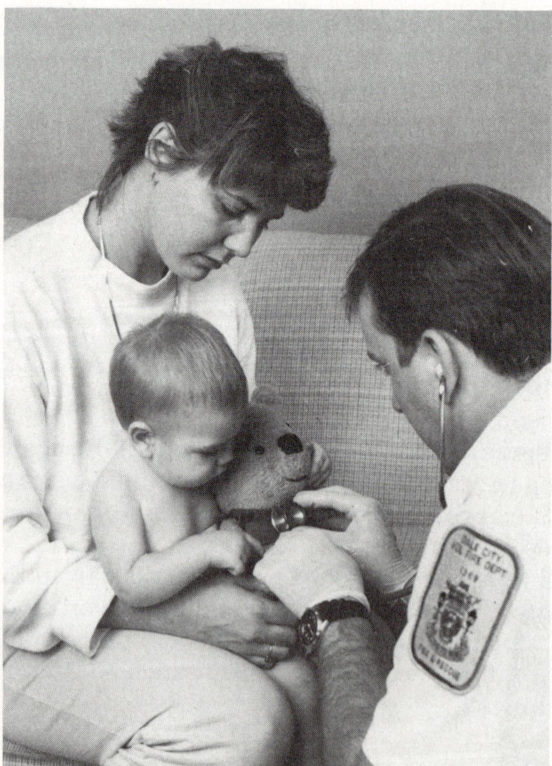

FIGURE 3.6 During the patient interview, speak to the child in a calm voice at the child's eye level. Provide a security toy which can be used to improve communication with the child.

Smile at the child frequently and project confidence. Look at your patient periodically, rather than staring at him or her. Children may perceive staring as threatening and become more afraid. Make sure young patients have their security toys or provide a toy to distract them. Keep the child with the parent for the examination, whenever possible.

Be honest when explaining, in simple terms, what you are going to do. If a procedure will hurt, explain this just prior to doing it, and say it will be over soon. However, do not inform the child about expected pain too soon, as the fear of pain increases with the length of the wait. Expect children to be distressed about a painful procedure, but most will cope better if informed. The child also benefits by learning to trust your honesty for the remainder of your care.

To gain the child's cooperation for the use of instruments during the examination, let the child handle or play with the equipment (Figure 3.7). Demonstrate how the equipment works on the parent, the EMT, or the child's toy. Try to explain the equipment in nonthreatening terms:

- A penlight is a candle that can be blown out.
- A stethoscope is a telephone.
- A blood pressure cuff is a balloon, and the dial is a clock.

Examine the child seated on the parent's lap, facing you (Figure 3.8). If an infant or toddler becomes distressed, place him or her over the parent's shoulder, facing away from you. Auscultation of the chest can be done successfully through the back because the chest wall is thin in children. You can then walk around the parent's back to look at the infant's face for other assessment parameters. When touching the child, begin at the feet, proceeding to the head. The child may develop more trust if less-threatening anatomy is examined first. Make sure your motions are slow and deliberate.

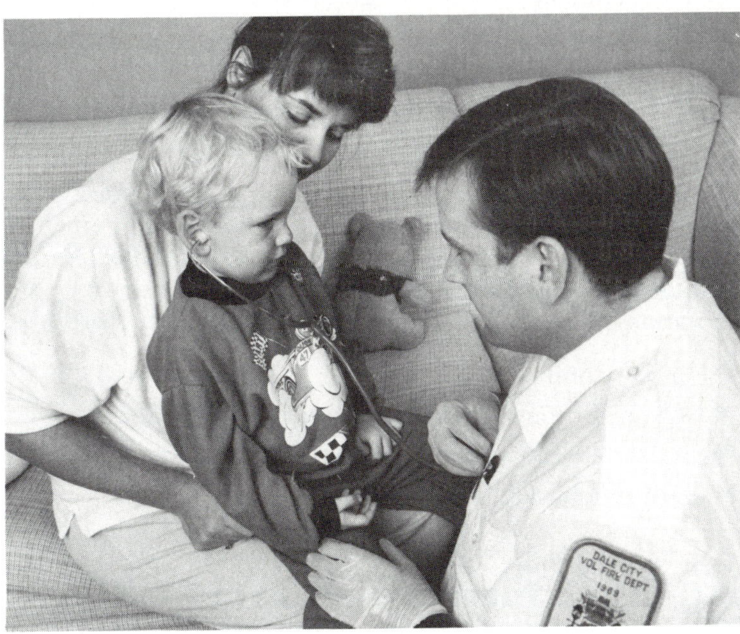

FIGURE 3.7 To enhance cooperation during the examination, permit the child who is not critically ill or injured to become familiar with the examining equipment.

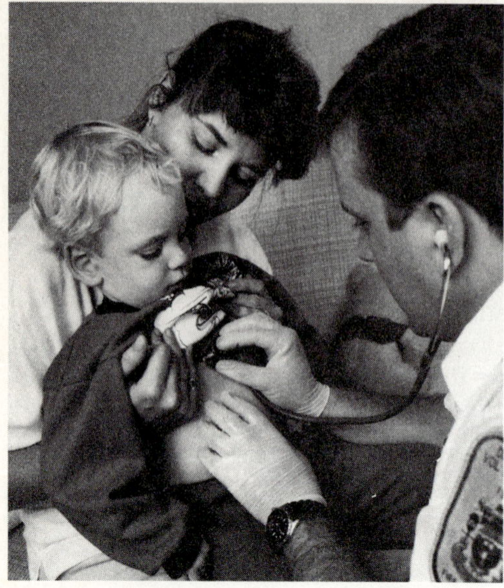 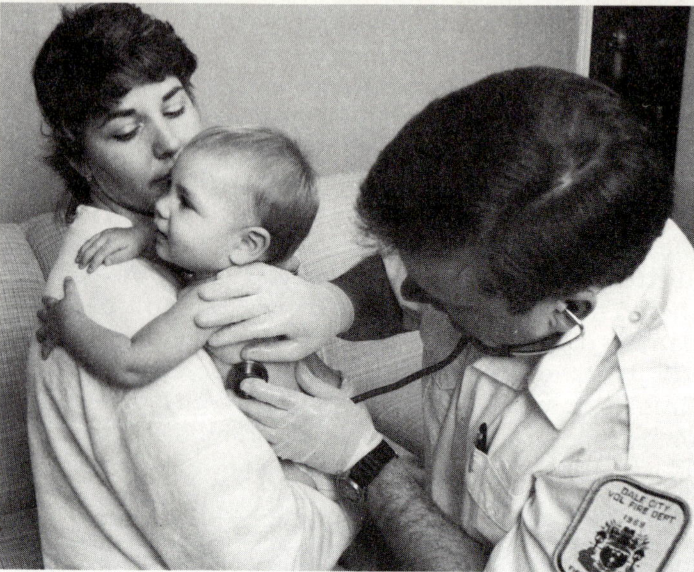

A   B

FIGURE 3.8　Encourage the child's sense of security during the examination by keeping the child with the parent. (A) Examine the toddler on the parent's lap. (B) Examine the infant who is held across the parent's shoulder.

A number of factors will contribute to your success in completing all aspects of the examination. Examination of the child will be more difficult in any of the following situations:

- If the child has had a bad prior experience with a health care provider;
- If the child is not old enough to understand the reasons for what you are doing;
- If a parent is not present to reassure the child;
- If the child has been taught that certain parts of his or her body should not be touched by a stranger.

If the child becomes uncooperative in spite of your best efforts to reduce the child's anxiety, you should complete what you can of the assessment and transport. It is fruitless to waste more time. Remember to take advantage of assessment opportunities, even if the child is uncooperative. Observation of the crying child will provide a lot of information:

- Quality of the cry
- An open mouth to evaluate color and hydration
- A deep breath as the child inspires to evaluate breath sounds
- Symmetry of facial expression.

Physical Examination and Interpretation of Findings

Inspection, auscultation, and palpation are the examination techniques most frequently used during the primary and secondary survey. In every case you will initially perform your ABCDEs to detect the presence of any life-threatening problem.

- Listening to the child's cry, voice, and breathing provides information about the status of the airway and ventilation.
- Observing the child's skin color and assessing capillary refill provides information about circulation.
- Observing the child's interest (orientation or mental status) during the assessment provides clues about the level of consciousness.

Weight of the Child

If the parent or caretaker is unable to provide you with an estimate of the child's weight, it will be necessary to make your own estimate. Parents generally know their child's weight in pounds, but drug dosages are calculated by weight in kilograms. The conversion factor is 2.2 lb = 1 kg, or refer to Table 3.2. While children come in various weights for their age, one formula to estimate the child's weight in kilograms is as follows:

$$8 + (2 \times \text{the child's age})$$

A 5-year-old child would then weigh approximately 18 kg.

$$8 + (2 \times 5) = 18 \text{ kg}$$

Skin Condition

The color of a child's skin provides clues about tissue perfusion. To best assess the generalized color in dark-skinned children, observe the palms of the hands and the mucous membranes in the mouth.

- Pallor may indicate poor tissue perfusion.
- Localized flushing or redness may indicate inflammation.
- A mottled appearance is associated with hypoxia or hypothermia.
- Cyanosis is most often associated with a congenital heart defect, but may be present in cases of severe hypoxemia associated with respiratory distress.
- During their transition to extrauterine life, newborns often have cyanotic feet and hands while the rest of the body is pink (acrocyanosis).
- Jaundice, yellowing of the sclerae of the eyes and skin, is associated with hepatitis and a congenital liver defect.

Look for signs of tissue injury, such as bruises, burns, abrasions, lacerations, bleeding, and inflammation. Note their distribution and any special characteristics.

The resilience of the skin (turgor) and dryness of the mucous membranes in the mouth provide clues about the hydration status of the child. Pinch some skin between your finger and thumb and let it go. The skin should immediately return to previous contour (Figure 3.9). Any delay in this return, or tenting, indicates poor skin turgor and moderate to severe dehydration. Dry or parched mucous membranes also indicate dehydration.

Moist skin may be related to perspiration associated with exercise, high external temperatures, and fever. The child with an uncorrected congenital heart defect may have profuse sweating with minimal activity, such as feeding.

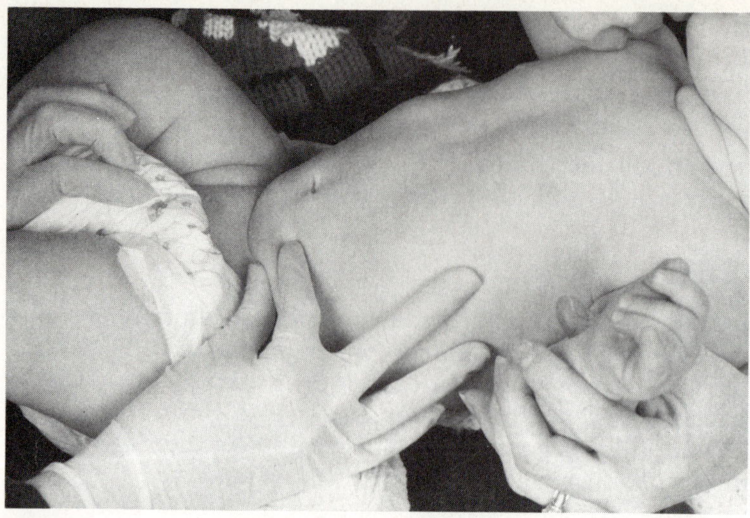

FIGURE 3.9 Testing for skin turgor. Pinch some skin between your finger and thumb and release it. Watch to see if the skin immediately returns as expected to its previous contour.

Skin temperature can be assessed by placing the back of your hand against the child's forehead and extremities. Cool, pale extremities are associated with shock and hypothermia. Flushed, warm skin is associated with a fever.

Respiratory Assessment

A crying or talking child has a patent airway, at least at that time. Listen to the quality of the child's cry or speech to gain other clues about the child's problems.

- Hoarseness may be caused by a foreign body or inflammation associated with an upper airway disease.
- Moaning is associated with shock and a decreasing level of consciousness.
- A high-pitched cry is associated with increased intracranial pressure.

Observe the child's face for nasal flaring, which is the body's attempt to expand the size of the airway to move more air. Also observe the child's facial expression. *Children who are anxious and focused on breathing, rather than demonstrating interest in what is happening around them, are in acute respiratory distress* (Figure 3.10). Listen for other sounds that can be heard without a stethoscope.

- Stridor is a hoarse voice or cry and a seal-like barking cough that is heard on inspiration and expiration. It is associated with a foreign body and inflammation in the glottic area of the trachea.
- Wheezing is the passage of expired air over mucous secretions that have collected in the bronchi during bronchospasm.
- Grunting is a sound in which an infant attempts to build back pres-

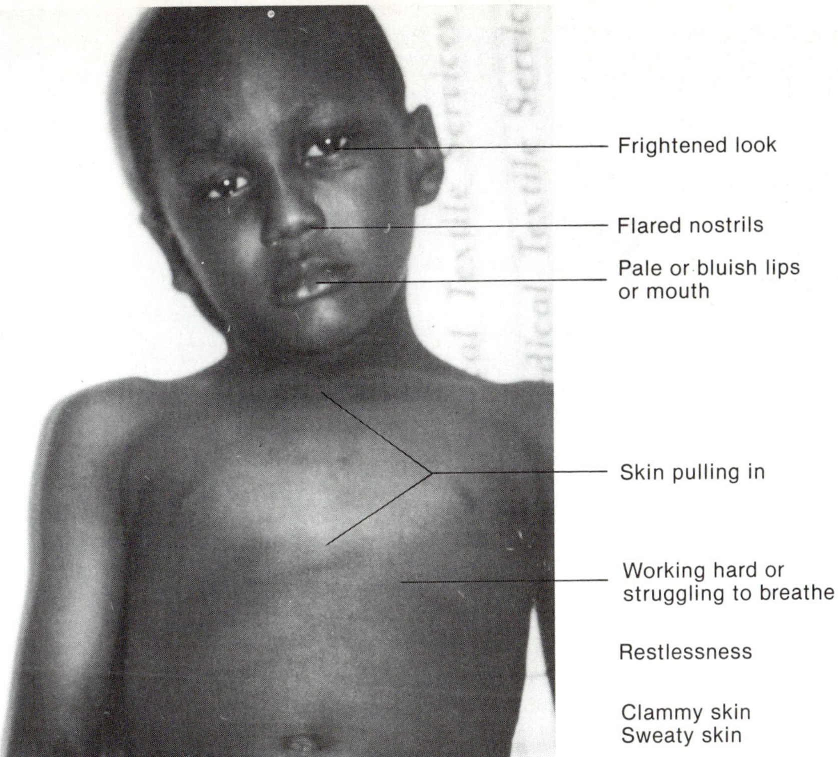

FIGURE 3.10 Observe signs indicating respiratory distress.

sure during expiration to keep the alveoli open. It indicates severe respiratory distress in newborns.

● Bubbling or gurgling may indicate an open chest wound.

Observe the movement of the chest with respirations. There should be bilateral chest rise with each breath, even if it is subtle. Note the presence of any retractions, and their location (intercostal, suprasternal, and sternal). These indicate increased effort with breathing. There should be a synchronized rise of the chest and abdomen with each breath. See-saw respirations, in which the child's chest falls (sternal retraction) as the abdomen rises and vice versa, indicate severe respiratory distress.

Count the respiratory rate by observing the abdomen rise. Make this assessment prior to touching the child to obtain the most accurate rate. Often touching the child will increase the child's anxiety and lead to an acceleration in the respiratory rate.

Listen to breath sounds with the stethoscope. A pediatric stethoscope is not necessary; the bell of an adult stethoscope pressed firmly to the skin so the skin fills the bell will create a pediatric diaphragm. Because the chest wall is so thin in children, breath sounds are disseminated from one side of the chest to the other. Place the diaphragm of the stethoscope in the axillae along the midaxillary line and just under the clavicles in the midclavicular line (Figure 3.11). Listening in these locations provides the best chance to hear local breath sounds rather than the sounds transmitted from the other lung. If a child is crying, be patient and listen for the breath sounds at the end of each cry when the child inspires. The breath sounds should be present bilaterally.

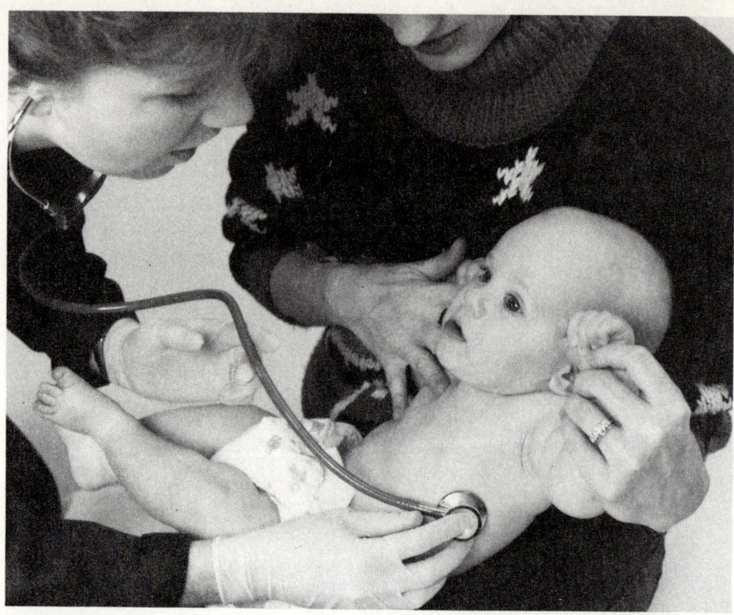

FIGURE 3.11   Assess breath sounds by placing the stethoscope along the mid-axillary line as demonstrated here and just under the clavicles in the midclavicular line.

Circulatory Assessment

Capillary refill is a good indicator of circulatory perfusion in children and one of the best indicators of early shock. Press on the child's nailbed and release. A pink return to the blanched tissue should occur within 2 seconds, or the time it takes to say "capillary refill." Alternate sites for capillary refill assessment are the forehead, sternum, or gums of the mouth (Figure 3.12). These alternate sites should be used in any child suspected of hypothermia, when vasoconstriction to the extremities is present.

Observe for any lacerations or bleeding. Assess the amount of blood loss in relation to the child's total blood volume, generally estimated to be 80 ml/kg (see Table 3.2, page 32).

Count the child's heart rate. For infants, palpate either the brachial or femoral pulse, or auscultate the apical pulse. The infant's neck is so short that it is difficult to palpate the carotid pulse. Older children can have their carotid pulse palpated. Because the chest wall is so thin, it is also possible to auscultate the heart through the back when the child is held over the parent's shoulder.

The quality of distal pulses should be assessed, but these sites are the least accurate to use when determining the heart rate of a child under 4 years of age. There is no tested association between the strength of distal pulses and blood pressure in children. (Children readily vasoconstrict blood vessels in their extremities, and distal pulses become hard to palpate.) If the brachial and femoral pulses are weak in a child, this is an indicator of severe shock.

Children's heart rates will vary by age and with respirations. Heart rate increases on inspiration and decreases on expiration. The child's myocardium is generally strong and dysrhythmias are uncommon. Bradycardia and asystole are the two most common dysrhythmias. Make sure to note any rate irregularities.

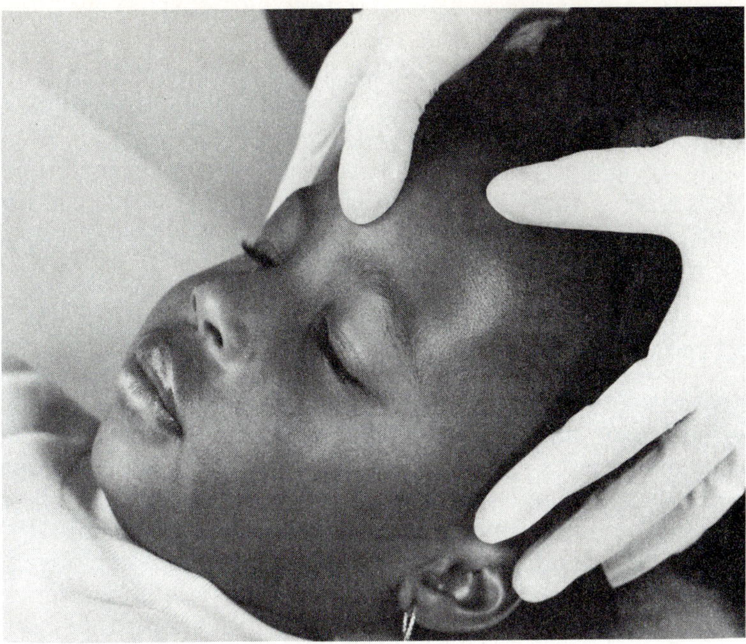

FIGURE 3.12 Assessment of capillary refill time by pressing the skin over a bony prominence (forehead, sternum, chin) or over a nailbed.

When taking a child's blood pressure, the cuff or bladder size is the most important variable in obtaining an accurate reading. Blood pressure cuffs come in numerous sizes; thus it is necessary to determine the one most appropriate for the child you are assessing:

- The bladder should not overlap when wrapped around the extremity, but should cover at least two-thirds of the circumference.
- The width of the cuff should be about two-thirds of the length of the long bone used (upper arm, lower arm, thigh).

If the cuff you have does not fit one extremity in the child, such as the upper arm, see if it can be used on the thigh.

It may be difficult to get an accurate blood pressure reading when the child does not cooperate. Emotional upset, fear, and anxiety will all increase the systolic reading. In some cases it will be difficult to auscultate the blood pressure because of extrinsic noise, unless an ultrasound doppler is available. The systolic reading may then be estimated by palpation. While there are ranges of blood pressure by age group, a formula to estimate the appropriate blood pressure in a child over 1 year of age is:

$$80 + (2 \times \text{the child's age [years]}) = \text{systolic BP}$$

The diastolic reading should be approximately two-thirds of the systolic reading.

Abdomen

The contour of the abdomen should be observed when the child is supine. It is usually rounded in children. A sunken or scaphoid abdomen in a newborn should alert you to the possibility of a hiatal hernia, a life-threatening congenital defect.

Observe for any discolorations on the abdomen such as bruises or bluish discoloration around the umbilicus (Cullen's sign) or along the flanks. These signs may indicate intra-abdominal bleeding.

Lightly palpate the abdomen, noting any expression of pain on the child's face or guarding as you palpate (Figure 3.13). Do not rely on the young children to tell you when it hurts. They will often say it hurts when they feel you touching or tickling them.

Extremities

Observe the alignment of the arms and legs, noting any deformity that might indicate a fracture. The alignment should be symmetric, when comparing extremities on each side. Carefully inspect for any open wounds in the area of a suspected fracture, which would indicate an open fracture.

Palpate each extremity, noting any deformity or pain. Palpate the distal pulse; check capillary refill time and the presence of sensation whenever a fracture is suspected prior to and immediately after any manipulation of the extremity. Compare your findings with those on the opposite extremity.

Neurologic Assessment

Level of consciousness is initially assessed by determining how alert the child is. Infants and young children who are not verbal must be observed for activity and interest in what is happening. The infant and young child who is irritable and cannot be consoled by the parent has an altered level of consciousness. Parents are often able to tell you if the child is not as alert as usual.

The *AVPU* mnemonic is useful in the initial assessment of conscious state.

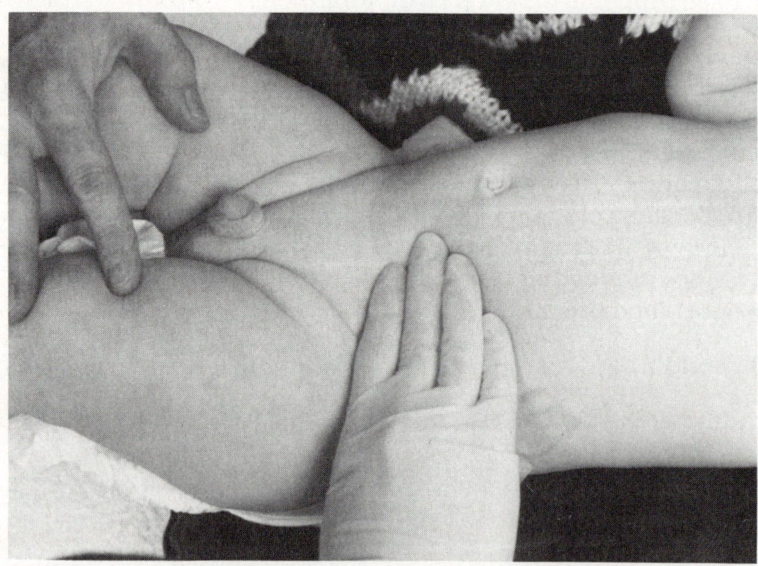

FIGURE 3.13   Lightly palpate the abdomen to detect any pain, guarding, or rigidity.

Alert—Children are curious and usually vigilant when approached by a stranger.

Responsive to *Verbal* stimuli—The child is uninterested in events or dozing (lethargic), but responds by turning the head or stopping activity in response to sound.

Responsive to *Painful* stimuli—The child is hard to arouse, (stuporous) but moans or moves when pinched.

Unresponsive—The child is comatose and does not respond to any stimuli.

Cranial nerves are important to evaluate in the child, especially in the case of head injury, because they originate in the brain. They control the movement and sensation of the head and neck, and special senses such as vision, hearing, smell, and taste.

- Observe the child's face for symmetry of facial features when the child smiles or cries.
- Observe eye movement by having the child look at a penlight or toy as you move it slowly from one side of the child's face to the other. Make sure the child's head does not move.
- Use the penlight to check pupils for size and reaction to light.
- A response to questions or turning the head to noise indicates the presence of hearing.
- Infants should be able to suck and swallow from a bottle in a coordinated way without choking. However, do not feed a head-injured infant to assess this cranial nerve.

The Glasgow Coma Scale can be used to quantify the level of consciousness. It must be slightly modified for use with infants. The two categories that have different criteria for scoring are *verbal response* and *motor response.* (See Table 3.3 for the recommended modification for infants.)

The integrity of the child's motor function can be tested by observing the voluntary, purposeful movement of the extremities. Infants under 4 months of age can have motor function tested by the palmar grasp reflex.

TABLE 3.3   Glasgow Coma Scale Modifications for Infants

Category	Response	Score
Verbal	Coos, babbles, or cries spontaneously	5
	Irritable crying	4
	Cries to pain	3
	Moans to pain	2
	None	1
Motor	Spontaneous movement	6
	Withdraws to touch	5
	Withdraws to pain	4
	Abnormal flexion	3
	Abnormal extension	2
	None	1
Eye Opening (same as adult)	Spontaneous	4
	To speech	3
	To pain	2
	None	1

Source: Adapted from James, H.E., (1986): "Neurologic evaluation and support in the child with acute brain insult," *Pediatric Annals,* 15(1):17.

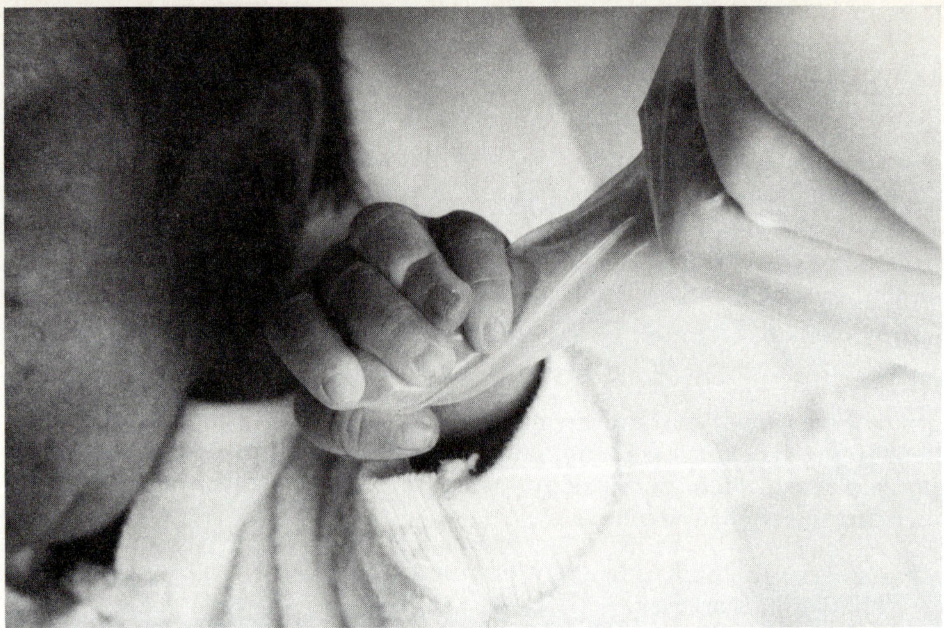

FIGURE 3.14 Test motor function in the young infant with the palmar grasp reflex. Place your finger into the palm of the infant's hands, which should be followed by an immediate grasp around your finger.

Place your finger into the palm of the infant's hands (Figure 3.14). There should be an immediate grasp around your finger, equal in strength on each side. Offer a toy to the toddler and watch him or her take it. Test strength by seeing how tightly the child holds on to the toy. The same information can be obtained by watching the child cling to the parent or attempt to get away from you. The child over 3 years of age will often follow directions and squeeze your finger or push your hand away if you approach this like a game.

Sensation can be tested by lightly stroking each arm and leg with your finger. This often stimulates a ticklish response from which the child attempts to withdraw. There should be equal movement bilaterally.

Signs Associated with Common Pediatric Emergencies

Once you have completed your examination of the child, it is then necessary to put signs together to determine what is wrong with the young patient and the severity of the problem. Some signs fall together in a classic pattern to assist you in making your assessment (see Table 3.4).

TABLE 3.4 Classic Patterns of Signs Indicating Various Physiologic Problems

Pain	*Respiratory Distress*
Shallow breathing	Nasal flaring
Irritable crying	Mottled, dusky skin color
Splinting	Tachypnea, shallow breathing

Pain	Respiratory Distress
Facial expression change when touched or moved Resists movement Rigid posturing	Altered level of consciousness Sounds—stridor, hoarseness, muffled voice, wheezing Tripod positioning Retractions Asymmetric chest movement "See-saw" respirations
Early Shock Tachycardia >130/minute Capillary refill >2 seconds Pale, cool skin Altered level of consciousness Normal systolic blood pressure	**Late Shock** Tachycardia >130/minute Capillary refill > 3–4 seconds Pallor, cold extremities Altered level of consciousness Systolic BP <80 mmHg (except infants whose systolic BP is often normally lower)
Moderate Dehydration Sunken fontanelle Pallor Doughy skin texture Dry mucous membranes	**Severe Dehydration** Sunken fontanelle Signs of shock Parched mucous membranes No tears Sunken eyeballs
Altered Level of Consciousness Combative Decreased responsiveness Lethargy Weak cry, moaning Personality change	**Increased Intracranial Pressure** Bulging fontanelle Altered level of consciousness High-pitched cry Change in vital signs Irritable cry, unable to distract or console child

Assessment References

CHAMEIDES, L., ed., *Textbook of Pediatric Advanced Life Support.* Dallas: American Heart Association, 1988.

DICK, T., and JENKINS, G., "Looking at little people: Tips on assessing young children in the field," *JEMS*, 6, no. 7 (July 1981), pp. 24–32.

JACKSON, P. L., "Assessing increased intracranial pressure in infants and young children," *Critical Care Update*, 10, no. 9 (September 1983), pp. 8–15.

JAMES, H. E., "Neurologic evaluation and support in the child with acute brain insult," *Pediatric Annals*, 15, no. 1, (January 1986), p. 17.

SEIDEL, H. M., and others, *Mosby's Guide to Physical Examination.* ed. 2, St. Louis: Mosby-Yearbook, Inc., 1991.

SEIDEL, J. S., and HENDERSON, D. P., eds., *Prehospital Care of Pediatric Emergencies,* Los Angeles: Pediatric Society of California, 1987.

Equipment and Procedures for Management of ABC's

OBJECTIVES

When you have completed this chapter you should be able to

✳ Describe the anatomic and physiologic considerations in the management of the child's airway.

✳ Describe effective airway management with basic life-support maneuvers.

✳ Identify techniques for packaging an injured child that protect the airway, breathing, and cervical spine.

✳ Describe advanced airway and respiratory management of the child to include the following:
- Orotracheal intubation
- Cricothyrotomy
- Pleural decompression

✳ Describe the procedures to obtain a fluid route in the pediatric patient to include the following:
- Peripheral lines
- Umbilical vein cannulation
- Intraosseous infusion

✳ List the steps in the procedure for defibrillation and cardioversion of the pediatric patient.

Airway and Breathing

The purpose of the respiratory system is to deliver oxygen to the lungs and body tissues and remove carbon dioxide. It maintains a delicate balance within the body, making adjustments on a continuous basis. The ability of the respiratory system to regulate change assures a constant and precise exchange of gases. The airway must be open for gas exchange to occur.

Therefore, it is essential for all emergency providers to master the skill of airway management. This is accomplished by having a thorough understanding of the anatomy and physiology of the airway and respiratory system, as well as those management techniques and adjuncts used in the assessment and treatment.

Anatomy and Physiology

The chapter on general pediatric assessment provides a thorough review of the pediatric respiratory system as well as all other body systems. It is suggested that a review of that chapter be completed prior to this section.

There are six anatomical features to know in order to manage the pediatric airway effectively (refer to Figure 3.3). They are as follows:

- Nasal openings are smaller.
- The tongue is large in proportion to the oral cavity.
- The trachea is short and narrow.
- The larynx is higher and more anterior.
- The nose and face are flat.
- The tracheal cartilage is more elastic.

With these six unique features of the pediatric airway committed to memory, you can next concentrate on management with the appropriate adjunct.

Plan of Action for Airway Control

The goal of airway management is to achieve adequate oxygenation. This can be accomplished with a variety of maneuvers and equipment, from very simple to very complex. In planning airway management, a solid plan of action needs to be established, which includes an assessment of the child's current airway status and the possible future needs of this patient. A six-step plan of action from simple to complex should be implemented for every child that presents with respiratory distress or an uncontrolled airway.

1. Reposition the airway
2. Suction
3. Bag-mask ventilation
4. Oral airway
5. Orotracheal intubation
6. Surgical intervention

After assuring the scene is safe and noting any mechanism of injury, opening the airway is the first step. The airway should be repositioned. Because of the child's large head, there is a tendency for the trachea to become flexed when the child is supine. A small pillow or towel placed underneath the shoulders raises the shoulders and straightens the neck, so the child is in "sniffing position" or neutral alignment (Figure 4.1).

Use the chin lift of the jaw thrust to reposition the airway. If a neck injury is suspected, the preferred method is the jaw thrust with in-line stabilization. The tongue is the most common airway obstruction in infants and children. The jaw thrust and chin lift move the tongue forward, opening the airway (Figure 4.2).

Suctioning is the next step if the airway is still uncontrolled. If the patient continues with inadequate air exchange then assist the patient with bag-mask ventilation with 100% oxygen. When the child is unconscious without a gag reflex, an oral or nasal airway may be inserted. Continued airway instability requires orotracheal intubation or, as a last resort, surgical intervention by cricothyrotomy.

This plan of action in anticipating the potential airway management needs of the patient works well by following the simple to the more complex management options. It is important to proceed from the most simple airway maneuver on up because of the potential complications associated with more complex maneuvers.

Airway Adjuncts

As a rescuer you are provided with an arsenal of equipment to manage the airway. By using this equipment, along with the knowledge you already possess and the information provided in this text, you will be optimally prepared to manage the pediatric airway.

Oxygen

Normal atmospheric concentration of oxygen is 21%. Prehospital providers have the ability to increase this concentration anywhere from 30% to 100%, depending on the selection of adjuncts. To start there must be an

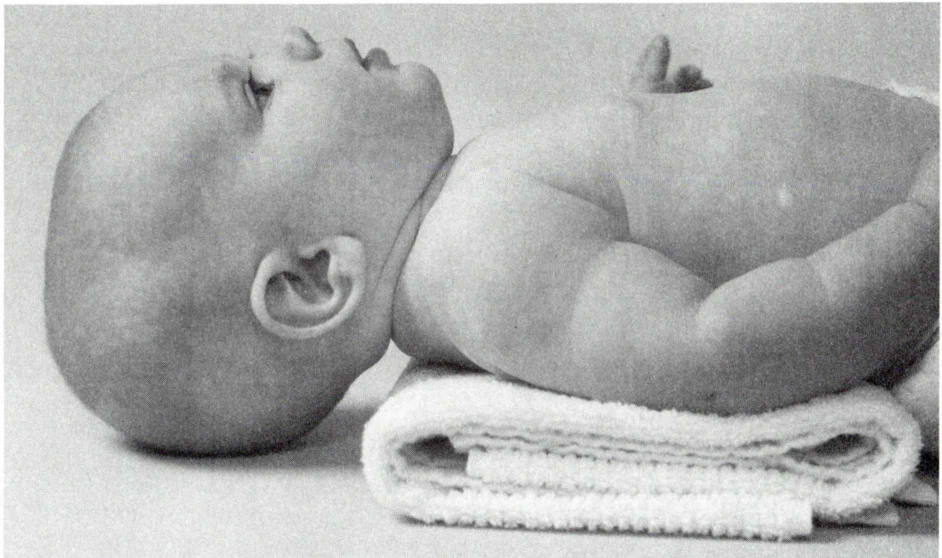

FIGURE 4.1   Head in neutral or sniffing position. Use a folded towel to keep the airway in alignment.

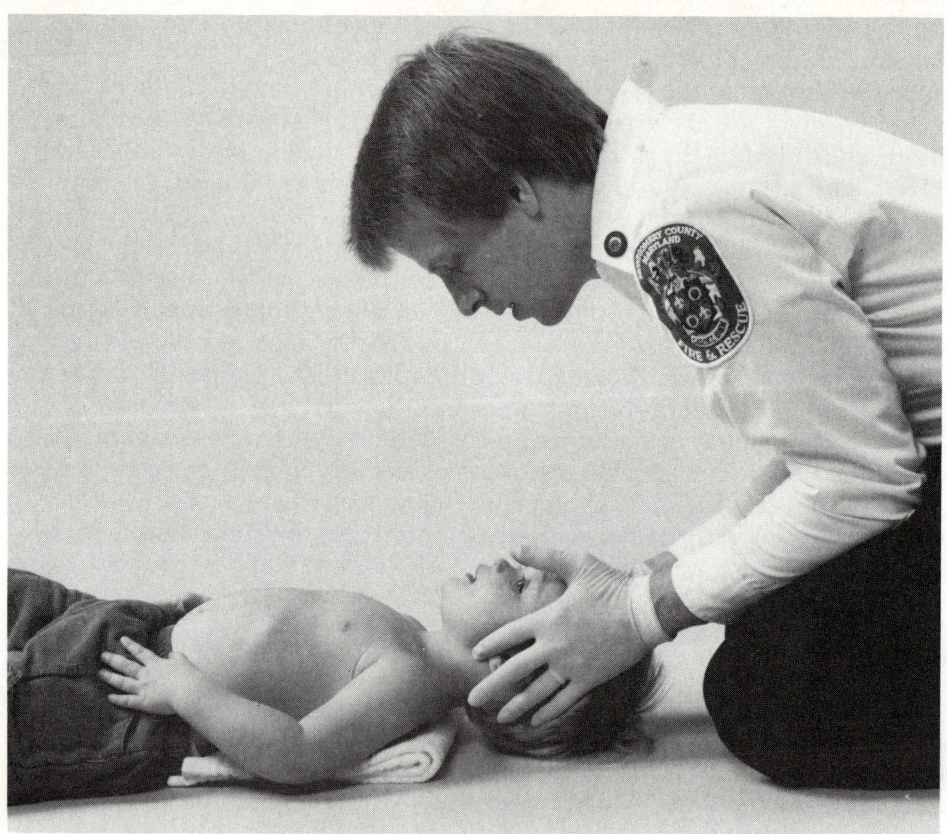

FIGURE 4.2 Jaw-thrust maneuver. Note the simultaneous in-line stabilization of the C-spine.

adequate supply of oxygen. Other highly desirable characteristics are humidified or heated oxygen.

- Humidified oxygen prevents the mucous membranes of the airway from drying and becoming thick with secretions.
- Heated oxygen is particularly beneficial in cold climates and management of children with hypothermia. When cold oxygen is blown on their faces in the distribution of the trigeminal nerve, newborns and young infants also have the diving reflex triggered causing apnea and bradycardia.

Unfortunately, warmed humidified oxygen is often unavailable in the prehospital setting. This should not preclude the rescuer from administering oxygen.

Oxygen Delivery Devices

The nasal cannula is a plastic tube with two plastic prongs that can be inserted into the anterior portion of the nares. With a flow rate of 4–6 l/min, a concentration of 30–50% is achieved. Increasing the flow rate will not increase the concentration, but will only lead to increased irritation of the nose and throat. Position the nasal cannula in the pediatric patient, making sure the prongs do not fit in the nostril too tightly. If blanching of the nostril is constant, then the prong is too large and should be removed. An alternate position might be to rest the prongs on the ridge of the lip,

Equipment and Procedures for Management of ABC's

pointed toward the nostril (Figure 4.3). The nasal cannula should be used in the older child or adolescent and is not adaptive to the younger child.

The simple face mask (Figure 4.4a) is a plastic mask designed to fit over the nose and mouth of the patient. The mask has vents on the side that allow for air to be exhaled. At a flow rate of 6–10 l/min, the concentration will vary from 30–60%. This variation is dependent on the patient's respiratory rate and depth of respiration. The more external air entering the mask, the lower the concentration. As a rule, this type of mask should have a minimum liter flow of 6 l/min to achieve higher levels of oxygen concentration.

The non-rebreather mask is equipped with a reservoir bag and a one-way valve that allows inspiration of oxygen and expiration of gases. With a flow rate of 10–12 l/min and a tight fit, this mask should deliver 90–100% oxygen (Figure 4.4b).

Special Considerations

Placing one of these adjuncts on a pediatric patient can be a test in itself. Some points to remember include the following:

- Always explain what you are doing to the patient. Children are afraid of everything involved in this situation. An explanation, and possibly a demonstration, can go a long way to comfort the young patient. Use the parents to demonstrate placement of the mask.

- Some children will not tolerate a mask because they feel it is suffocating them. In this case, the mask can be held in front of the child by the parent, or perhaps even the child if he or she is able to do so.

- If the child still resists, try a nasal cannula. Some oxygen is better than no oxygen.

FIGURE 4.3 Delivery of oxygen via nasal cannula in the school-age child.

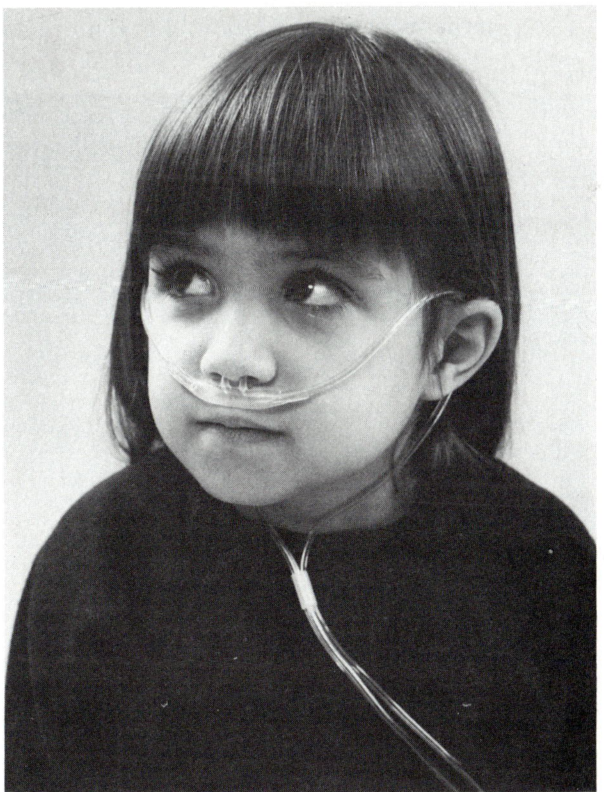

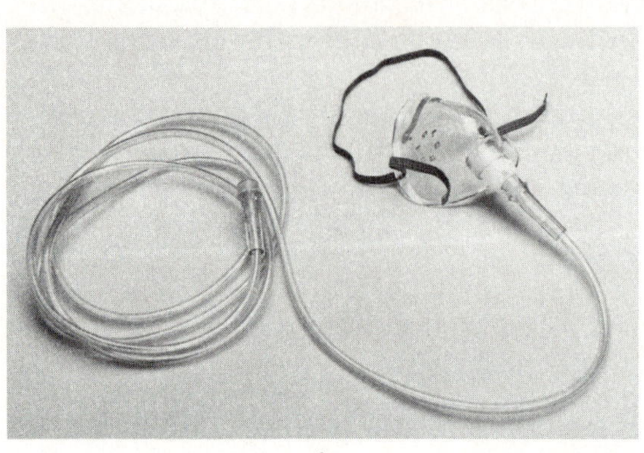

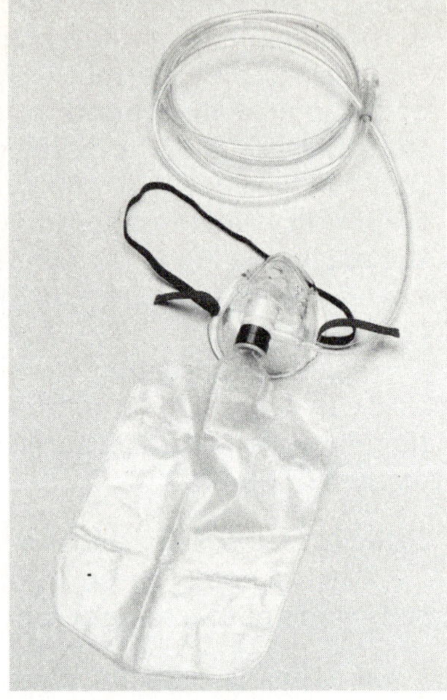

A   B

FIGURE 4.4   (A) Simple face mask. (B) Non-rebreather mask.

- In delivering oxygen to an infant, care should be taken not to blow the oxygen directly onto the face. The infant has an immature nervous system, and stimulation of the nerves around the mouth and nose with cold oxygen could trigger a slowing of the respiratory and heart rate. The recommended method of delivering oxygen is the blow-by method. This can be done by placing the oxygen tubing through the bottom of a paper cup, and holding the cup to one side of the infant's face, about 4 to 6 inches away (see Figure 4.5).

FIGURE 4.5   Delivery of oxygen using blow-by method.

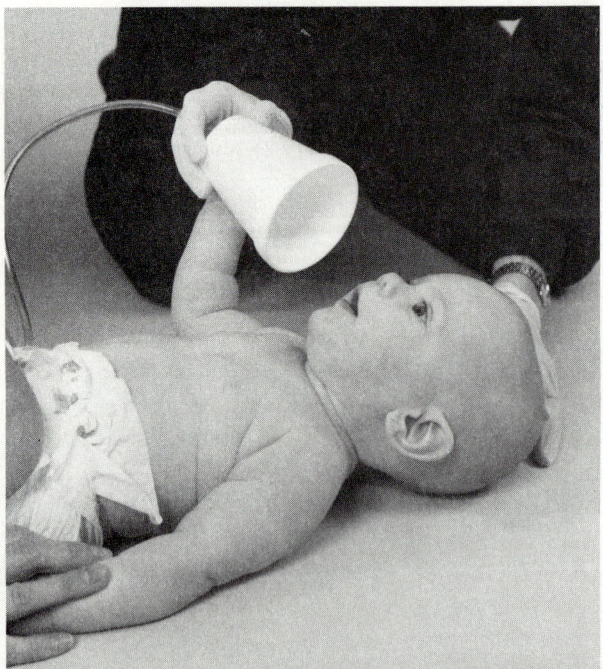

Equipment and Procedures for Management of ABC's

Oral and Nasal Airways

The oropharyngeal airway is a curved plastic tube that can be inserted into the mouth to lift the tongue off the back of the throat. It should be used only in the unconscious patient who has an absent gag reflex. Pediatric sizes range from 000–4.

Measurement of the oral airway is the most important step in the process. An oral airway that is too long will rest against the epiglottis, obstructing the airway completely. An oral airway that is too short will push the tongue back into the posterior pharynx, resulting in a completely obstructed airway. The proper method of measurement and insertion is as follows:

- To select the proper-size oral airway, place it near the face between the ear and mouth. Choose the oral airway that most closely fits in the space from the angle of the jaw to the crease of the mouth.

- Using a tongue depressor, press down the tongue while inserting the airway. Insertion should be done in the position of function. There is potential for damage to the soft tissues of the mouth if the oral airway is inserted upside down and rotated.

- Assess for good air exchange (Figure 4.6).

The nasopharyngeal airway is a soft rubber tube that is inserted through the nose into the posterior pharynx. This allows air to pass from the nose to the lung. The airway is available in sizes 12 to 36 French. A 12 French is about the size of a 3 mm endotracheal tube and should fit a full-term infant. This adjunct is not widely recommended for pediatric prehospital management because of the possibility of laceration of the adenoids, which are much larger in children than in adults. The nasopharyngeal airway should be inserted as follows:

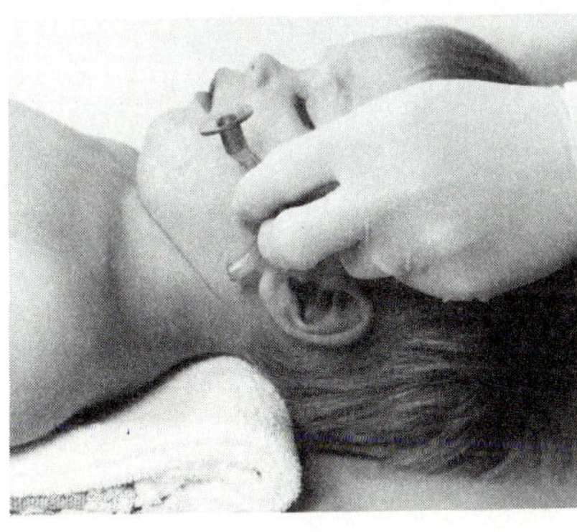

A

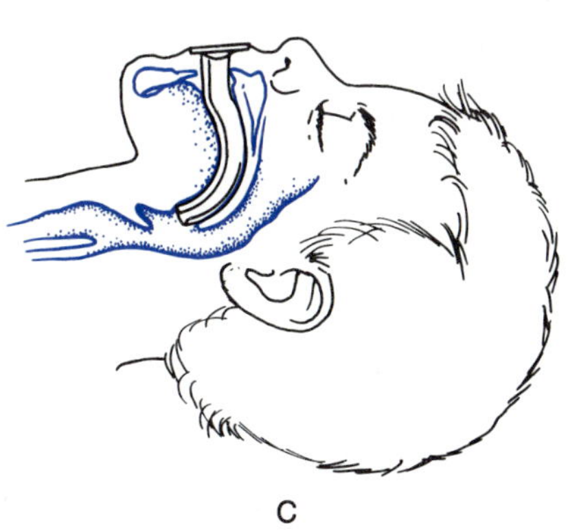

C

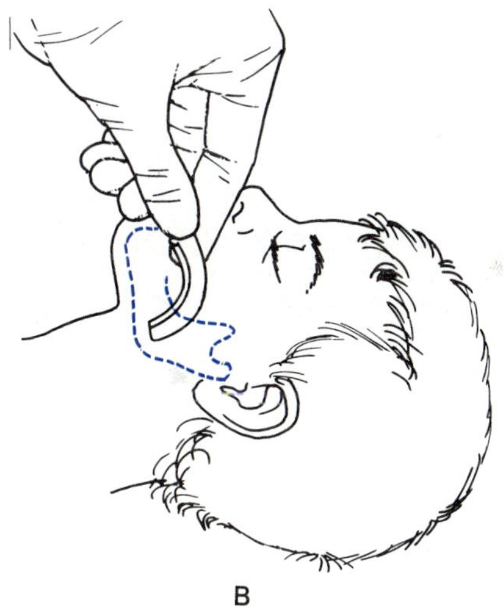

B

FIGURE 4.6 (A) Selecting correct size of oral airway: Length should equal distance from crease of mouth to angle of jaw. (B) Insertion of oral airway in anatomically correct position using a tongue blade. (C) Proper placement of the airway.

- Select the appropriately sized airway. The length should fit the space from the tip of the nose to the tragus of the ear. The size of the airway can be determined by the size of the child's little finger or external naris opening.
- Lubricate the airway with a water-based lubricant.
- Insert the airway gently into the nostril in the position of function and slide it along the floor of the nasopharynx.
- If resistance is felt, don't force the airway. This may lacerate the tissues, resulting in hemorrhage that will further complicate airway management.
- The diameter of the airway is too large if it causes blanching at the naris. If this occurs remove the airway and replace it with a smaller size (Figure 4.7).

Suction

Achieving good air exchange often requires suctioning secretions from the airway. Suctioning can be provided by manual or electrical sources. The two types of manual suction are the bulb syringe and the DeLee suction trap. Both are the method of choice for suctioning the narrow fragile airways of the infant.

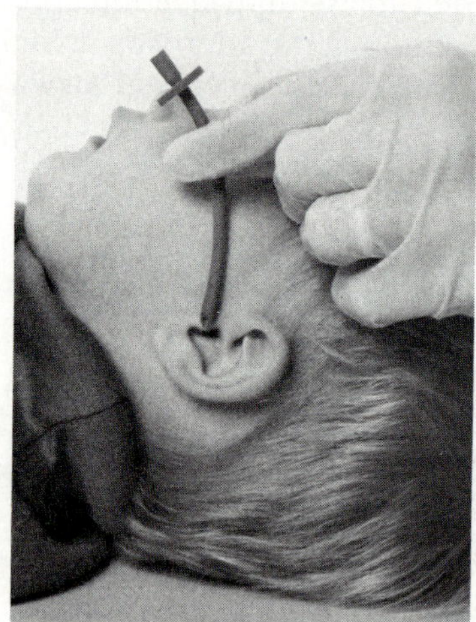

A

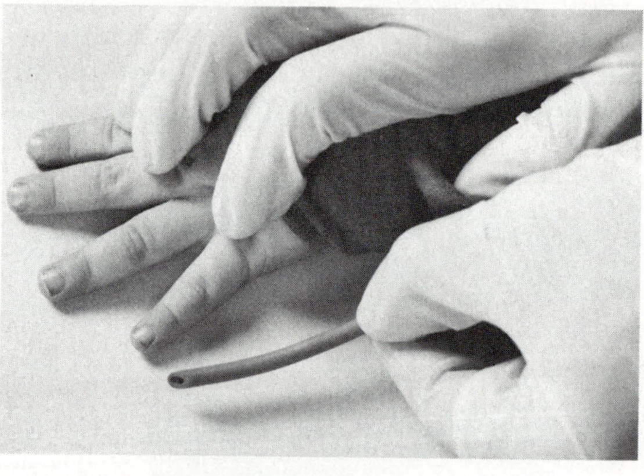

B

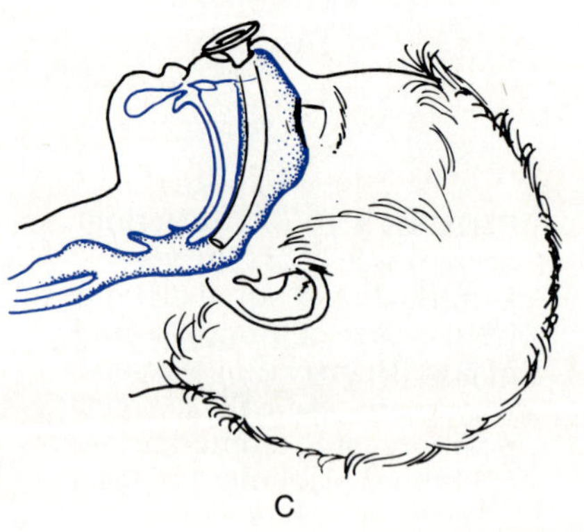

C

FIGURE 4.7 (A) Selecting the correct size of the nasopharyngeal airway length should equal the distance from the nasal opening to the tragus of the ear. (B) Circumference of the nasopharyngeal airway should equal the size of the child's small finger. (C) Proper placement of the nasopharyngeal airway.

Bulb Syringe Technique

- Place the bulb syringe in your hand and squeeze out the air.
- Place the nipple of the bulb into either the nostril or the mouth. Secure a form-fitting seal and release.
- Remove the syringe and expel the contents.
- Repeat the procedure as needed (Figure 4.8).

DeLee Suction Trap

The DeLee suction trap allows the rescuer to generate the suction source. It is excellent for suctioning the airway of a newborn or infant.

- Place the mouthpiece into your mouth.
- Place the suction tube into the infant's mouth or nose.
- Apply gentle suction with mouth.
- Watch the 10 cc chamber fill. Withdraw the catheter while actively suctioning for about 10 seconds.
- Monitor the child for decreasing respirations or slowing heart rate as a result of vagal stimulation (Figure 4.9).

FIGURE 4.8 Bulb-syringe suctioning of infant. Squeeze the bulb prior to placing the nipple to the infant's nose.

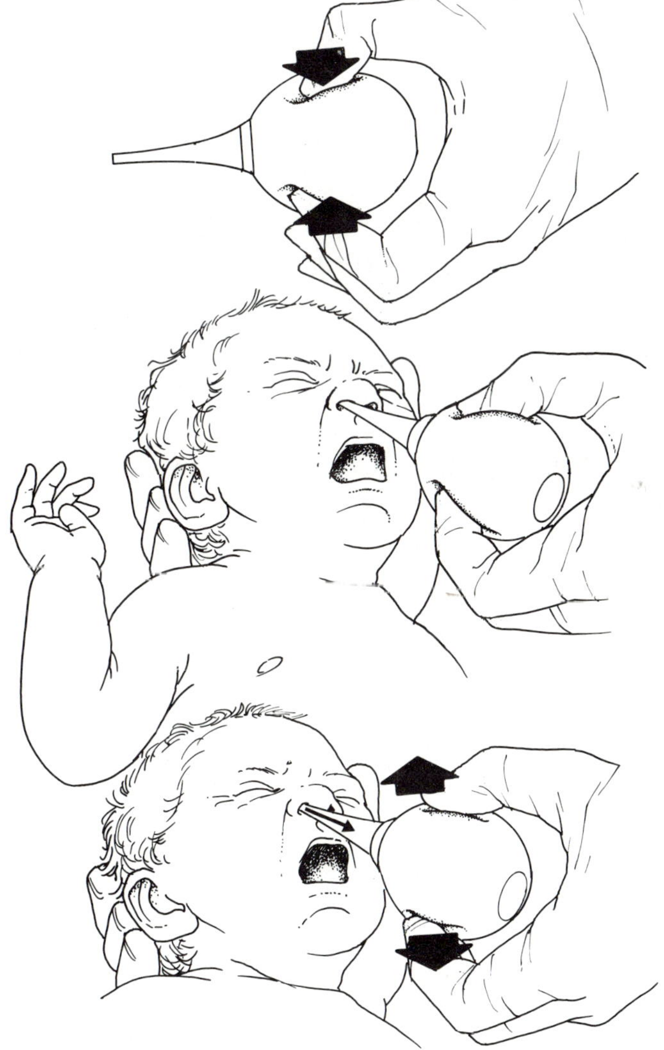

Mechanical Suction

- Select the appropriate suction device. A flexible catheter should range in diameter size from 10 to 16 French. A hard catheter is not recommended in infants and should only be used to clear obstructions in the mouth (Figure 4.10).
- Flexible catheters can be placed either in the nose or the mouth, but hard catheters should be used only in the mouth.
- Apply suction for no more than 5 to 10 seconds, withdrawing the catheter in a circular motion. Suctioning the infant or child for longer time periods may stimulate a vagal response, thus slowing the heart and respiratory rates.
- Oxygenate between each suctioning attempt, and closely monitor the vital signs.

Assisting Ventilation

Bag-Mask Ventilation

The objective in bag-mask ventilation is to augment respirations or provide complete assistance in respiratory failure. The inspired oxygen concentration should be as close to 100% as possible. The bag-valve mask is the preferred ventilatory equipment for infants and children. You can

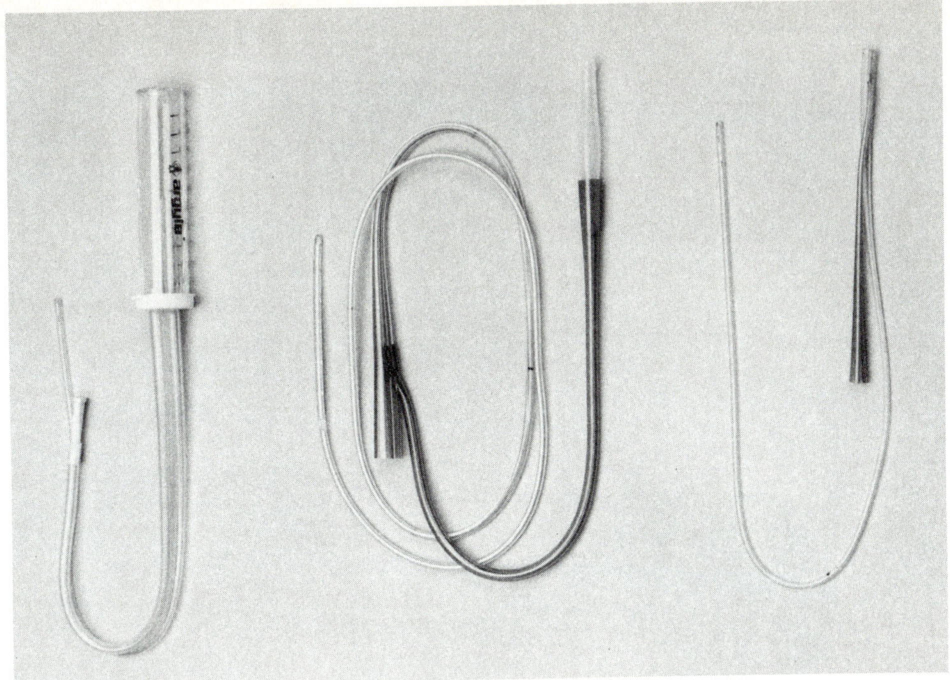

FIGURE 4.10   Suction devices: DeLee Suction trap, soft suction catheter, feeding tube.

manage the airway more effectively by assessing the rise and fall of the chest, securing a constant mask seal, and providing constant supervision of the airway. The importance of bag-mask application cannot be overemphasized. You must be familiar with the parts of the bag mask and assembly and select an appropriate-size mask (Figure 4.11).

- Make sure the bag has a constant source of 100% oxygen. This oxygen reservoir tubing system, or a pressure demand valve should be hooked into the bag to ensure refilling of oxygen (Figure 4.11a,b).
- Select a clear mask. This will enable you to watch for vomitus, blood, or other secretions that may cause airway obstruction.
- Select the appropriate-size mask with an air cushion. The mask should fit over the bridge of the nose to the cleft of the chin (Figure 4.12).
- Position the head in neutral or ''sniffing'' position.
- Securing the mask to the face with a tight seal is essential for ventilation. To assure a tight seal with the mask:
  1. Wrap the index finger and thumb around the mask where it connects with the bag.
  2. Place the middle, ring, and little fingers along the lower jaw and hook them underneath it. Infants and smaller children only require that the middle finger be used in hooking the jaw. The ring finger and little finger should be folded out of the way (Figure 4.13).
- Do not press on the soft tissue underneath the chin. This will cause the tongue to obstruct the airway.
- Gently pull the patient's face up to the mask while maintaining a neutral or sniffing position.

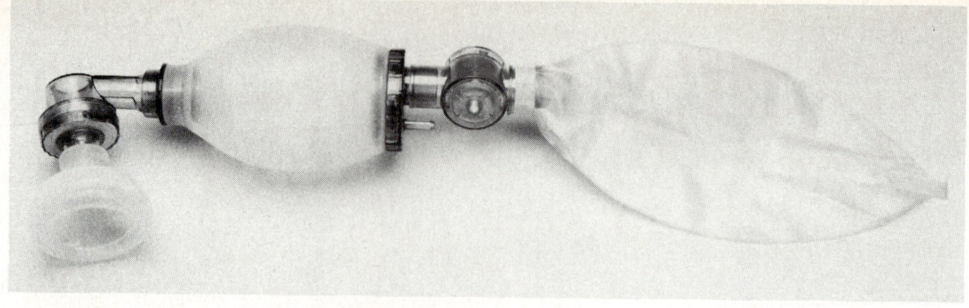

A

B

FIGURE 4.11 Self-inflating bag. (A) With an oxygen reservoir. (B) Without an oxygen reservoir.

- Squeeze the bag and ventilate the patient, assessing the quality of respiration and making adjustments as needed.
- If an adequate seal is not maintained, you may need to place both hands on the mask to assure a tight seal.

Ventilate the infant or child with only enough pressure to make the chest rise at a rate equivalent to their expected respiratory rate, or higher if the patient's condition warrants it. Use even, gentle pressure to ventilate; only enough to see chest rise. Provide ventilation with a 1:1 inspiration:expiration ratio. This provides an optimal time for oxygen exchange to occur.

Oxygen-Powered Breathing Devices

These devices are not recommended for use in the pediatric patient because of the difficulty in regulating tidal volume and the amount of force used. Complications from these types of devices include gastric distention and trauma to the pulmonary system.

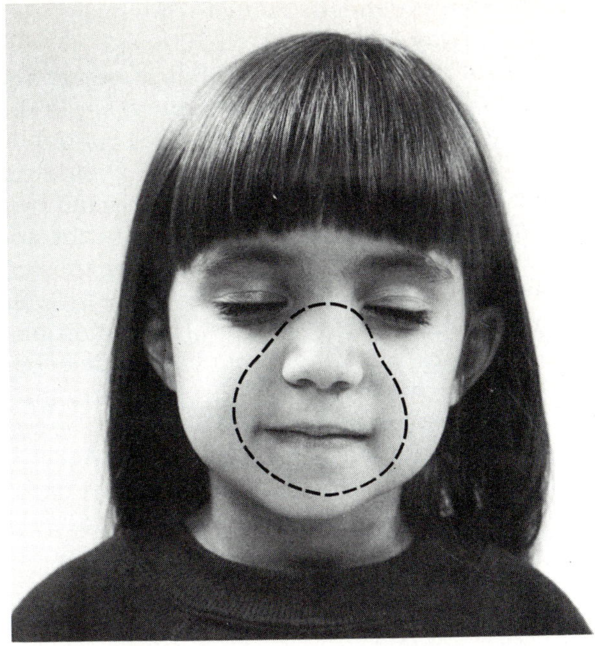

Orotracheal Intubation

When basic life-support methods of airway management have failed or the child needs complete immediate respiratory control, the method of choice is orotracheal intubation. Its advantages include the following:

- Complete and accurate airway control by visualizing the airway and placing the endotracheal tube directly into the lungs.
- Ability to suction the airway while protecting it from the contents of aspiration.
- A route for medications to be administered when IV access cannot be achieved.

The preferred method of intubation in the child is the orotracheal route. The nasotracheal route may cause massive hemorrhage or the tube may become obstructed by adenoid tissue. The blind nasotracheal method

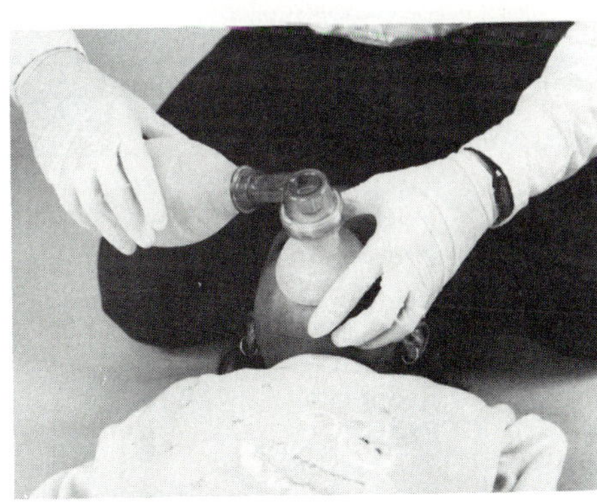

A

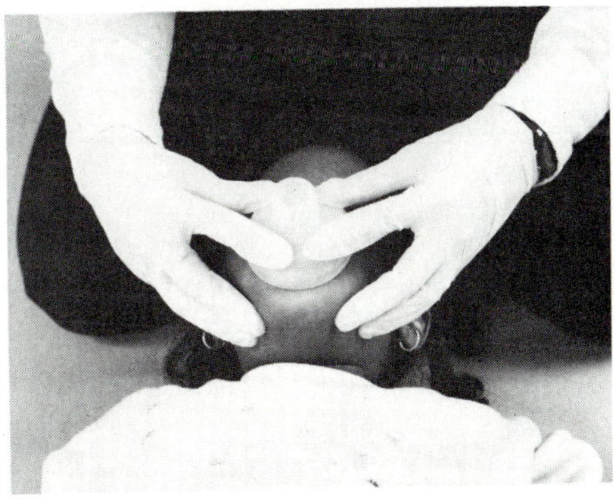

B

FIGURE 4.13 Proper hand and finger placement to hold a face mask in position for ventilation. (A) One-handed technique. (B) Two-handed technique; a second person is needed to ventilate.

is not recommended, owing to the complexity of the anatomy in the child's nasal airway.

Prior to the intubation attempt, select and prepare the equipment. Because of the child's small anatomy, some special considerations in equipment selection are important.

Children under 8 years of age should not be intubated with a cuffed tube. In infants and children, the cricoid ring is the site with the smallest diameter, not at the glottic area as in the adult. The cricoid ring will provide a natural and sufficient seal for the tube. The size of the tube used should be equal to the diameter of the little finger or external nares. Tubes come in sizes 2.5 to 9.0 mm. Have additional tubes one size smaller and one size larger available should they be needed.

The decision to use a curved or straight laryngoscope blade is one of preference and comfort. Use Table 4.1 as a guide for the size of the blade. After the blade has been selected, connect it to the laryngoscope handle and check the power and light source (Figure 4.14).

Additional equipment to have available includes a bag-valve mask with reservoir and endotracheal tube, suction apparatus, and tape or one of the commercially available devices for securing the endotracheal tube.

The procedure for orotracheal intubation of infants and children is as follows:

- Preoxygenate the child with positive-pressure ventilation for 30 seconds prior to intubation.

- Place the child's head in a "sniffing" position, avoiding hyperextension of the neck because of the high, anterior position of the larynx. Maintain in-line immobilization if cervical trauma is suspected (Figure 4.15).

- Time the length of the intubation effort. Each attempt should not exceed 30 seconds to prevent hypoxia and bradycardia. The child should be reoxygenated between attempts. Either hold your breath as you begin intubation or have an assistant keep time. When you need to take a breath, it is time to reoxygenate the patient.

- Insert the laryngoscope blade to the right side of the mouth and

TABLE 4.1 Guidelines for Appropriate Sizes of the Endotracheal Tube, Laryngoscope Blade, and Suction Catheter to Use in Infants and Children

Age	Laryngoscope Blade	Endotracheal Tube	Suction Catheter	Distance (cm): Midtrachea to Teeth
Preterm	Miller 0	2.5 or 3.0	5 or 6 French	8
Newborn	Miller 0–1	3.0	6 French	10
6 Months	Miller 1	3.5	8 French	12
18 Months	Miller 1–2	4.0	8 French	13
3 Years	Miller 2	4.5	8 French	15
5 Years	Miller 2	5.0	10 French	16
6 Years	Miller 2	5.5	10 French	16
8 Years	Miller 2	6.0	10 French	18
	Macintosh 2			
12 Years	Macintosh 3	6.5	10 French	20
16 Years	Miller 3	7.0	12 French	22
	Macintosh 3			

Source: Adapted from "Standards for CPR and ECC," *JAMA,* 255 (21):2962, June 6, 1986, and Chameides, L., ed., *Textbook of Pediatric Advanced Life Support,* Dallas, American Heart Association, 1988.

Equipment and Procedures for Management of ABC's

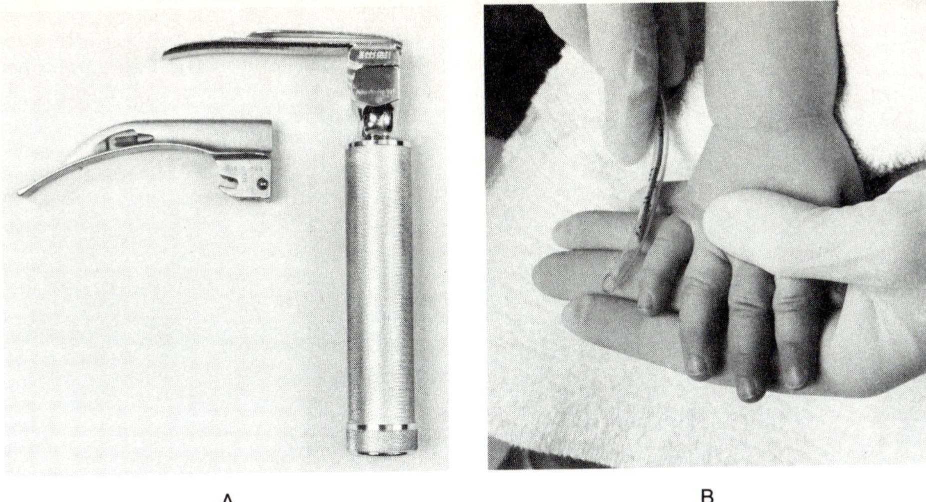

A   B

FIGURE 4.14   (A) Selection of a laryngoscope blade for intubation, either curved or straight and the appropriate size for the age of the child. (B) Selection of the correct-size endotracheal tube. Note the vocal cord marking. Select a tube closest in size to the child's little finger.

sweep the tongue to the left side. Use a lifting motion to expose the vocal cords. The blade should not press on the teeth or gums of the maxilla (Figure 4.16a,b).

- Introduce the tube on the right side of the mouth. Pass the tube through the vocal cords to about 2–3 cm below the vocal cords. Confirm this by numbers on the tube.

- Auscultate the chest to make sure the tube is in the trachea, not in the esophagus or in the right main stem bronchus. Listen at each lung apex and midaxillary area. Listen in the stomach area for gurgling associated with esophageal intubation. Signs of proper tube placement include:

FIGURE 4.15   Positioning the child before intubation. Note the relationships among the oral, tracheal, and pharyngeal axes (a) before and (b) after placing the child in neutral position. Intubation is easier to accomplish when the axes are in close relationship with each other.

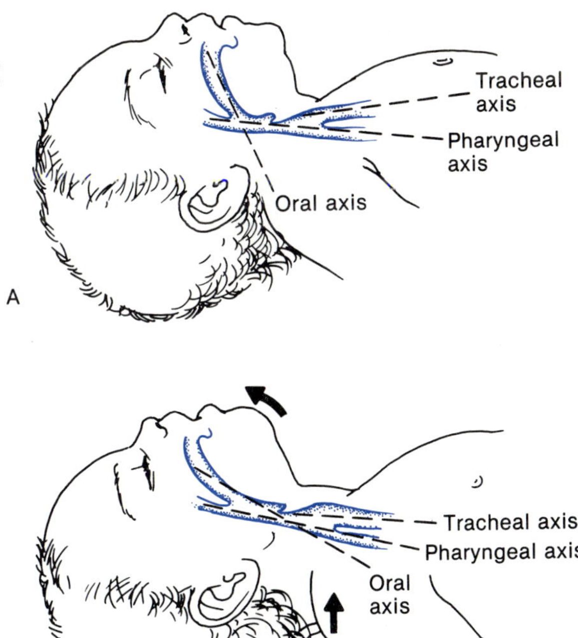

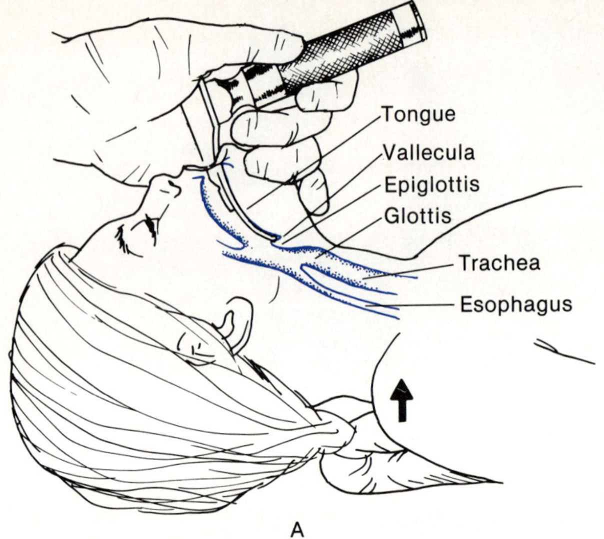

FIGURE 4.16 Intubation of the child. Slowly insert the laryngoscope blade. To visualize the vocal cords, pull the handle upwards without touching the teeth. (A) Introduction of the laryngoscope. (B) Exposing the vocal cords and other internal anatomy.

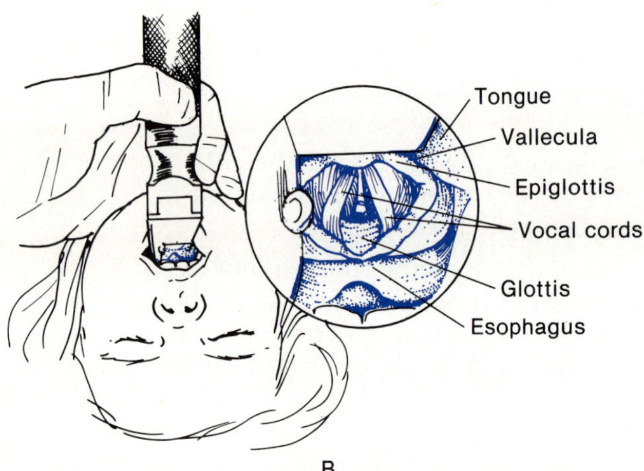

1. Augmented breath sounds on auscultation
2. Condensation in the tube with exhalation
3. Bilateral chest wall movement with positive pressure ventilation
4. Improved heart rate and color.

- Tape the endotracheal tube securely to the child's face. Recheck the numbers on the tube at the mouth to make sure the position of the tube has not changed. Do not release the tube until the tape is securely attached (Figure 4.17a–d).

- Reconfirm the tube placement frequently, as the airway is short in infants, and minimal head movement is needed to displace the tube (Figure 4.18a–d).

Cricothyrotomy

Cricothyrotomy is a temporary life-saving procedure for an obstructed airway. It creates an opening through the cricothyroid membrane into the larynx. The procedure should only be used by trained personnel when all other procedures to open the airway fail. It is particularly difficult to perform in children, especially those under 3 years of age, because the airway

Equipment and Procedures for Management of ABC's

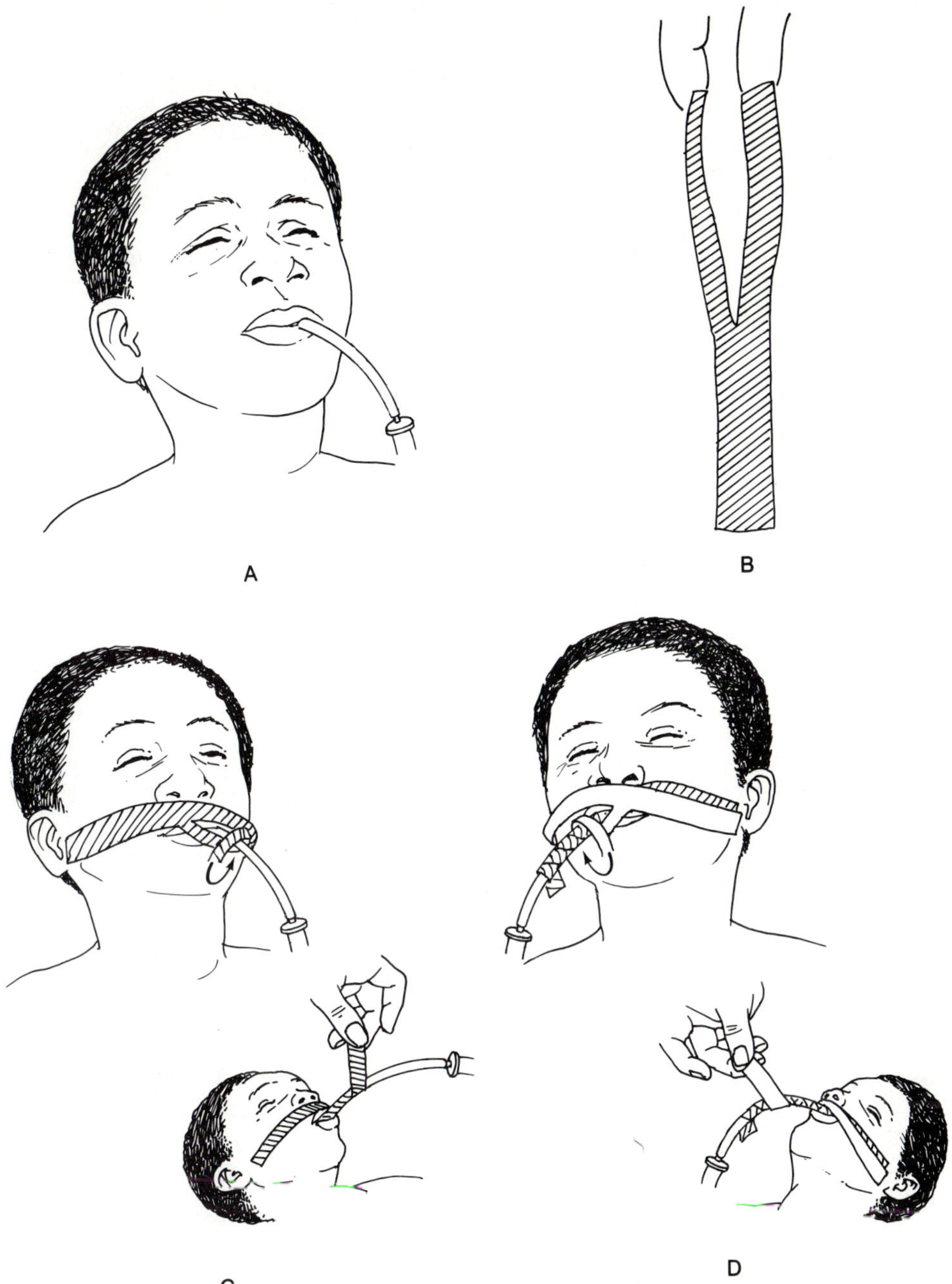

FIGURE 4.17 (A) Once the endotracheal tube is in place, hold the tube to keep it from becoming dislodged. (B) Tear two strips of tape, each with a Y configuration. (C) Apply the tape across the maxillary area of the face, wrapping the lower half of the torn tape around the tube. (D) Repeat the taping with the second strip of tape, wrapping it around the tube in the opposite direction.

is narrower, landmarks are less easily palpated, the infant's neck is short, the larynx is higher than an adult's, and the vocal cords are just above the cricothyroid membrane.

Indications for cricothyrotomy include the following:

- A child in respiratory or cardiac arrest with an obstructed airway
- Facial trauma with anatomic disruption that prevents other airway management

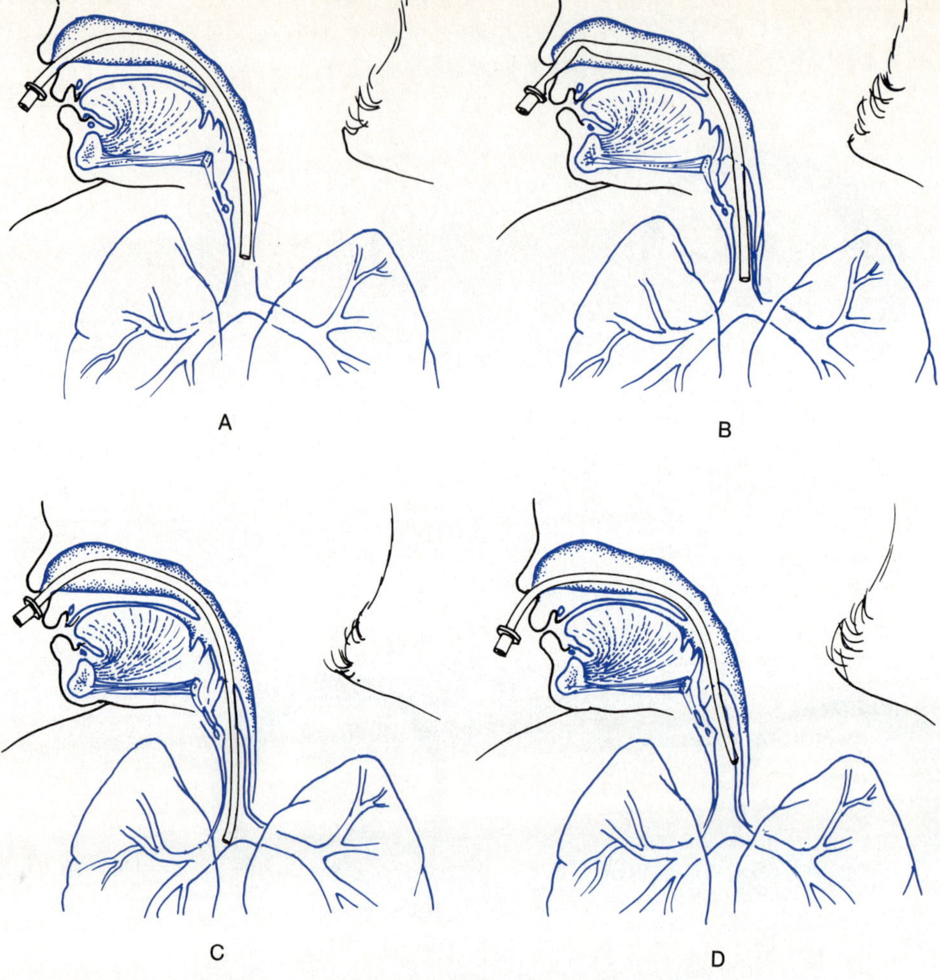

FIGURE 4.18 Note possible endotracheal tube placements. (A) Ideal positioning in the trachea. (B) Kinked ET. (C) ET in right mainstem bronchus. (D) ET tube displaced against tracheal wall. Nasotracheal intubation was used in this case on a child older than 8 years.

- All other methods of airway control have failed.

Cricothyrotomy should not be performed when there is an airway obstruction below the level of the cricoid cartilage; when there is a complete expiratory obstruction; when there is gross infection over puncture site; when there is a primary laryngeal injury; or when there is an inability to locate landmarks for puncture. Complications to the procedure include hypoxemia and CO_2 toxicity, esophageal perforation, subcutaneous emphysema, bleeding, infection, and damage to tracheal cartilage with possible vocal cord disruption.

The following equipment is needed to perform the cricothyrotomy: angiocath (14 or 16 gauge), a syringe filled with 1–2 cc of saline, an adapter to the infant endotracheal tube (size 3.0), oxygen, and a bag-valve-mask with oxygen reservoir. Once the equipment is assembled, the following procedure may be used:

- Position child with slight neck extension, unless C-spine injury is suspected.

- Locate the cricothyroid and thyroid cartilages in the neck. The thy-

roid cartilage has a notch along the bottom edge, and the cricoid
ring is the cartilage just beneath the thyroid cartilage.

- Once the thyroid notch is identified, move your fingers down to the
  cricothyroid membrane, between the two cartilages.

- Prepare the area with alcohol or other antiseptic solution.

- Insert the needle into the cricothyroid membrane at less than a 90°
  angle to the longitudinal axis of the neck. Maintain suction with the
  connected syringe until bubbles of air are noted. Then advance the
  catheter over the needle and reconfirm air flow with the syringe. Remove the needle.

- Attach the 3.0 endotracheal tube adapter to the hub of the catheter,
  and begin ventilation with the bag mask.

- Secure the cannula with tape after confirming correct placement by
  auscultating for breath sounds over the lungs and stomach. Observe for kinking of the cannula.

- High-pressure oxygen should be provided (50 psi) for long-term ventilation because of the high resistance of the small tube.

- Bag-mask ventilation will give some time (about 40 minutes) until
  either intubation or a tracheostomy can be performed.

- If ventilation is inadequate, occlusion of the nose and mouth may
  decrease the upper airway leak (Figure 4.19).

Pleural Decompression

This is a life-saving technique to relieve a *tension pneumothorax*. It is a
procedure that should only be performed by personnel who have had
proper training and experience. Tension pneumothorax develops following a chest injury that permits the progressive entry of air into the pleural
space, elevating the pressure in the space above the atmospheric pressure
level and causing the lung to collapse. See Chapters 9 and 11 for more de-

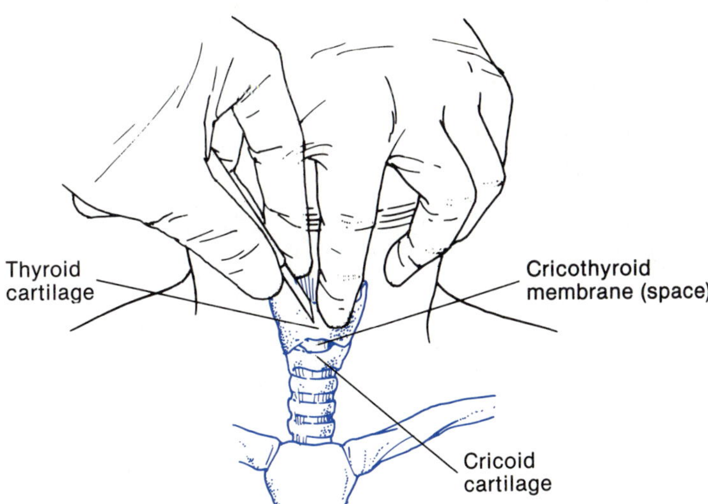

FIGURE 4.19 Cricothyrotomy, location of the cricothyroid
membrane for needle insertion.

tails. Indications of the development of a tension pneumothorax and the need for pleural decompression include rapid deterioration in the child's heart rate, blood pressure, and perfusion (bradycardia, hypotension, delayed capillary refill, and decreased level of consciousness). Potential complications to this procedure include a collapsed lung if a pneumothorax is not present; trauma to the pulmonary artery or vena cava, resulting in hemothorax; and a lacerated lung.

The following equipment is needed for pleural decompression: An angiocath (14–18 gauge) and a flutter valve assembly. A McSwain dart may be used in older children, in place of an angiocath with flutter valve. The procedure for pleural decompression is as follows:

- Identify the side of the chest affected.
- Identify the landmarks for needle insertion. Use the 4th intercostal space at the level of the nipple line, along the anterior, midaxillary line for infants and young children. Use the 2nd intercostal space at the midclavicular line for older children (Figure 4.20).
- Prepare the skin with antiseptic.
- Advance the needle under the skin over the rib below the intercostal space selected and on into the intercostal space until air is expelled under pressure.
- Remove the needle and tape the catheter in place. The flutter valve should be attached, or connect the catheter to IV tubing and place it under water.
- Successful decompression is indicated by an immediate improvement in the child's heart rate, blood pressure, and perfusion.

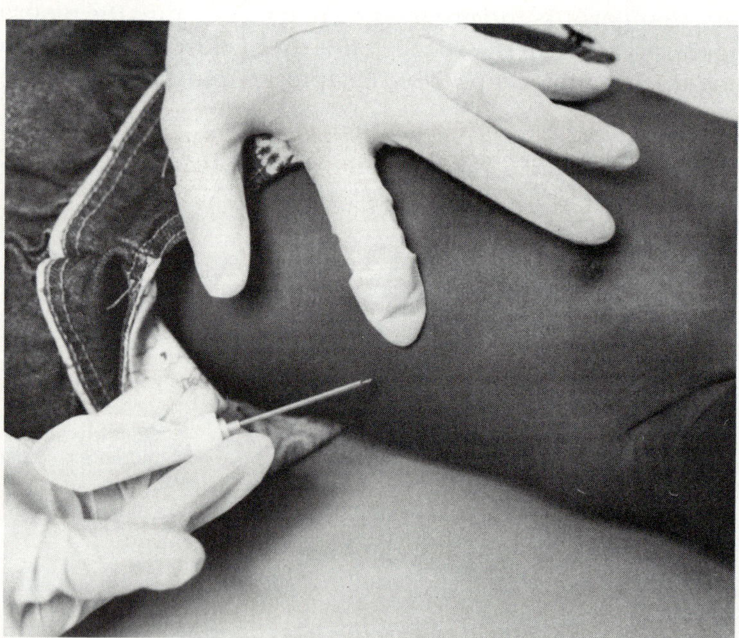

FIGURE 4.20 Location for needle thoracostomy is at the fourth or fifth intercostal space in the mid-axillary line for infants and young children.

Establishing Intravenous Access

The decision to initiate intravenous (IV) therapy should be based on an assessment of the patient's immediate needs. This assessment should establish criteria that identify those patients that require immediate therapy, intermediate therapy, or no therapy. Below is a list of questions that should be considered before initiating therapy:

- What benefits will be gained? Fluids, medications?
- How much time is involved in the procedure?
- Is transport to the intended facility more appropriate?
- What is the rescuers' experience and skill level?
- How many resources will have to be committed to manage the patient?

While these criteria are not absolute, they are intended to be used as guidelines. When a decision has been made to establish IV therapy, it is essential for the rescuer to be familiar with the equipment and specific techniques to achieve IV access. Some tips for successful insertion include the following:

- Rubbing or patting the site may enhance local vein filling.
- Use warm packs to the area to enhance vein presentation.
- Elevate the lower extremities.
- Application of Pneumatic Anti-Shock Garment (PASG) may increase vein presentation in the upper extremities.

IV Equipment

Various types of equipment are used in establishing IV therapy. Thus, it is absolutely essential that the rescuer have a working knowledge of this equipment. In attempting to achieve IV placement in the pediatric patient you will only make two attempts. Therefore, it is essential that you select the appropriate equipment for the job.

Types of Needles

The *butterfly* is a needle with attached catheter supplied in sizes 25 to 16. It is used for establishing an IV line using a scalp vein. The benefit of this device is its stability, but it is not recommended for peripheral lines, owing to infiltration.

Over-the-needle catheters can be inserted in the back of the hands and feet, the antecubital fossa, and external jugular, saphenous, and femoral veins. These catheters range in size from 26 to 10. They are more difficult to insert but are much more likely to survive taping and patient movement.

The recommended IV solution for infants and children is Ringer's Lactate or Normal Saline for medical and trauma patients. These crystalloid solutions stay in the vascular space longer when compared to other solutions.

Antiseptic cleaner, saline, small syringe, tape, and an arm board for immobilization are also required for IV therapy.

Establishing a Peripheral Line

The procedure for insertion of a peripheral line is as follows:

- Restrain the child.
- Place a rubber band tourniquet around the head for a scalp vein; a regular tourniquet for an extremity.
- Clean the skin with antiseptic.
- Check the patency of the catheter by injecting sterile saline through it.
- Stick the needle through the skin just below the vein, and advance the needle toward the vein until flashback occurs. For angiocatheters, advance the catheter and pull out the needle.
- Remove the tourniquet and inject a small amount of saline into the vein to test for patency.
- Tape the needle in place and begin the infusion.

External Jugular Placement

Placement of an external jugular line in the pediatric patient should be used in cases where all other means of vascular access have failed. There is the potential complication of puncture to the lung or great vessel because of the proximity of these structures to the neck. To insert a catheter into the external jugular vein, use the following technique:

- Place the child in a 20–30° Trendelenburg position with the head turned away from the side to be punctured. The right side is preferred.
- Restrain the child.
- Identify the external jugular vein and scrub the area with antiseptic.
- Insert an over-the-needle catheter into the vein for peripheral cannulation.
- When free blood flow is obtained, make sure that no air bubbles are in the tubing and attach the infusion set.

Umbilical Vein Cannulation

This method of establishing a lifeline should be used only in infants less than 5 days old. The procedure involves placing a catheter into the umbilical vein. This vein leads directly into the liver. This procedure is to be used only as last resort for administering fluids or medications to an acutely ill or injured newborn. It should only be attempted by a rescuer who has been trained and is experienced in the procedure. The following equipment is required for this procedure: a scalpel blade; a 5.0 French umbilical catheter; feeding tube, or a 24–20-gauge angiocath; and a 3-way stopcock and sterile saline-filled syringe.

The procedure for umbilical vein cannulation includes the following:

- Trim the cord to 1–2 cm above the skin attachment and hold it firmly to prevent bleeding. A piece of umbilical tape can be tied around the umbilical stump to control bleeding.
- The umbilical vein is identified as the single thin-wall vessel. The arteries are paired, thick-wall vessels.
- Attach the umbilical catheter or angiocatheter filled with saline to a stopcock. Advance the catheter so the tip is just below the surface of

the skin, just until blood return is apparent. Insert the catheter no
further so as to avoid infusion directly into the liver.

- If there is no free blood flow then the catheter is most likely wedged
  against the liver and should be pulled back some until free flow occurs.
- Place a tie around the umbilical stump to hold the catheter in place
  and prevent bleeding. Attach the IV and begin infusion. Tape the
  catheter and tubing to the child's stomach (Figure 4.21a–c).

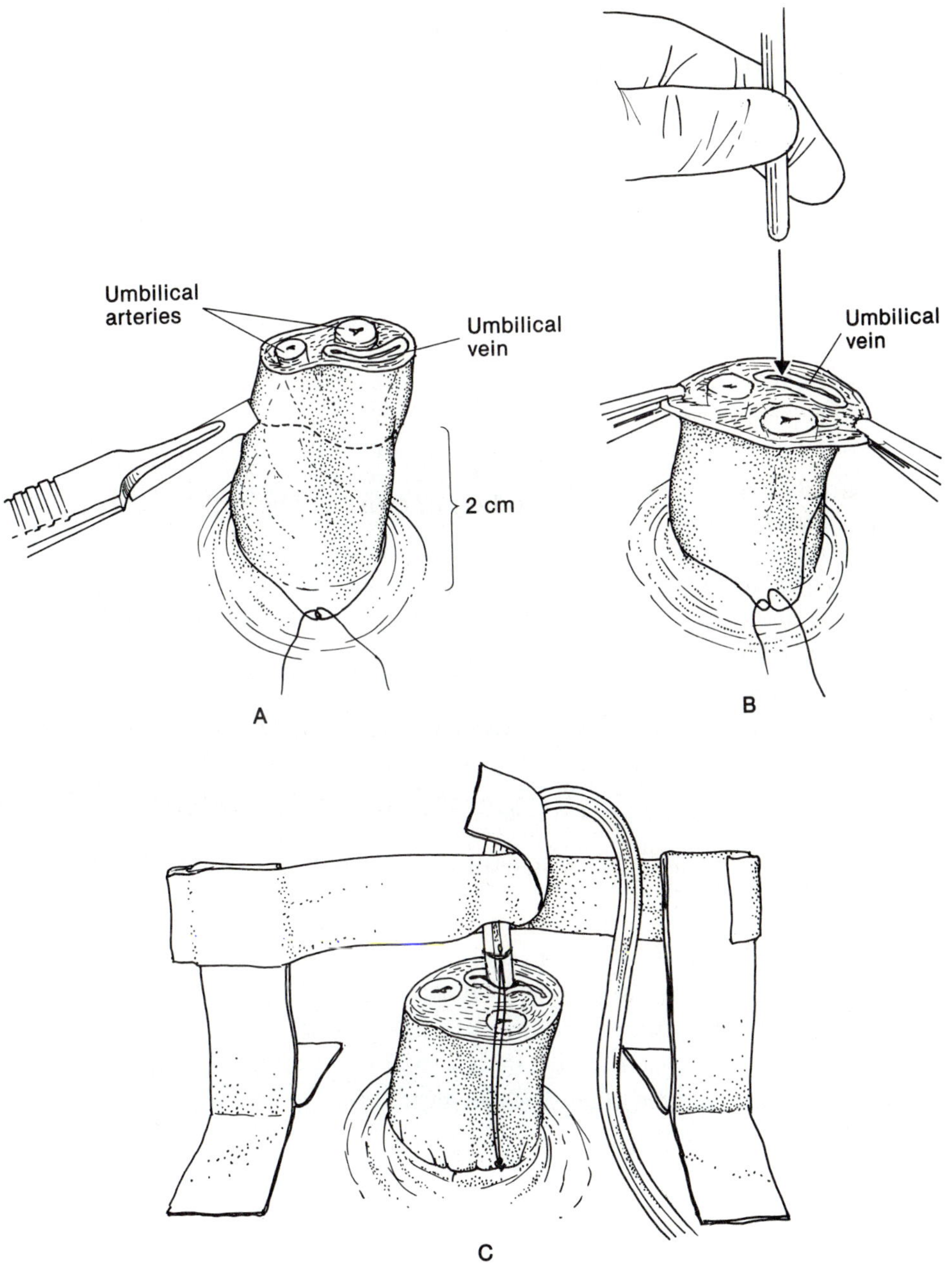

FIGURE 4.21 Umbilical vein cannulation procedure. (A) Identify the umbilical
vein after trimming the cord. (B) Insert an umbilical catheter or angiocath into
the vein, advancing the tip just until blood return is apparent. (C) Place a tie
around the base of the cord to hold the catheter in place. Stabilize the catheter
with tape as illustrated and begin IV infusion.

Intraosseous Infusion

The technique of intraosseous infusion was first described 60 years ago. It was used extensively in the 1930s and 1940s for administration of fluids and blood. It has gained widespread use in emergency resuscitation over the past 8 years. The major advantage of the intraosseous (IO) infusion is that the bone shaft acts as a non-collapsible vein through which medication and fluids can be administered. While the IO technique is a proven means of establishing a lifeline, it should not be the first choice.

Indications for IO insertion include the following:

- Attempts at establishing a peripheral line has failed. As a rule the rescuer is allowed 3 sticks or 90 seconds.

- Drugs and fluids need to be given to a child with unstable vital signs who is unconscious or nonresponsive.

- The child is under 3 years of age, although IO infusion is now performed on older children.

Equipment to have available for IO infusion includes Betadine, disposable gloves, adhesive tape, gauze 4 × 4's, a 10-cc syringe, a 15–19-gauge bone marrow needle or 18–20-gauge short spinal needle with a stylet. The procedure for establishing an intraosseous line is as follows:

- Place infant or child in a supine position.

- Identify and locate the bony landmarks. The preferred site is the proximal tibia, 1 to 2 finger breadths below the tibial tuberosity on the anteromedial surface (Figure 4.22a). An alternate site is 1–2 cm proximal to the medial malleolus on the anteromedial surface of the distal tibia.

- Prep the site with Betadine.

- Direct and insert the needle, with the stylet in place, perpendicular to the bone or angled away from the joint, avoiding the epiphyseal plate. Insert with pressure and in a boring motion until penetration into the bone marrow, which is marked by a sudden lack of resistance.

- Remove the stylet and attach the syringe with stopcock. If the needle is properly placed in the bone marrow, aspiration of blood with marrow may be possible, but does not always occur. Another sign of proper placement is lack of resistance to infusion and no sign of infiltration. The needle stands without support (Figure 4.22b).

- Attach the IV tubing, with or without stopcock, and pressure-infusion bag. A pressure bag is needed to infuse fluids.

- Stabilize the needle on both sides with sterile gauze and secure with tape (Figure 4.22c).

Pneumatic Anti-Shock Garment

The use of the Pneumatic Anti-Shock Garment (PASG) has engendered much controversy in the field of emergency medicine. Although many studies have assessed the effectiveness of this piece of equipment, the question still remains as to its benefit and where, if at all, it should be used in augmenting circulation in children. The advantages that have been demonstrated by the PASG in adults are:

Equipment and Procedures for Management of ABC's

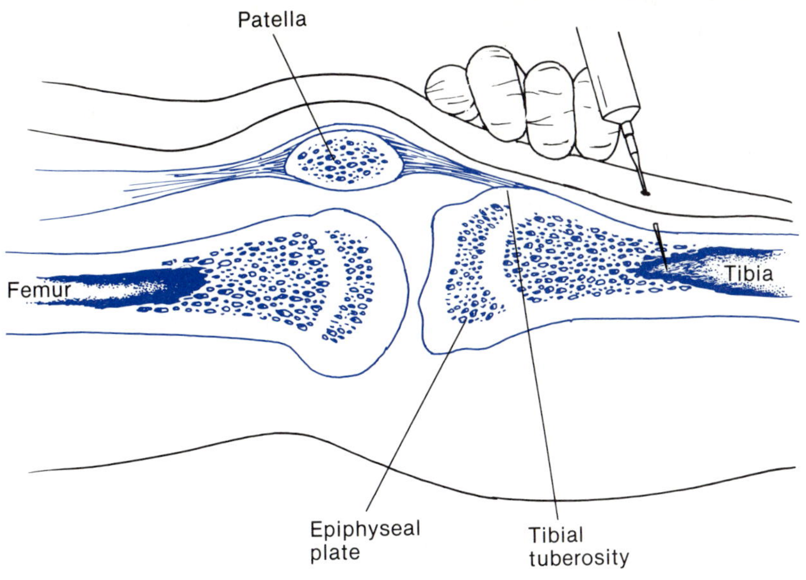

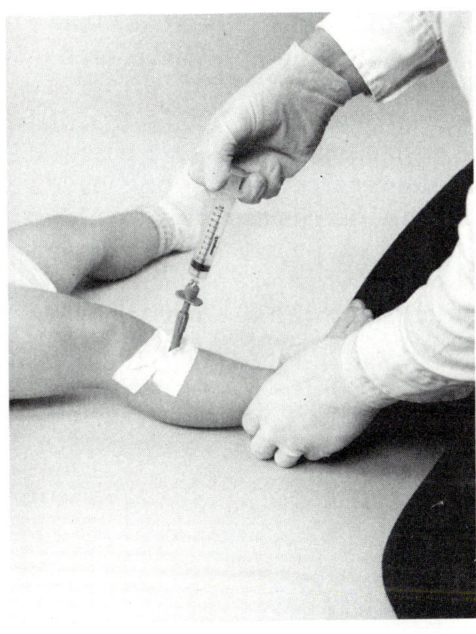

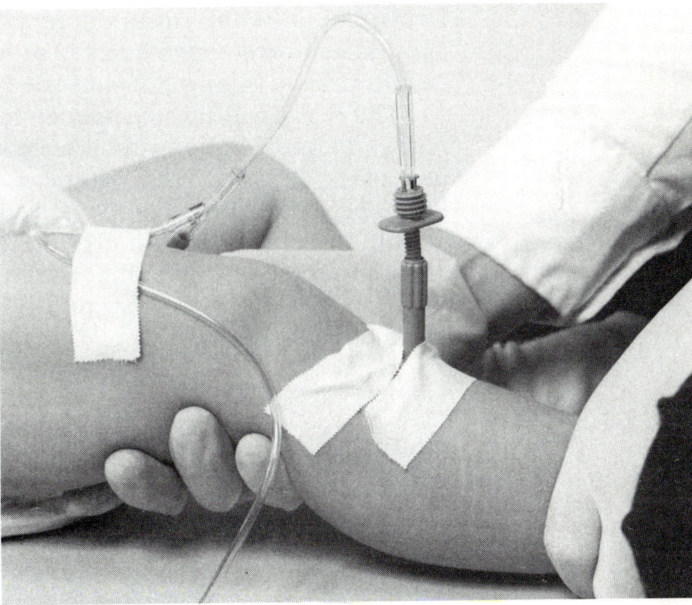

FIGURE 4.22 Intraosseous infusion technique. (A) Locate the site for intraosseous needle insertion, two finger breadths below the tibial tuberosity on the anteromedial surface of the tibia. Insert the needle at an angle toward the foot. (B) After needle insertion, attach a syringe with saline to the needle. Try to aspirate blood from the marrow or infuse a small amount of saline through to needle. No resistance to infusion should be noted. (C) Tape the needle and IV catheter for stabilization during transport.

- Increased peripheral vascular resistance.
- Improvement of blood flow to the heart, lungs, and brain.
- Tamponading effect to areas underneath the garment.

The PASG cannot and should not be used as a long-term support device; its use constitutes a life-saving, hemorrhage controlling, short-term technique. Use of the PASG in pediatric patients should be done at the direction of the medical control.

Application Criteria

The systolic blood pressure reading is the criteria used for application and inflation of the PASG. Place the garment on the child when the systolic blood pressure is less than 80 mm Hg and when signs of shock are present (tachycardia, pallor, diaphoresis, delayed capillary refill time). Do NOT inflate it until consultation with medical control or the patient's systolic blood pressure drops to under 60 mm Hg.

Inflate the leg compartments only (Figure 4.23). The abdominal compartment is only inflated in the presence of a pelvic fracture and hemorrhage. The pressure placed against the abdomen may cause the diaphragm to stop functioning, resulting in ventilatory compromise and respiratory arrest. The trousers are inflated adequately when the Velcro attachments begin to separate. Monitor the patient's vitals signs. Application of the PASG in children is no different from the procedure used for adults.

Defibrillation and Synchronized Cardioversion

Defibrillation is the untimed depolarization of cardiac cells that allow a spontaneous organized heart beat to return. The same principle is used in cardioversion, but in that case the charge delivered is timed.

The exact paddle size needed for children of different body size is not currently known. As a rule the electrode or paddle that covers the largest area of the chest is the correct size. The paddle or electrodes should have a space between them to allow for conduction. The position of the paddles should be below the right clavicle and just below the left nipple more lateral than medial. In small children the one paddle may be placed on the anterior chest and the other on the posterior chest with the heart between them (Figure 4.24).

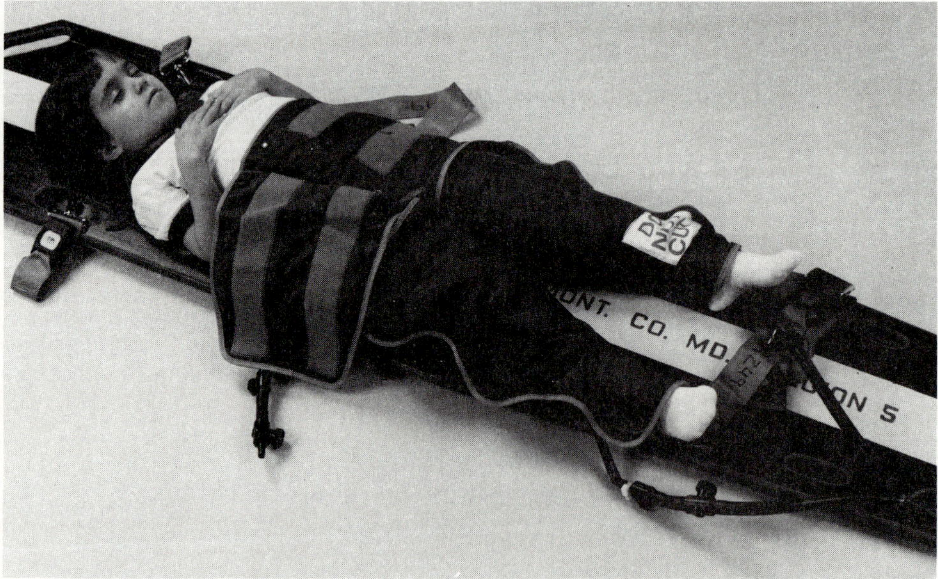

FIGURE 4.23 Application of Pneumatic Anti-Shock Garment (PASG).

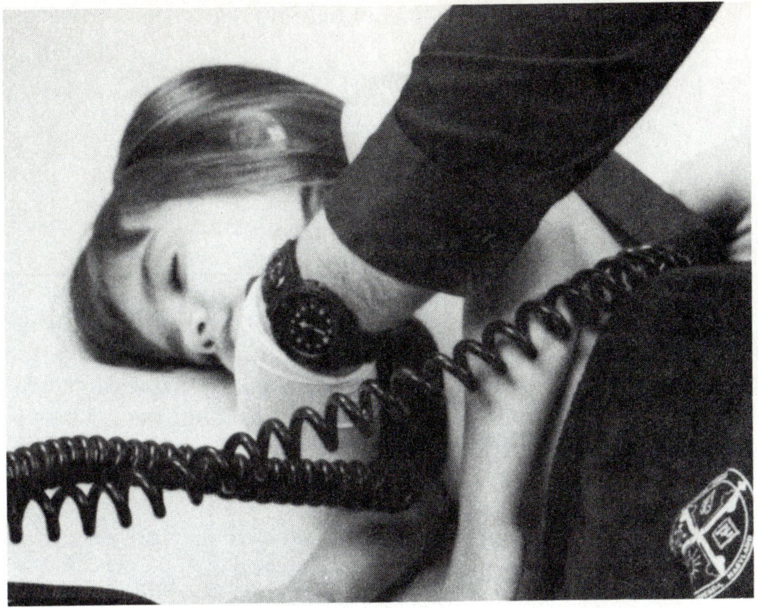

FIGURE 4.24 Anterior-posterior placement of defibrillator paddles.

Defibrillation

The sequence for defibrillation should be as follows:

- Continue CPR with as little interruption as possible.
- Apply conductive gel to the appropriately sized paddles.
- Turn the defibrillator on and check to see that it is not in the synchronous mode.
- Select the energy dose and charge the capacitor (2 J/kg).
- Stop chest compressions and place the paddles in the proper position.
- Recheck the rhythm.
- Clear the area to ensure that no personnel are in direct contact with the patient.
- Apply firm pressure to the paddles while depressing both discharge buttons simultaneously.
- Reassess the rhythm and pulse. If ventricular fibrillation (VF) persists, repeat countershock at twice the initial dose (4 J/kg). If an organized rhythm has been established, check the pulses and continue CPR as needed. If VF recurs, immediately repeat the countershock, using the same dose.

Synchronized Cardioversion

This procedure is the same as that outlined for defibrillation except as follows:

- If the paddles are the monitor type, the ECG must be connected to a defibrillator.
- The synchronizer circuit must be activated.

- The discharge buttons must be held until the countershock is delivered.
- Initial dose of energy is 0.2–1.0 J/kg.
- Reassess the ECG and pulse.

Spinal Immobilization

The objective of spinal immobilization is to protect the injured spinal column from further injury. This can be achieved in a variety of ways and with a wide array of equipment. Because every situation is unique, it is not the intent to address every conceivable possibility. Therefore, general guidelines will be presented.

- Select the appropriate equipment for the situation. This includes cervical collars, immobilization devices, and all other equipment designed or routinely used on children.

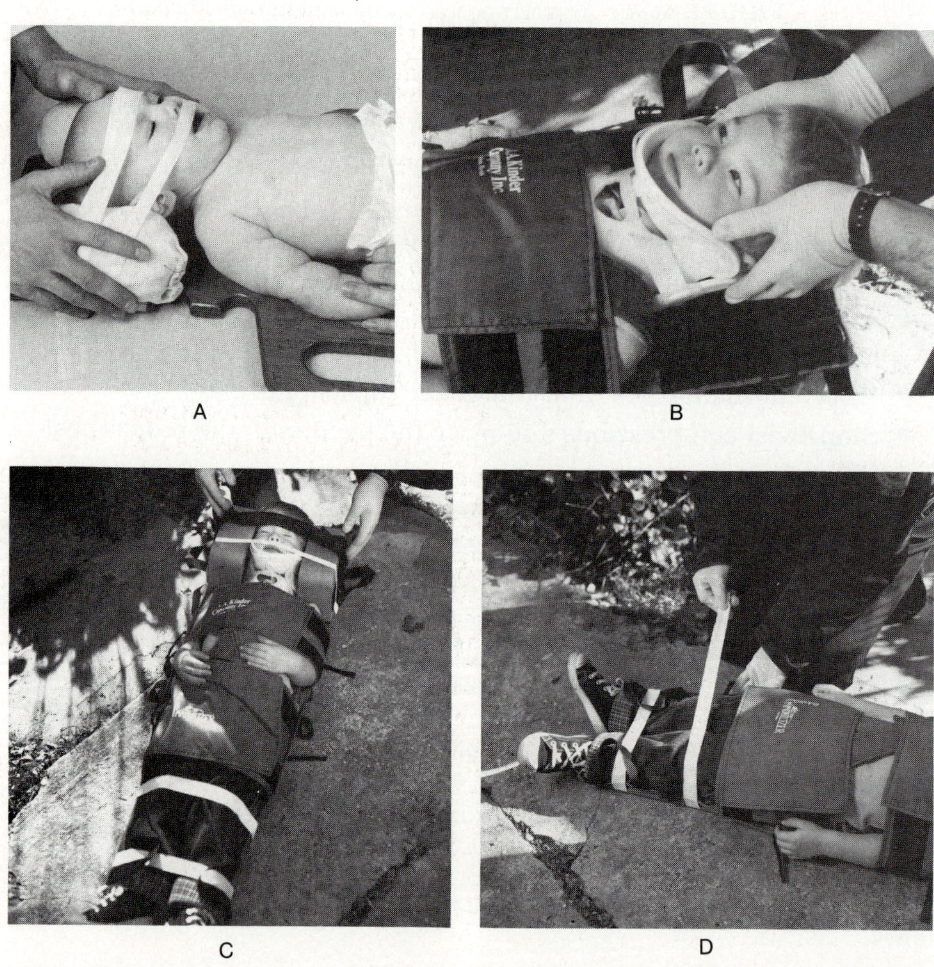

FIGURE 4.25   Spinal immobilization techniques. (A) Immobilize the infant's head with a towel roll and tape across the forehead and maxilla. (B) Cervical collars can be used in older children. (C) Immobilization of a child on a pediatric immobilizer. (D) Restraint of the legs: Use tape across the knees and lower legs.

- Assess the scene for safety of the rescuer and the child.

- Assess the ABC's and treat accordingly.

- Apply manual stabilization.

- Measure and apply the appropriate-size cervical collar. The correct-size collar should limit the amount of cervical movement.

- Select the appropriate immobilization device, long board, papoose board, Kendricks Extrication Device (KED), etc. This device should limit the majority of body movement. This is not easily achieved unless matched with an equally limiting strapping device or system.

- When immobilizing children, they will not sit still to allow you to place a device on them. Skill, patience, and practice are all necessary to achieve success (Figure 4.25a–d).

References for Management of ABC's

CHAMEIDES, L., ed., *Textbook of Pediatric Advanced Life Support.* Dallas: American Heart Association, 1988.

EICHELBERGER, M., STOSSEL-PRATCH, G., eds., *Pediatric Emergencies Manual.* Rockville, MD: Aspen Publishing Co., 1984, pp. 13–31.

GRANT, H., MURRAY, R., BERGERON, J., *Emergency Care.* Englewood Cliffs, N.J.: Prentice Hall, 1990, pp. 418–448.

5

Pediatric Cardiopulmonary Resuscitation

OBJECTIVES

When you have completed this chapter you should be able to

✳ Identify the most frequent causes of cardiac arrest in the newborn and the child.

✳ Describe the technique for ventilations and compressions in CPR for the following age groups:
  - newborns
  - infants
  - children

✳ Describe signs that indicate CPR is effective in the pediatric patient.

✳ List the steps in the procedure to relieve airway obstruction for infants and children.

✳ Describe appropriate management of specific conditions leading to cardiac arrest in children:
  - foreign body airway obstruction
  - drowning
  - anaphylaxis

Overview of Respiratory and Cardiac Arrest in Children

The child's heart is generally healthy and strong, undamaged by smoking and dietary abuse. Cardiac arrest in children is usually the result of progressive deterioration in respiratory and cardiac status, rather than a sudden event. The usual sequence is a long period of hypoxemia resulting in respiratory arrest. With no intervention, progression to full cardiopulmonary arrest occurs.

Because there is a long period of hypoxia, and accompanying metabolic acidosis and tissue damage, the resuscitation of children who have progressed to cardiac arrest is frequently unsuccessful by both prehospital or hospital providers. Thus, it is important to identify infants and children with respiratory compromise and intervene early. Provision of adequate support for respiratory failure will often prevent respiratory arrest.

In children, common causes of hypoxemia that result in cardiac arrest include the following:

- Asphyxia from suffocation or drowning
- Airway obstruction from a foreign body, infection, congenital defect, or smoke inhalation
- Sudden infant death syndrome
- Trauma

Other causes of cardiopulmonary arrest in children include:

- Poisoning by a central nervous system depressant, which decreases the respiratory rate to the point of hypoxia and apnea;
- Metabolic disorders involving an electrolyte imbalance such as that associated with dehydration from vomiting and diarrhea;
- Shock (poor tissue perfusion) that results in hypoxia and tissue damage when managed inappropriately; shock may occur with burns, severe dehydration, blood loss, sepsis, and anaphylaxis.

Respiratory Failure

Respiratory distress, preceding respiratory failure, occurs when the child attempts to compensate for hypoxia by increasing the work of breathing. Signs include tachypnea, retractions, nasal flaring, and tachycardia. If hypoxia is not managed (i.e., by supplemental oxygen), the carbon dioxide tension in the blood increases, leading to metabolic acidosis and respiratory failure.

Respiratory failure results from prolonged impairment of pulmonary gas exchange in which there is inadequate oxygenation of the blood and inadequate elimination of carbon dioxide.

Ventilatory failure results when an infant or child tires from the increased work of breathing. The child does not have the ability to sustain a rapid respiratory rate for lengthy periods and will begin breathing ineffectively at a lower rate. Other causes of a slow respiratory rate include hypothermia and poisoning by a central nervous system depressant.

History

Important information to obtain during the history:

- How long has the child been experiencing breathing difficulty?
- Could the child have possibly choked on something (like a small toy object or food item)?
- Has the child had any respiratory infection (cold, pneumonia, bronchitis, croup) recently? Has it gotten any better or worse?
- Has the child ever had asthma or another lung condition?
- Has the child sustained any recent injuries (hypovolemic shock, chest injury, or head injury)? How long ago did it happen?

Assessment

You should recognize the potential for respiratory failure in the child with diminishing level of consciousness, respiratory rate over 60 per minute, mottled or cyanotic color, and poor muscle tone. This is a child in need of rapid intervention to prevent further deterioration to ventilatory failure and respiratory arrest. A decreasing respiratory rate may be an indicator of ventilatory failure, especially when no intervention has been provided for respiratory distress (see Table 5.1).

Management

Basic life support (BLS) management for respiratory and ventilatory failure includes the following steps:

- Monitor the airway, ventilations, the circulatory status, neurologic status, including vital signs and body temperature.
- Maintain the child with respiratory distress in a position of comfort. The child will generally find the best position to maintain the airway.
- Administer high-flow oxygen by face mask.
- Do not create any additional anxiety in the child with invasive procedures. Do not inspect the mouth or tongue with a tongue blade.
- Transport rapidly.

 **CAUTION!**

If the child's respiratory rate is greater than 60/min, and oxygen alone does not result in a lower respiratory rate, it may be necessary to bag-mask ventilate with high-concentration oxygen at a rate slightly higher than the child is breathing. Once you have control of the child's ventilations with the bag valve mask, begin slowing the manual ventilation rate to less than 60/min. Then maintain the ventilation rate at 40–45/min.

If the respiratory rate begins decreasing, and the child's level of consciousness deteriorates, assist ventilations (by bag mask with high-concentration oxygen). Maintain ventilations at 35–40/min and monitor the patient's vital signs. 

Advanced life support (ALS) treatment additionally will include:

- Orotracheal intubation, and
- Establishing a peripheral IV line with Ringer's Lactate at a keep-open rate. Transport should not be unnecessarily delayed to accomplish this.

Respiratory Failure	Ventilatory Failure
Altered level of consciousness	Altered level of consciousness
Tachycardia	Tachycardia
Tachypnea, greater than 60 per minute	Respiratory rate below lowest normal rate for age
Weak, limp	Weak, limp
Retractions	Retractions
Mottled or cyanotic color	Mottled or cyanotic color
Head bobbing with each breath	
Diminished breath sounds	Diminished breath sounds
Weak central pulses	Weak central pulses
Absent peripheral pulses	Absent peripheral pulses

Rescue Breathing

If the child is found to be unresponsive, shake patient gently to determine the level of response. Protect the cervical spine if trauma is suspected. Call for additional help if the child is not breathing. Position the child with the head in neutral or "sniffing" position (the slight extension of the neck associated with sniffing a flower) prior to opening the airway. Make sure you do not hyperextend the neck. (Refer to Figure 4.1, page 49).

The muscles in the mouth and throat will relax when the child is unconscious, allowing the tongue to fall back into the throat and to occlude the airway. Manually open the airway with either the chin lift or jaw thrust maneuver. The modified jaw thrust maneuver should be used with both hands, keeping the neck stabilized whenever a cervical spine injury is suspected. A second rescuer must ventilate when the airway cannot be maintained or a good seal is not achieved with one rescuer ventilating.

Once the airway is opened, check again for breathing. Place your ear close to the child's nose and mouth, listening and feeling for exhaled air flow (see Figure 5.1). Look at the chest and abdomen for movement. If

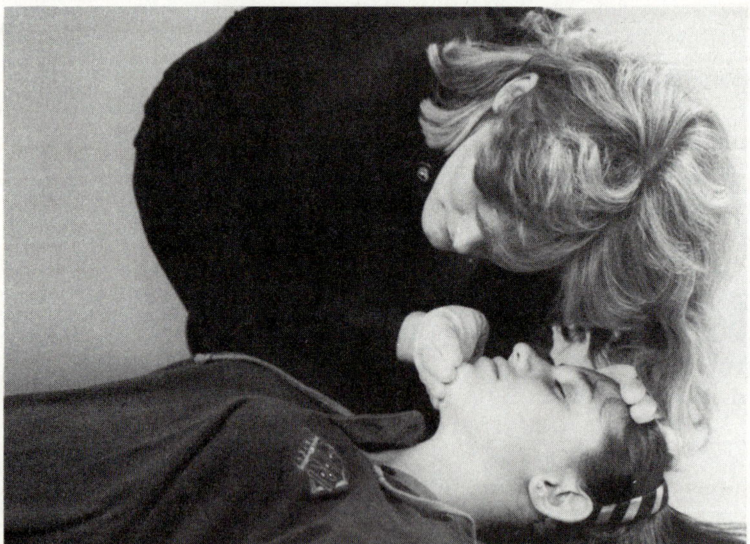

FIGURE 5.1   Assess for breathing after opening the airway by placing your ear close to the child's nose and mouth. While you listen and feel for exhaled air, look at the patient's chest and abdomen for movement.

there is no obvious spontaneous breathing, begin rescue breathing or manual ventilation.

Use mouth-to-mask breathing (mouth-to-mouth if no mask is available to fit the child) for children. If mouth-to-mouth ventilation is performed, pinch the patient's nose tightly. For infants, use the mouth-to-mouth and nose technique (Figure 5.2). Give two *slow* breaths (1 to 1.5 seconds/breath) to keep the pressure low and avoid gastric distention. Use enough pressure and volume to make the chest rise. The rate of rescue breathing, when chest compressions are not performed, should closely approximate the normal respiratory rate of the child. Rates are shown below:

- Newborns—40/min
- Infants—20–30/min, every 2 to 3 seconds
- Children—20/min, every 4 seconds.

The rescuer can increase the oxygen concentration delivered during rescue breathing from 16% to 28% by wearing nasal prongs with oxygen flowing at 10 l/min. As soon as possible, switch to a bag-valve-mask with an oxygen reservoir to continue manual ventilation of the child. The ALS provider will want to consider intubation if spontaneous breathing does not resume quickly.

If there is a high resistance to airflow and the chest does not rise, assume there is an airway obstruction. Reposition the child's head with the chin lift or jaw thrust maneuver. If there is still an obstruction, suspect an occlusion by a foreign body. See guidelines for airway obstruction management (pp. 84–87). Once the first two breaths have been successfully given,

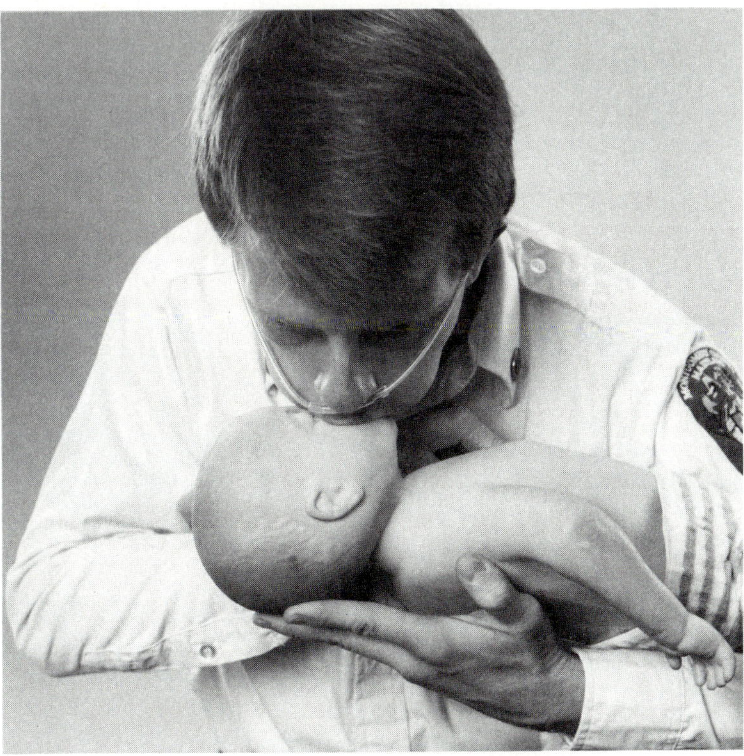

FIGURE 5.2 Use the mouth-to-mouth and nose technique of rescue breathing for infants. Use nasal cannula to increase oxygen delivery to the infant.

check for the presence of a pulse in a central artery. The brachial pulse is recommended for infants because their neck is short, making the carotid pulse difficult to palpate. Children over 1 year of age can have their carotid or brachial pulse palpated (see Figure 5.3). If the pulse is absent, initiate chest compressions. If a pulse is present, continue rescue breathing, checking for the presence of a pulse periodically.

Chest Compressions

Chest compressions are indicated when there is no central pulse palpated or there is a pulse rate less than 60 beats/min (bradycardia) unresponsive to ventilation and oxygenation (see Table 5.2).

When initiating CPR, make sure the child is supine on a hard surface. Hand position for performing compressions varies with the age of the child (Figure 5.4).

- *Newborns.* Place both thumbs on the sternum just below the imaginary line across the nipples, with the fingers around the torso supporting the back. This hand position requires an additional rescuer to provide ventilation. When an extra rescuer is unavailable, the hand position used for the infant is also effective.

- *Infants.* Position the hand by placing the index finger of the hand farthest from the infant's head just below the nipple line on the sternum. The area of compression is 1 finger breadth below this imaginary line, at the location of the middle and ring fingers. Make sure the fingers are not on the xiphoid.

- *Children over 1 year of age.* Position the hand by following with your index and middle finger the rib cage margin to the notch where the ribs and sternum meet. Place the middle finger in this notch with the index finger next to it. Visually identify the position of the index finger and place the heel of the same hand next to it, with the long axis of the heel parallel to that of the sternum.

- *Children over 8 years of age.* Position the hands as you do for children over 1 year of age. Use both hands interlocked for compressions.

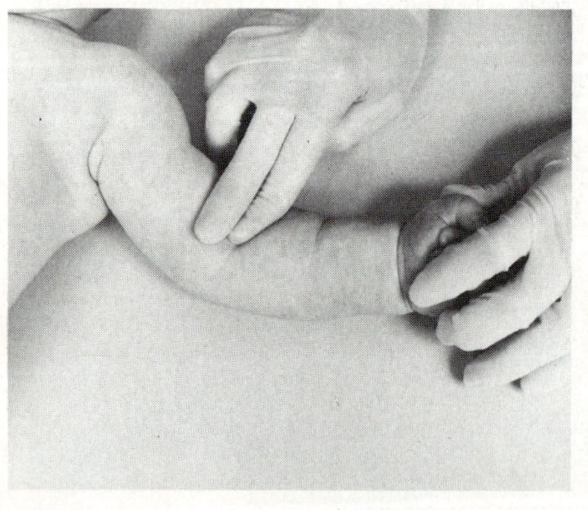
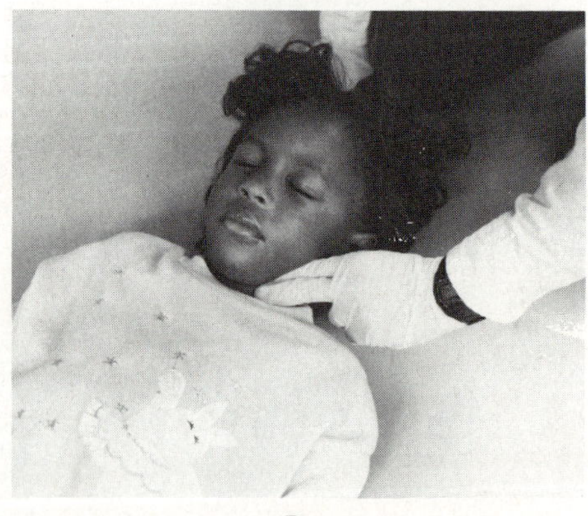

A   B

FIGURE 5.3 Palpate the pulse after breathing for the child. (A) Assess the brachial pulse in infants and young children. (B) Assess the carotid pulse in older children.

Pediatric Cardiopulmonary Resuscitation

TABLE 5.2 Rate and Depth of Chest Compressions for Children of Different Ages

Age	Rate	Depth*
Newborns	120/min	0.5–0.75 inch
Infants	100/min	0.5–1.0 inch
Children (1–8 years)	80–100/min	1.0–1.5 inches
Children (over 8)	80/min	1.5–2.0 inches

*Make sure femoral or brachial pulses are periodically checked to assure adequate chest compressions.

Chest compressions should be smooth rather than jerky. Allow the chest to resume normal position without removing the fingers or hand from the sternum. Develop a compression-relaxation rhythm with equal time for each. Both the rate and the depth of compressions vary with the age of the child.

Compressions must be coordinated with rescue breathing. At the end of every fifth compression, a pause (of no more than) 1 second should be allowed for ventilation. A 5:1 compression-to-ventilation ratio should be maintained for both infants and children: 20 breaths/min for infants and

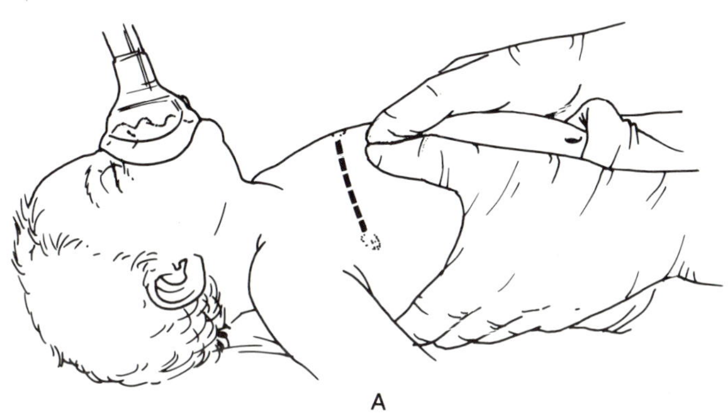

A

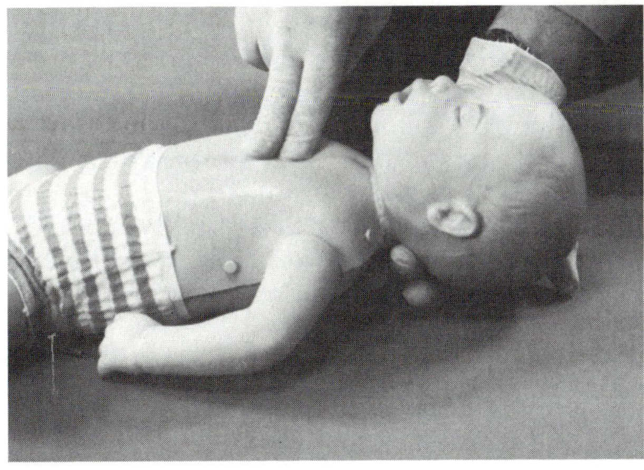

B

Infants: Use tips of fingers and light pressure.

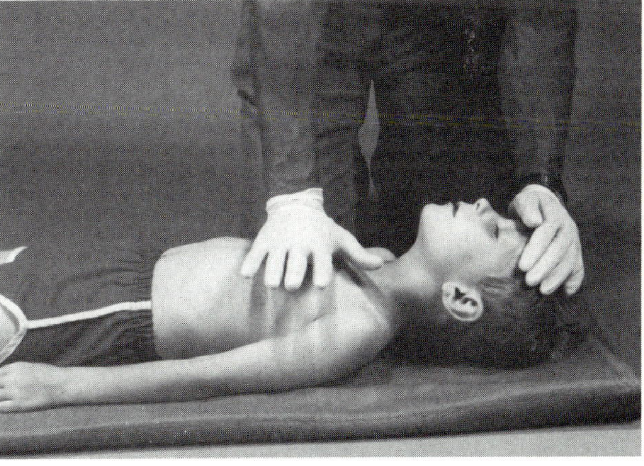

C

Children: Use heel of one hand only.

FIGURE 5.4 Positioning the hands for chest compressions differs according to the age and size of the child. (A) Newborn, (B) Infant, (C) Children between 1 and 8 years of age. (Parts B and C reproduced with permission from Grant et al. *Emergency Care,* Fifth Ed., © 1990 Prentice Hall.)

15 breaths/min for children. Reassess the child after 10 full cycles, and every few minutes after that. Controversy continues regarding the adequacy of this rate of ventilation, especially with infants and small children who are already hypoxic. However, achieving the optimal number of chest compressions and allowing 1 second for each ventilation is not an easily accomplished task.

When there is only one rescuer, even more compromises are necessary to coordinate compressions and ventilation. If the rescuer hopes to provide the optimal number of compressions and ventilations each minute, time is inadequate either to move the hand from the chest for the chin lift or to physically identify the landmarks for compression after each ventilation.

- In infants, head tilt should be used *without the chin lift* to maintain airway patency after the initial two ventilations. The rescuer should observe the patient's chest to make sure it rises with each breath, repositioning the patient's head if chest rise is not apparent.
- In children, the chin lift and head tilt are both needed to maintain an open airway for ventilations. The hand performing the compressions must be used for the chin lift, and then be returned to the chest position for compressions using only visual recall of position.

Signs of effective CPR include the following:

- The heart resumes beating, and there is a palpable spontaneous pulse.
- There is improved color as the child pinks up.
- There is spontaneous movement of the arms and legs.
- There are spontaneous respiratory efforts, such as gasping with chest rise.
- The pupils constrict to light.

Management of Parents

When a child needs CPR, the parent is in crisis. It is important to be gentle, but firm, with the parent so you can proceed with resuscitation. Parents will be most reassured if you demonstrate how you are helping the child and convey control of the situation. When available, another pre-hospital provider, police, or bystander should be employed to support the parent. If no one is available, it may be helpful to enlist the parent's support in caring for the child. Direct the parent to perform simple tasks (get the child's favorite toy or the parent's own wallet or purse in preparation for the trip to the hospital). Remember, any instructions you give should be clear and brief. *Parents will tend to hear the instructions but not listen to them.* Anxiety also produces a short-term memory loss, so instructions will usually need repeating.

Airway Obstruction

Aspiration of a foreign body is a common problem in children under 3 years of age. In 1989, it was the second leading cause of unintentional injury death in infants between 1 month and 1 year of age (18.5% of accidental deaths) and the fifth leading cause of unintentional injury death in children 1 to 4 years of age (2.1% of accidental deaths in this age group). However, many more such events occurred that did not result in death.

Infants and young children explore the environment by putting objects in their mouth such as pins, coins, and parts of toys. They also have few or no teeth, and have yet to develop full control of swallowing. For this reason, foods are often aspirated as well. Commonly aspirated foods include hot dogs, peanuts, grapes, and candy. Their size, shape, and consistency contribute to greater severity of symptoms. If the object is large enough, complete occlusion of the airway can occur.

History

Important information to obtain upon arrival:

- Did the child have a sudden episode of coughing, choking, wheezing, and cyanosis that was observed by the child's parent or care provider? Was this episode associated with eating any particular food or did it occur with play activities?
- Was there a sudden onset of respiratory distress not associated with an illness?
- Is the child still coughing and choking?

Assessment

The child who has aspirated a foreign object may be in any stage of respiratory distress. During the primary survey, note the ability of the child to talk, cry, cough, or wheeze. In this case, the child has a partial obstruction. The child may also be unresponsive with no spontaneous breathing, in which case there may be total occlusion of the airway. Infections such as croup and epiglottitis also cause airway obstruction, but the onset is longer, over hours or days. Management of airway obstruction for these infections is outlined in Chapter 6.

Management

BLS management for an *incomplete* airway obstruction is the same as that for a child with respiratory failure.

- Permit the child to find the best position to keep the airway open, and maintain the child in that position.
- Do not discourage the child from coughing.
- Administer high-flow oxygen by face mask if the child will tolerate it.
- Do not create any additional anxiety in the child by performing invasive procedures.
- Transport rapidly.
- Attempt to open the child's airway if the child's coughing becomes ineffective or if there is increased respiratory difficulty accompanied by stridor.

Attempts to clear the occluded airway should be made when the aspiration of a foreign body was witnessed or strongly suspected in the following cases:

- There is a conscious child who cannot talk or cry.
- There is an unconscious, nonbreathing child after usual attempts to open the airway are unsuccessful.

BLS management for the infant with an *obstructed airway* includes the following steps (see Figure 5.5):

- Perform a series of 4 back blows and 4 chest thrusts. (The Heimlich maneuver is not recommended because of the potential for intra-abdominal injury.)
- Position the infant face down, with head lower than the body, on one arm
- Use one hand to deliver 4 forceful blows between the shoulder blades of the back
- Sandwich the infant between both arms and turn the patient's face upwards. Support the infant on your thigh with head lower than the body.
- Deliver 4 chest thrusts in the same location where chest compressions are performed
- Open the airway with the tongue-jaw lift and look for the foreign body. Remove any foreign material observed. Make NO blind finger sweeps in the mouth; this could cause the foreign body to be pushed back even farther into the airway.
- If no spontaneous breathing is observed, perform rescue breathing. If the airway is still obstructed, repeat the sequence of back blows, chest thrusts, inspection of the mouth, and rescue breathing until the airway obstruction is removed.
- Transport patient rapidly to the nearest hospital.

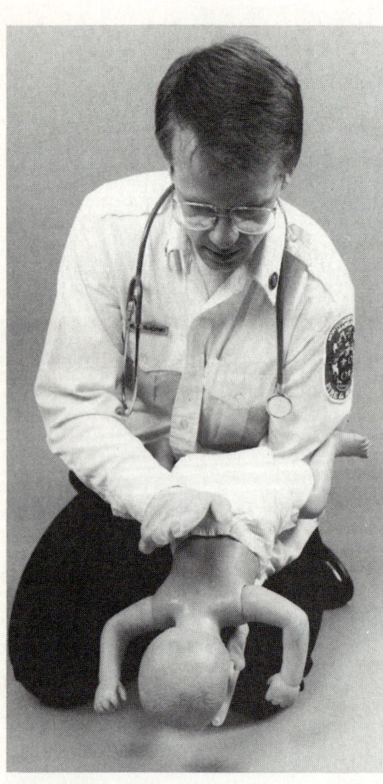
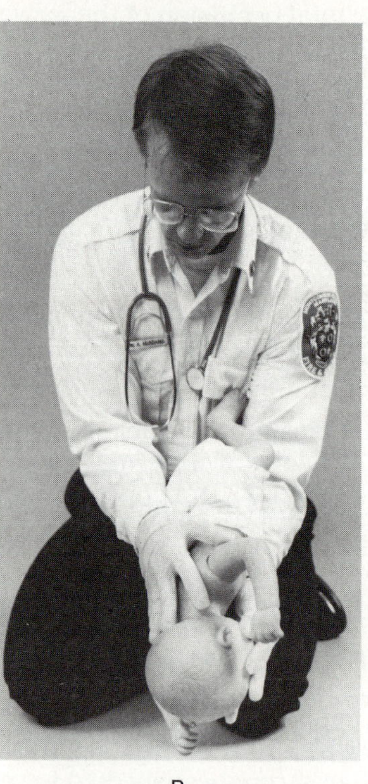
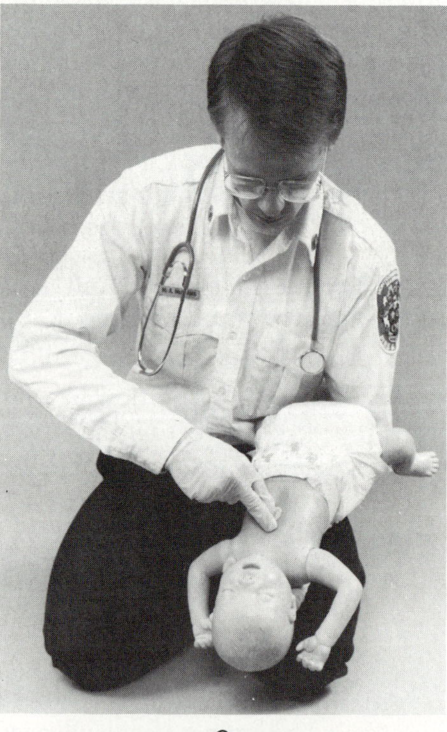

ABC

FIGURE 5.5 Management of an obstructed airway in infant. (A) Perform 4 back blows with the infant face down, head lower than the body. (B) Turn the baby face upward, sandwiched between both of your arms. (C) Perform 4 chest thrusts.

Pediatric Cardiopulmonary Resuscitation

BLS management for the child with an *obstructed airway* includes the following steps (see Figure 5.6):

- Use subdiaphragmatic abdominal thrusts (the Heimlich maneuver).
- When the child is conscious, perform this maneuver standing behind the child who is sitting or standing:
  1. Make a fist with one hand, placing the thumb side against the middle of the child's abdomen, slightly above the navel.
  2. Grasp the fist with the other hand and press into the child's abdomen with a quick upward thrust. Take care not to press on the xiphoid or the rib cage.
- When the child is unconscious and lying on the floor:
  1. Position yourself at the child's feet or straddle the child.
  2. Place the heel of one hand in the middle of the child's abdomen above the navel. Place the other hand on top of the first and press the abdomen in the midline with quick upward thrusts.
- Individual thrusts should continue until the foreign body is expelled or 10 abdominal thrusts have been delivered.
- Check for the foreign body in the mouth and remove it if seen. *Caution:* NO BLIND FINGER SWEEPS.
- Check for spontaneous breathing and if not present, attempt to perform rescue breathing. If no ventilation is possible, repeat the sequence until the airway is open or the child loses consciousness.
- Transport patient rapidly to the nearest hospital.

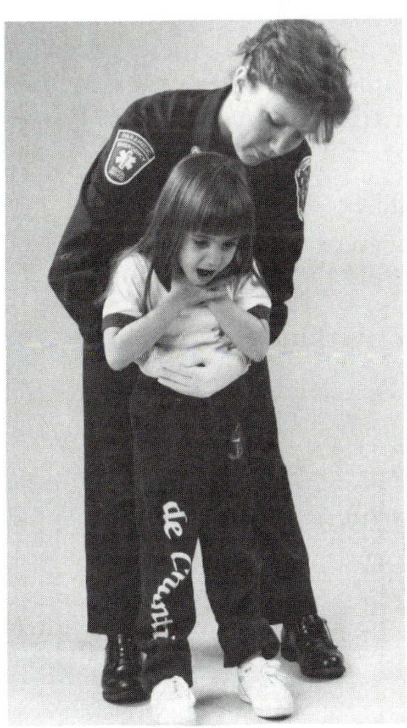

A

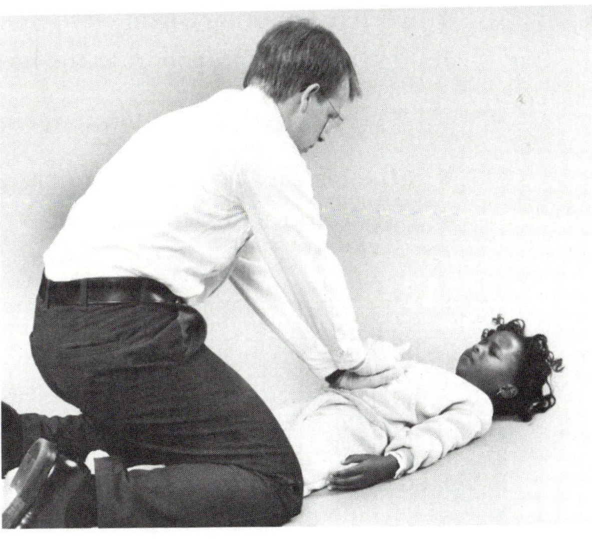

B

FIGURE 5.6 Management of an obstructed airway in the child. (A) Perform subdiaphragmatic abdominal thrusts when the child is conscious and sitting or standing. (B) Straddle the unconscious child and perform abdominal thrusts.

Bradycardia

This is the most common dysrhythmia in children. It usually develops as a result of hypoxia, hypotension, and acidosis. Bradycardia also develops with vagal stimulation, caused by suctioning or intubation that is too aggressive without adequate reoxygenation. The newborn will become apneic and then hypoxic if cold oxygen is directed to the baby's face in the distribution of the trigeminal nerve (mammalian diving reflex).

Assessment

The child will have signs of hypoxemia and a slower heart rate than expected for his or her age (under 80/min in infants, or 60/min in young children). The rhythm strip will show a slow rate, the P wave may or may not be present, and the QRS duration may be normal or prolonged (see Figure 5.7).

Management

BLS management for bradycardia includes the following:

- Control the airway with oxygenation and good ventilation to prevent progression to asystole.

- Assist ventilations prior to respiratory arrest with a bag mask and high-concentration, high-flow oxygen; hyperventilate (at a rate of 10 breaths more/min than normal for age group) if bradycardia persists. Make inspiratory and expiratory phases of each breath equal in length.

- Initiate CPR if child is unconscious and the heart rate is less than 80/min in infants or 60/min in young children when there is no response to ventilation with high-concentration oxygen.

- Keep the patient warm.

- Provide rapid transport to the hospital.

The ALS provider should additionally initiate the following care:

- Attach a cardiac monitor and record a rhythm strip.

- Begin orotracheal intubation.

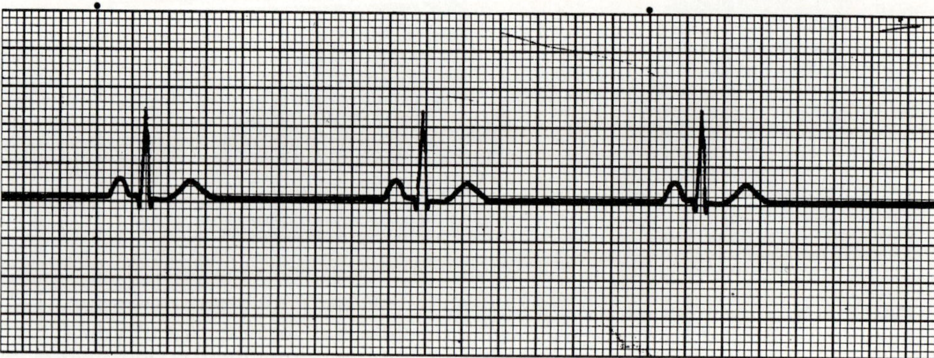

FIGURE 5.7   Rhythm strip indicating bradycardia in the child with a rate of 40 per minute.

- Establish an IV or intraosseous line. Do not delay transport to establish the line.

- Epinephrine and atropine administered by endotracheal tube or IV may be ordered by medical control or protocols, when oxygen and ventilation do not restore the heart rate to more adequate levels. (Refer to Table 5.3 for drug dosages.)

Asystole and Ventricular Fibrillation

Asystole is the absence of a palpable pulse in a nonbreathing child. It is a terminal rhythm that generally results from poorly managed bradycardia. Children with bradycardia who progress to asystole have a poor outcome. Studies have indicated that no more than 10% of these children are successfully resuscitated, and many survivors have neurologic damage. For such children to have a chance, effective resuscitation during transport is essential.

Ventricular fibrillation is a disorganized dysrhythmia without a detectable pulse. It rarely occurs in children unless a metabolic condition is present such as acidosis or an electrolyte imbalance.

History

In this case, assessment and management will proceed without an extensive history. Questions about what happened to the child, and then more specific questions related to the mechanism of injury should follow.

Assessment

The child in asystole and ventricular fibrillation will be unconscious, have no pulse or spontaneous respirations, and lack perfusion. The rhythm strip in asystole is generally a straight line, with an occasional P wave. It is important to check for a loose electrode wire that might also give a straight-line reading. The rhythm strip in ventricular fibrillation will have waveforms varying in size, shape, and rhythm, with no identifiable P, QRS, or T waves (see Figure 5.8, page 92).

Management

BLS management of asystole and ventricular fibrillation includes the following steps:

- Initiate CPR.
- Control the airway and ventilate with high-flow, high-concentration oxygen by bag-valve mask.
- Keep the child warm.
- Provide rapid transport to the hospital.

ALS providers should additionally manage the child with the following care:

- Orotracheal intubation.
- Attach a cardiac monitor and defibrillate as soon as possible at 2 Wsec/kg (200 Wsec maximum) initially. If there is no success in establishing a rhythm, double the energy dose (360 Wsec maximum) for the second defibrillation. Defibrillation may be repeated once more at the higher energy dose if no rhythm is established.

Drug Preparations Available	Dose/Route of Administration	Indication	Action	Adverse Effects
First-Line Drugs				
Epinephrine 1:10,000 Do not mix with sodium bicarbonate	0.1 ml/kg/dose IV 0.2–0.3 ml/kg/dose ET up to 10 ml maximum Repeat every 5 min	Asystole, ventricular fibrillation, electromechancial dissociation	Alpha & beta adrenergic, increased heart rate, vasoconstriction, force of contraction increased, increased myocardial irritability	Tachycardia Dysrhythmia Hypertension *Contraindicated* for irritable rhythms, ventricular tachycardia
Atropine 0.1 mg/ml Do not mix with sodium biocarbonate	0.02 mg/kg/dose IV or ET Minimum dose 0.1 mg Maximum single and cumulative doses: 1.0 mg in children 2.0 mg in teens	Bradycardia Asystole Increased vagal tone	Increases the heart rate	Tachycardia Dysrhythmia Dry mouth Dilated pupils *Contraindicated* for tachycardia, either sinus ventricular or atrial
Sodium Bicarbonate 50 mEq/50 ml	First dose: 1 mEq/kg Second dose: 0.5 mEq/kg IV push slowly Maximum dose 3 mEq/kg Dilute 1:1 with D5W	Metabolic acidosis	Neutralizes acid pH, leads to CO_2 production	Metabolic alkalosis *Contraindicated* in cases of inadequate ventilation
Lidocaine 10 mg/ml Concentration varies by drug company	1.0 mg/kg/dose IV or ET Maximum dose of 50 mg 20–50 mcg/kg/min continuous drip	Ventricular tachycardia, hyperexcitable myocardium, cardiac arrest by ventricular fibrillation	Depresses ventricular electrical activity, raises electrical stimulation threshhold, stabilizes ventricular arrhythmia	Hypotension Bradycardia Seizure Drowsiness Muscle twitching *Contraindicated* for asystole, heart block
Dextrose D 50 W	0.5–1.0 g/kg IV only Dilute D50W 1:1 with sterile water to D25W (2–4 ml/kg)	Unresponsive without mechanism, and no response to initial round of drugs, suspected hypoglycemia	Raises blood sugar level, needed for vigorous myocardia	Causes scarring of peripheral veins *Contraindicated* if known to be in diabetic ketoacidosis
Second-Line Drugs				
Bretylium 50 mg/ml	5 mg/kg/dose IV push Repeat q 15 min 10 mg/kg/dose to maximum dose 30 mg/kg	Ventricular dysrhythmias, lidocaine is not effective	Antiarrhythmic agent makes fibrillating heart susceptible to defibrillation	Hypotension Bradyrhythmias Nausea Vomiting Transient hypertension
Dopamine 200 mg/5ml Do not mix with sodium bicarbonate	2–20 mcg/kg/min IV drip (6 mg × kg in 100 ml D5W) 1 ml/hr = 1 mcg/kg/min	Cardiogenic shock Hypotension Poor peripheral perfusion Stable rhythm	Renal vasodilation at low doses (2–5 mcg/kg), beta adrenergic effect, increases heart rate, cardiac contractility, and cardiac output	Tachycardia Dysrhythmia Hypertension *Contraindicated* in hypovolemic shock

Drug Preparations Available	Dose/Route of Administration	Indication	Action	Adverse Effects
Valium (Diazepam) 5 mg/ml Do not mix or dilute with other drugs or solutions	0.2–0.3 mg/kg IV slow push over 3 min Inject as close to vein as possible Maximum total dose: child, 10 mg adult, 30 mg Repeat dose in 5–10 min if seizures continue	Persistent seizure activity	Rapid action anti-convulsant	Respiratory depression, be prepared to assist ventilations
Epinephrine 1:1000	0.01 mg/kg/dose Subcutaneous Maximum single dose 0.3 ml May be repeated every 20–30 min × 3 if heart rate is <180	Asthma, expiratory respiratory distress, anaphylaxis	Rapid-acting bronchodilator, induces relaxation of bronchial smooth muscle	Tachycardia Dysrhythmia Hypertension
Aminophylline 1 mg/ml Do not mix with epinephrine, demcrol, or morphine	Loading dose 6–7 mg/kg IV over 20 min, if previously receiving theophylline Maintenance dose 0.8–1.2 mg/kg/hr IV drips if >1 yr	Status asthmaticus unresponsive to epinephrine Medical control order—identify the time and dose of theophylline taken	Bronchodilator—relaxes smooth bronchial muscles	Tachycardia Dysrhythmia Irritability Seizures Nausea, vomiting, abdominal pain *Caution:* Toxic effects may occur, especially if child is maintained on oral theophylline
Narcan (Naloxone) 0.4 mg/ml	0.1 mg/kg/dose initially Maximum dose 0.8 mg IV push, may give ET If no response in 10 min give 2 mg IV when narcotic overdose suspected	Coma, respiratory depression, hypotension, known or suspected narcotic overdose	Antidote for narcotics	None listed
Racemic Epinephrine 2.25% solution	0.25–0.5 ml diluted in 2–3 ml normal saline, by nebulizer Dose/kg ratio 0.25 ml if <20 kg 0.5 ml if 20–40 kg	Croup, severe dyspnea, and a long transport time is anticipated	May reduce respiratory distress	*Contraindicated* For marked tachycardia

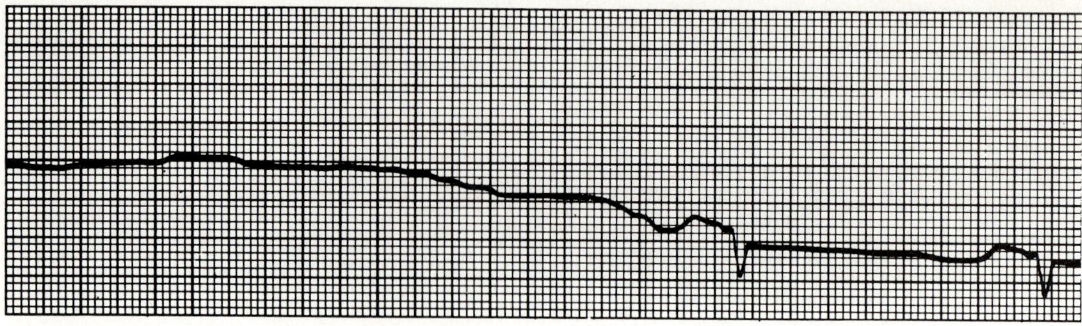

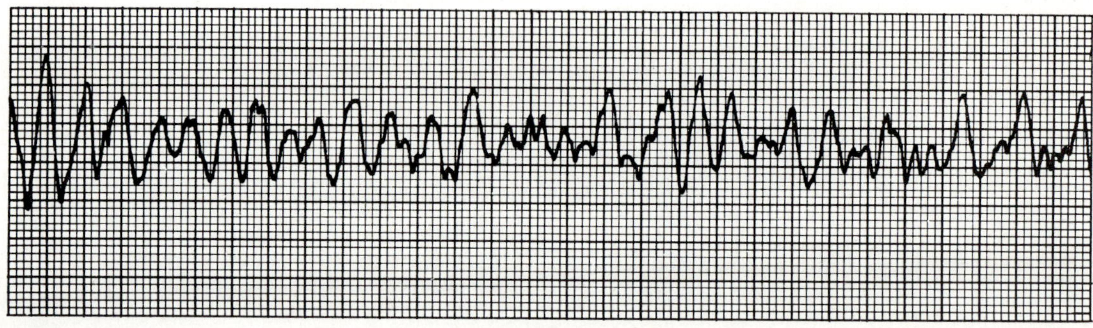

FIGURE 5.8 (A) Asystole, (B) Ventricular fibrillation. (Reproduced with permission. *Textbook of Pediatric Advanced Life Support,* 1987. Copyright American Heart Association.)

- Establish an IV peripheral or intraosseous (IO) line without delaying transport to the hospital.
- Administer drugs ordered by medical control or protocol either endotracheally or IV (epinephrine, atropine, dextrose, sodium bicarbonate, and naloxone if mechanism of injury is present). Lidocaine, bretylium, or dopamine may be indicated if a rhythm becomes established. (Refer to Table 5.3 for recommended drug dosages and routes of administration.)

Supraventricular Tachycardia

Supraventricular tachycardia is an episodic, serious dysrhythmia occurring in infants or older children, often near puberty. It is a rare but frightening disorder for parents and providers to treat, with an occurrence of 1 in 25,000 children. These children experience sustained heart rates in excess of 200/min, and often up to 300/min. It has been linked to prior cardiac surgery, but usually occurs in otherwise healthy children. There is no known trigger to the episode.

Children can sustain these heart rates for a while, but after several hours they may develop congestive heart failure. *It is a true medical emergency!*

History

Important information to obtain during the history includes:

- Does the child have a heart defect? Has the child ever had heart surgery?

- Has the child had any illness or injury recently? (This is to differentiate from shock of another cause.) Has the child experienced vomiting or feeding problems?
- Has the child's behavior changed to more anxious or irritable?

Assessment

Infants with supraventricular tachycardia will be pale or cyanotic, irritable, sweating, breathing rapidly, and feeding poorly or vomiting. They will have a regular heart rate too fast to count, about 220–350/min. Signs of shock may be present.

Older children will complain of feeling bad and have a fainting spell. Adolescents will have a regular heart rate between 150–250/min. Perfusion is poor so there will also be pallor or cyanosis and signs of shock. The child may recognize what is happening if this is a recurrent problem.

Supraventricular tachycardia will be exhibited by a rapid rate, no detectable variation in the R–R interval, lack of identifiable P waves, and narrow QRS complexes on rhythm strip (see Figure 5.9).

Management

BLS field care for supraventricular tachycardia includes the following:

- Monitor ABC's and vital signs.
- Maintain airway control and administer high-flow oxygen by face mask.
- Prepare to administer CPR, and
- Transport immediately.
- Medical control may recommend stimulation of the diving reflex by placing an ice pack over the child's face.

ALS providers can provide the following additional care as medical control or protocols direct:

- Attach a cardiac monitor and record a rhythm strip.
- Perform cardioversion at 0.25–0.5 Wsec/kg, or the lowest energy setting (minimal setting on the Lifepack is 5 Wsec). If the attempt is unsuccessful, repeat doubling the energy charge.
- Start an IV of Ringer's Lactate at a keep-open rate.
- Intubate the child if his or her level of consciousness deteriorates.

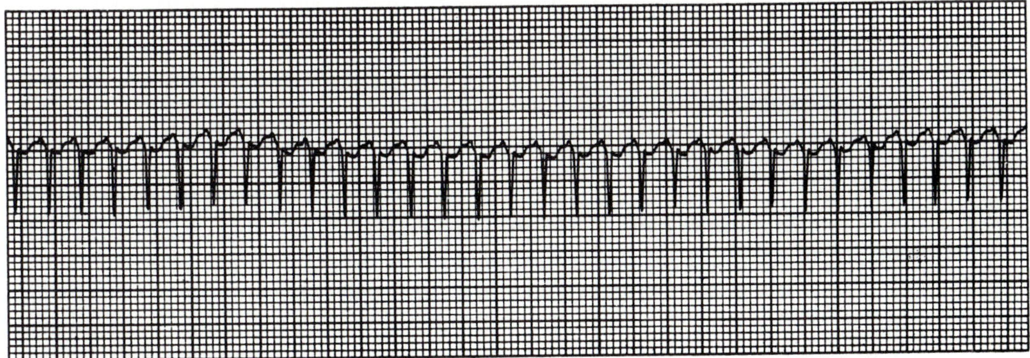

FIGURE 5.9 Supraventricular tachycardia with a rate of 320 beats per minute. (Reproduced with permission. *Textbook of Pediatric Advanced Life Support*, 1987. Copyright American Heart Association.)

There are five first-line drugs used during the resuscitation of children. There are also some additional drugs used for specific circumstances (see Table 5.3).

The intravenous route is preferred for drug administration during a cardiac arrest; however, establishing a peripheral line is not easily accomplished in children, particularly those in shock. Often prehospital providers are directed to obtain an IV line during transport rather than delay transport for this procedure. The endotracheal tube and intraosseous site are alternate routes for drug administration.

It is currently recommended that the *same* drug dosage used for the IV route be used for endotracheal administration, except epinephrine, which should be given at a dosage double or triple that used for the IV route. Other changes may be recommended as studies compare drug absorption between the two routes of administration. Unless special care is taken when giving small doses of the drugs through the endotracheal tube, some of the drug remains on the tube, never making contact with the lung tissue for absorption. Drugs administered to children through the endotracheal tube should be diluted in 1–2 cc of Normal Saline. The drug should then be injected into the endotracheal tube as deeply as possible, and followed with several positive pressure ventilations.

Drug absorption from the bone marrow is considered as good as an IV injection. When administering drugs by either of these routes, it is important to flush the IV line with saline (1–2 cc in infants, 5 cc in children) to make sure all of the drug is delivered and that drug interactions are also avoided.

Life-Threatening Conditions

Drowning and Near Drowning

Drowning is defined as death within 24 hours following a submersion accident. *Near drowning* describes a submersion incident in which the child survives at least 24 hours, but death may ultimately occur. Drowning is the third leading cause of preventable death to children in the United States, accounting for 1200 deaths to children under 15 years of age in 1989.

Among young children, the majority of drowning episodes occur when they are inadequately supervised, usually in fresh water (pools, lakes, bathtubs, buckets, toilets, and fish tanks). Children under 3 years of age are helpless in the water, and because they are top-heavy, often cannot extricate and save themselves when falling head first into buckets, bathtubs, pools, etc. Drowning incidents in older children and adolescents are often related to boating accidents, exhaustion after attempting to swim long distances, and alcohol use. Children with seizures are also at a higher risk of drowning if permitted to swim unsupervised.

The child who is trapped in water panics and struggles, initially holding his or her breath. Then the child swallows water, vomits, and cannot avoid aspirating water and vomitus. Some children develop laryngospasm, and if it persists beyond loss of consciousness and cessation of respiratory effort, there is no aspiration of water (dry drowning). During the submersion, the child develops hypoxemia, acidosis, and cardiac arrest, leading to the initial brain damage. Factors associated with the child's outcome following a submersion accident include the maximum submersion time, how quickly resuscitation efforts began following rescue, and the temperature of the water. The child who drowns in cold water becomes hypothermic very quickly because of the large body surface area. This reduces the metabolic rate and demand for oxygen, resulting in bradycardia. The diving reflex is triggered by cold water on the face, a protective mechanism that preferentially shunts blood to the brain and heart. This may partially protect children from significant brain damage. Children have been successfully resuscitated after submersion in cold water for 40 to 60 minutes.

History

Important information to obtain during the history:

- How long was the child submerged?
- Did the child have any spontaneous respiratory effort upon rescue? Was there a heart rate?
- How quickly did resuscitation begin following rescue?
- Was the child diving in shallow water?
- Does the child have a history of seizures?

Assessment

During the primary survey, note the presence of spontaneous respiratory effort and a heart rate, even if very slow. If spontaneous respirations are present, there may be crackles or wheezing. In most cases, the child will be unconscious, pulseless, and have no spontaneous respiratory effort.

Management

BLS management for drowning and near-drowning victims includes:

- Assess ABC's and vital signs.
- Clear the airway if obstructed.
- Control the airway and protect the C-spine, especially if trauma is suspected.
- Begin mouth-to-mouth or mouth-to-mask ventilation if no spontaneous breathing is apparent (see Figure 5.10). Ventilate by bag-valve mask with high-flow, high-concentration oxygen as soon as the equipment becomes available.
- Begin CPR if no heart rate is palpable.
- Remove wet clothing and wrap in blankets.
- If hypothermic, wrap in dry blankets and initiate rewarming measures while en route. Place heat packs along the torso of the body, protecting the skin from burns (if local guidelines permit). Follow BLS care guidelines in Chapter 7.
- Transport patient immediately to a hospital with pediatric intensive care, when available.

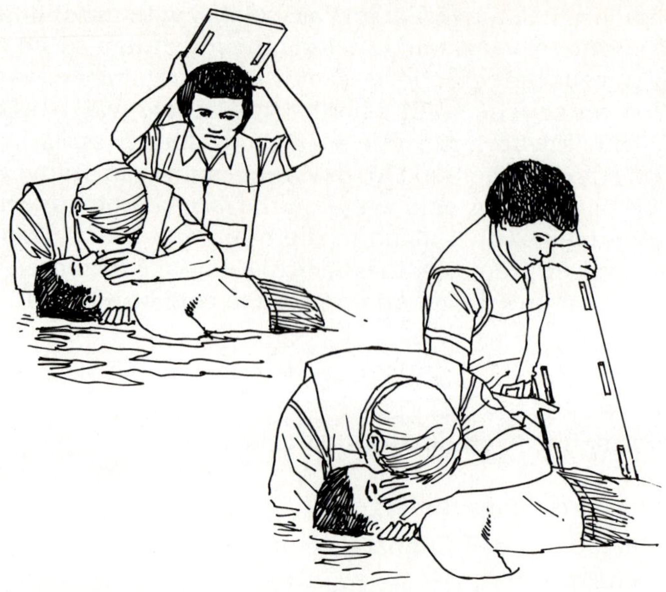

FIGURE 5.10 Begin rescue breathing to the drowning victim as soon as you have access to the child.

ALS providers should additionally initiate the following care:

- Intubate the child if there is no heart or respiratory rate.
- Establish an IV line with Ringer's Lactate (warmed if available) at a keep-open rate. Intraosseous infusion may be used for children who have no pulse or respiratory effort.
- Initiate the ACLS (advanced cardiac life support) drug protocol if the child is not hypothermic. (See dosages on Table 5.3.) Sodium bicarbonate should be used with caution in the child having spontaneous cardiac activity.

CAUTION! 

Drowning with Severe Hypothermia

If a heart rate is present, even if very slow, no invasive management should be attempted, such as intubation. Such a maneuver may irritate the vagus nerve, resulting in asystole. With severe bradycardia, some perfusion of the brain is occurring, and the hypothermia stimulates the body to shunt blood only to the major organs. In this case, it would be better to bag-mask-ventilate with high-concentration oxygen during transport.

Anaphylaxis

Anaphylaxis is a rare, acute, and generalized allergic reaction. The reaction may occur within minutes to hours after an exposure to the substance by mouth, inhalation, or injection. Common substances triggering this allergic response include bee stings, antibiotics, drugs, and foods. (See Figure 5.11). Generally, the child has had one prior exposure to the sub-

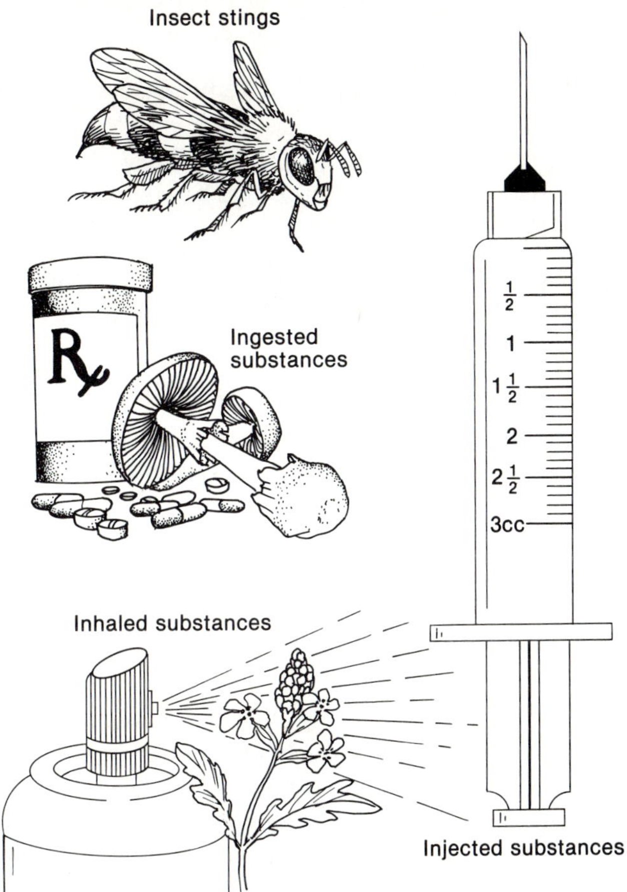

FIGURE 5.11   Common substances that trigger anaphylactic allergic responses.

stance, at which time the child became "sensitive." Subsequent expo-
sures to the same substance result in the severe allergic reaction.

Generally, four body systems are affected (skin, respiratory system,
cardiovascular system, and gastrointestinal tract). However, the response
is individual to the patient. Any or all systems can be affected initially.

History

Important questions to ask during assessment and transport of patient:

- What was the possible substance (food, bee sting, drug, etc.) that
  triggered this reaction?
- How much time was there between exposure and onset of symptoms? (The more rapid the reaction, the more severe the shock.)
- Is there any prior history of anaphylaxis or serious allergic reactions?
- Does the child have epinephrine for such allergic episodes? Has it
  already been injected? If so, how long ago? If not, is it available?

Assessment

During the primary survey, look for signs of respiratory distress and
altered level of consciousness. When you arrive at the scene, the child may

be in acute distress with shock and an airway obstruction. Look for a medic alert tag. Signs of a generalized allergic reaction by body system include:

Skin. Hives, itching, and redness; swelling of the face, mouth, and tongue.

Respiratory. Wheezing, respiratory distress, and tightness in the chest; stridor, choking, and hoarseness.

Gastrointestinal. Nausea and vomiting; diarrhea and abdominal cramps.

Circulatory. Flushed skin; hypotension; bradycardia and/or cardiac arrest.

Neurologic. Seizures; loss of bladder and bowel control.

Management

BLS management for anaphylaxis includes the following steps:

- Assess ABC's and vital signs.
- Administer high-flow, high-concentration oxygen.
- Prepare to administer rescue breathing and CPR.
- If patient carries epinephrine for anaphylaxis, and has not yet injected it, assist patient or family member to give it.
- Transport patient rapidly to the emergency department.
- If the allergy results from a bee sting or other injected venom, delay absorption of substance by cold pack over the site.
- If hypotension is present, child should be placed in Trendelenburg position or have pneumatic anti-shock garment leg compartments inflated.

ALS providers should additionally provide the following care:

- Orotracheal intubation. Remember that the endotracheal tube may need to be a size or two smaller than usual because of laryngeal edema.
- Epinephrine 1:1000 (0.01 ml/kg every 15 min × 3) subcutaneously is the treatment of choice for anaphylactic reactions.
- An IV of Ringer's Lactate. Administer a bolus of fluid IV push, 20 ml/kg. If there is no change in vital signs after the first bolus of fluid and epinephrine administration, the bolus of fluid can be repeated.
- For severe reactions, medical control may recommend that epinephrine 1:10,000 be administered IV at a dose of 0.01 mg/kg, very cautiously. Monitor for hypertension and bradycardia. If the IV cannot be established, epinephrine may be administered by endotracheal tube. Repeated dosages of IV or endotracheal epinephrine should be directed by medical control or local protocol.

Pediatric CPR References

Accident Facts. Chicago: National Safety Council, 1990.

Ballenger, M. J., "Pediatric cardiac arrest," *Emergency,* 18, no. 1 (January 1986), pp. 48–52.

BRILL, J. E., "Cardiopulmonary resuscitation," *Pediatric Annals*, 15, no. 1 (January 1986), pp. 24–29.

CHAMEIDES, L., ed., *Textbook of Pediatric Advanced Life Support*. Dallas: American Heart Association, 1988.

FRIESEN, R. M., and others, "Appraisal of pediatric cardiopulmonary resuscitation," *Canadian Medical Association Journal*, 1, no. 126 (May 1982), pp. 1055–1058.

GILLIS, J., and others, "Results of inpatient pediatric resuscitation," *Critical Care Medicine*, 14, no. 5 (May 1986), pp. 469–471.

HARRIS, C. S., and others, "Childhood asphyxiation by food," *Journal of the American Medical Association*, 251, no. 17 (1984), pp. 2231–2235.

HAZINSKI, M. F., "New guidelines for pediatric and neonatal cardiopulmonary resuscitation and advanced life support. Part 1: Basic CPR for adults and children," *Pediatric Nursing*, 15, no. 5 (September/October 1986), pp. 373–376.

HAZINSKI, M. F., "New guidelines for pediatric and neonatal cardiopulmonary resuscitation and advanced life support. Part 2: Pediatric advanced life support," *Pediatric Nursing*, 15, no. 6 (November/December 1986), pp. 445–448.

JANAKIRAMAN, N., "Cardiopulmonary resuscitation in children," *Emergency Medical Services*, 13, no. 4 (April 1984), pp. 42–46.

JONES, S., and BAGG, A. M., "Lead drugs for cardiac arrest," *Nursing 88*, 18, no. 1 (January 1988), pp. 34–42.

LOSEK, J. D., and others, "Prehospital care of the pulseless, nonbreathing pediatric patient," *American Journal of Emergency Medicine*, 5, no. 5 (May 1987), pp. 370–374.

SEIDEL, J. S., and HENDERSON, D. P., eds., *Prehospital Care of Pediatric Emergencies*. Los Angeles: Pediatric Society of California, 1987.

SILVERMAN, B. J., ed., *Advanced Pediatric Life Support*. Dallas: American College of Emergency Physicians, 1989.

STICHLER, J. F., and SHOWMAN, T., "A child drowns: A nursing perspective," *Journal of Maternal Child Nursing*, 6, no. 5 (September/October 1981), pp. 324–328.

TODD, I. K., "Anaphylaxis: Guidelines for prehospital management," *The EMT Journal*, 5, no. 2 (1981), pp. 97–99.

Pediatric CPR References

Respiratory Emergencies

6

OBJECTIVES

When you have completed this chapter you should be able to

✳ List the four most common respiratory emergencies in children.

✳ Describe the findings that differentiate asthma vs. bronchiolitis, and croup vs. epiglottitis.

✳ Describe the management of acute respiratory distress in the child with asthma, bronchiolitis, croup, or epiglottitis.

Introduction

Because of their association with acute respiratory distress and hypoxemia, conditions involving the respiratory tract should immediately alert you to be especially vigilant in assessing the child, monitoring the respiratory rate, and evaluating the progression of symptoms.

Children have lower resistance to viruses and bacteria; consequently, infants and small children are at greater risk of respiratory infections. The small diameter of their airway is susceptible to obstruction from foreign bodies and swelling. In addition, the smooth muscle in their airway is more reactive to pollutants and foreign bodies, also resulting in acute respiratory distress.

The most common respiratory disorders you will treat in the prehospital setting include croup, epiglottitis, asthma, bronchiolitis, and foreign-body aspiration. See Chapter 5 for information on foreign-body obstruction of the airway.

Asthma

Asthma is a chronic recurrent lower airway disease producing moderate to severe respiratory distress. The most common age of onset is the preschool years, but it may be diagnosed in children as young as 1 year of age. It is the most serious allergic disease in children.

The obstruction of the lower airways is caused by a sensitivity reaction to foods, inhalants, pollens, mold spores, or a combination of these allergens. Other factors contributing to the episodes of asthma include changes in temperature, physical exertion, psychologic stress, and respiratory infections.

The allergic response produces edema, increased secretion of thick mucous from the bronchial glands, and spasm of the bronchioles and bronchi (Figure 6.1). The mucous, bronchial spasm, and edema decrease the size of the bronchioles, causing a lower airway obstruction. The child develops respiratory distress and hypoxia. The expiratory phase of breathing becomes prolonged and forceful with noticeable wheezing as the child attempts to expire air beyond the obstructions. Dehydration of the airway, caused by breathing through the mouth, increases the thickness of the mucous and respiratory distress.

History

Important information to obtain during the history includes the following:

- Has the child ever had an asthma attack or other allergic problems?
- Does the child have any other illnesses or fever? Has it been treated?
- Does the child take medicine for asthma, either oral or inhalants?

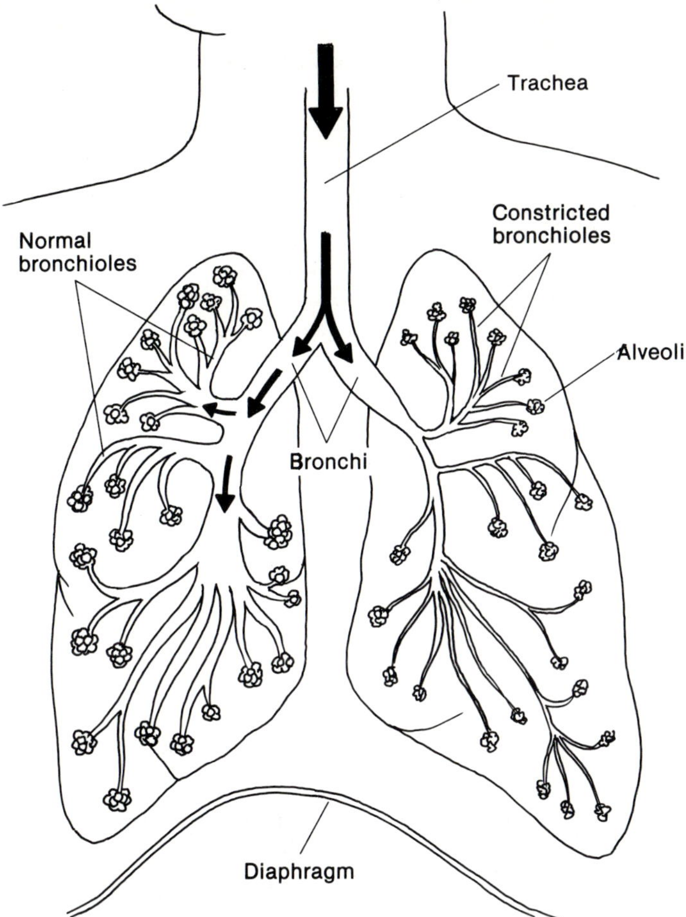

FIGURE 6.1 In asthma the lower airways are narrowed by constriction of bronchiole muscles and secretion of thick mucous, causing a lower airway obstruction.

Have any medications been used for this attack? Did the medications relieve any of the symptoms?

- Has anyone in the family ever had asthma or other allergy problems?
- How much has the child been drinking?
- How concerned is the parent about this attack in contrast to previous ones?

Assessment

The child with an acute asthma attack is in respiratory distress with shortness of breath, tachypnea, tachycardia, noticeable expiratory wheezing, intercostal retractions, and nasal flaring. The child has coughing episodes, attempting to clear the obstructing mucous. These episodes often trigger vomiting.

The patient often appears pale or mottled. The lips may be a deep, dark red color that progresses to cyanosis as the hypoxemia increases. The child is generally apprehensive and restless, and mental status may further deteriorate if hypoxemia is not controlled. The young child may be

most comfortable in the tripod position. Older children might brace themselves over a chair to facilitate the use of accessory muscles (Figure 6.2).
Breath sounds are usually bilateral with coarse rhonchi and generalized
inspiratory and expiratory wheezing.

Breath sounds may diminish, indicating progression of the obstruction
and little movement of air. Expiration is prolonged as the child attempts to
move inspired air beyond the obstruction. Shallow or irregular respirations, or a decrease in respiratory rate, are serious signs of imminent ventilatory failure.

Management

BLS field care for asthma includes the following:

- Assess and monitor ABCDE's.
- Administer high-concentration, high-flow oxygen by face mask.
  Use humidified oxygen if available.
- Maintain the child's airway, and be alert to the possibility of vomit-
  ing and need for suctioning.
- If the child has an inhaler or bronchodilator, encourage the parent
  or child to administer it.
- If the child will take oral fluids, encourage him or her to drink some
  water or clear liquid while en route to the hospital.
- Be prepared for ventilatory failure. Administer positive pressure
  ventilation and CPR if indicated.
- Transport patient immediately. Let the child determine position of
  comfort during transport.

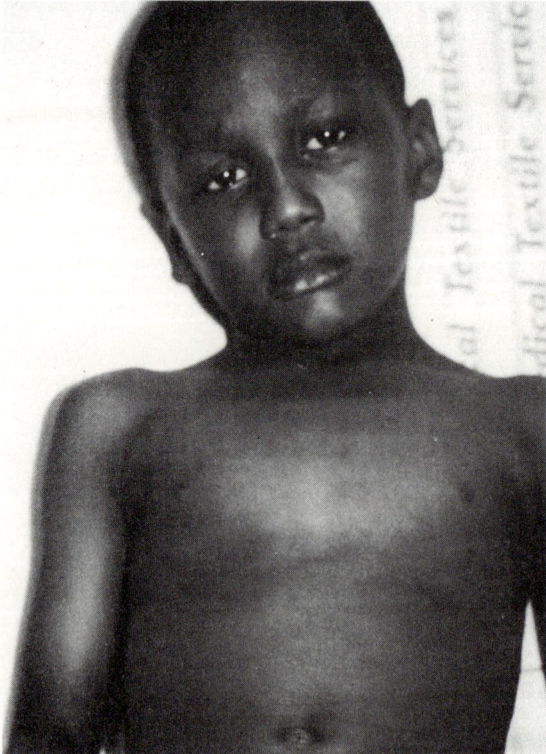

FIGURE 6.2   Child in respiratory distress from asthma.

ALS personnel may want to provide additional treatment as directed by medical control or protocol:

- Administer epinephrine 1:1000 (0.01 mg/kg subcutaneous route). *Caution: DO NOT give more than the maximum single dose of 0.3 mg.*
- Epinephrine may be repeated q 20–30 min × 3, if the heart rate is less than 180 beats/min.
- Start an IV with Ringer's Lactate or Normal Saline at a keep-open rate.
- Orotracheal intubation should be performed if airway management becomes difficult or ventilatory failure occurs.

Status Asthmaticus

Children who continue with acute signs of respiratory distress despite injections of epinephrine are considered to be in *status asthmaticus.* The child can move only a small amount of air. So little air is moved that wheezing may not be heard. The patient is cyanotic, pulse rate is elevated, and breathing obviously is labored. Humidified oxygen is required and transport to the hospital is immediately needed.

Bronchiolitis

Bronchiolitis is an infection of the lower respiratory tract, most often caused by the respiratory syncytial virus (RSV), or parainfluenza virus. The illness usually begins with a mild fever, runny nose, and cough that gradually progresses to respiratory distress. The bronchioles in the lower airway become obstructed with edema and increased mucous secretion due to the inflammatory process of the viral illness. It most often affects infants between 2 months and 18 months of age, and may recur. Recurrence may be associated with a different viral infection in the infant with a sensitive airway.

History

Important information to obtain during the history includes the following:

- When did the child become ill? Has the infant been to the doctor for this illness?
- What symptoms does the infant have, and how have they changed over time? When did symptoms become this severe?
- Has the child ever had symptoms like this before?
- Has the child had any fever and has it been treated?
- What medications and/or treatments have been given?

Assessment

When you arrive at the scene, the infant is in acute respiratory distress with difficulty breathing and irritability. In the older infant, it is difficult to distinguish between bronchiolitis and asthma.

The child may have a mild fever and a dry cough. Nasal flaring, tachypnea, tachycardia, and intercostal and suprasternal retractions will all be present. Inspiratory and expiratory wheezing is heard bilaterally when auscultating the chest. The infant will be restless and anxious when respiratory distress is severe. Mild dehydration may be present, lasting a few days as a result of the fever and the generalized illness.

Management

BLS field care for bronchiolitis includes the following:

- Monitor ABCDE's and vital signs.
- Clear nasal passages and maintain airway.
- Administer high-flow, high-concentration oxygen by face mask.
- Be prepared for increased respiratory distress. If this occurs, administer high-concentration oxygen.
- Transport patient and contact medical control. Keep child calm and with parent during transport.

ALS providers may additionally institute the following care:

- Start an IV with Ringer's Lactate or Normal Saline at a keep-open rate or rate as ordered by medical control.

Croup

Croup, a viral upper respiratory infection, commonly occurs in children between 6 months and 3 years of age. The infection localizes in the upper airway, leading to swelling of the larynx and subglottic tissue, and occasionally the trachea and bronchi (Figure 6.3a). The child usually has cold symptoms (runny nose, nasal congestion, sneezing, and mild fever) with an onset over 1 to 3 days. The child then develops the characteristic barking (seal-like) cough. The disorder tends to occur more commonly in the spring and fall, and may recur in the same child.

History

Important information to obtain during the history includes the following:

- How long has the child been ill? Has the child recently been to the doctor for this problem?
- What symptoms does the child have (fever, cough, runny nose, sore throat, etc.)? Have these symptoms changed over the last few hours or days?
- Has the patient ever had symptoms like this before?

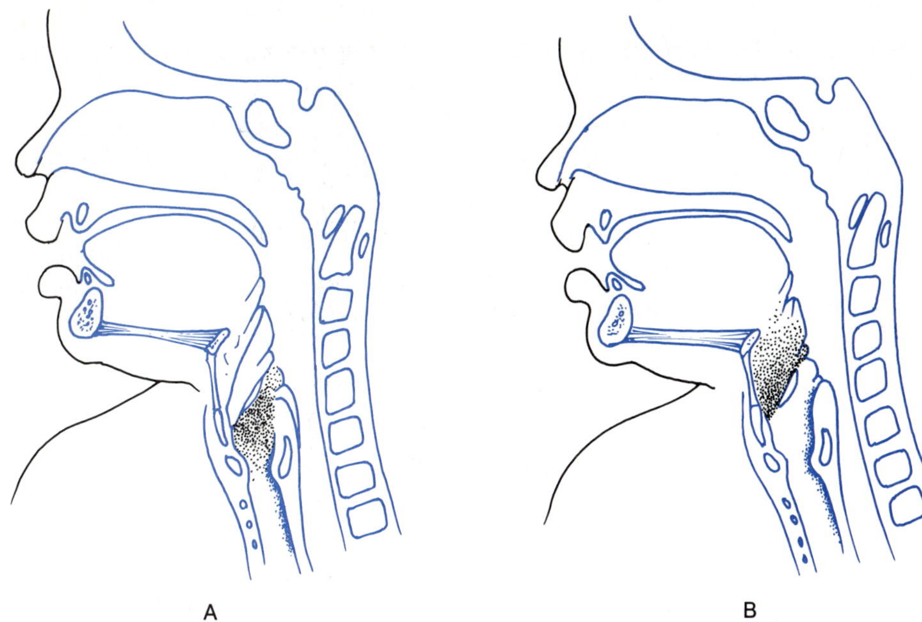

FIGURE 6.3 (A) Croup; note the swelling of the larynx and subglottic tissue in contrast to (B) epiglottitis with swelling of and above the epiglottis.

- Does the child have any difficulty swallowing liquids or is he or she drooling saliva?
- What medications has the child been given?
- What other treatment has been tried at home (vaporizer, steam in bathroom, exposure to cold night air)? How effective was the treatment?

Assessment

In most cases you will be summoned for a child in moderate to severe respiratory distress. Signs and symptoms of the child with croup include the following:

- Signs of respiratory distress, such as nasal flaring, tachypnea, retractions (intercostal, suprasternal, and sternal in severe cases), tachycardia, tachypnea, and pallor or cyanosis.
- The characteristic seal-like barking cough that worsens as the airway obstruction increases.
- Hoarse cry or hoarse voice
- Inspiratory stridor and expiratory stridor in severe cases.
- Anxious, restless, noticeable decrease in activity level.
- Altered level of consciousness in severe cases.
- A low-grade fever may be present.

On physical examination the infant or child appears anxious and in respiratory distress. Breath sounds may be decreased in severe distress. In less severe cases, you may hear expiratory and inspiratory wheezing, or harsh rhonchi. Use Table 6.1 to assess and describe the severity of croup to medical control.

TABLE 6.1 Croup Scale to Identify the Severity of Croup

	Severity Score			
Signs	**0**	**1**	**2**	**3**
Stridor	None	Mild	Moderate at rest	Severe, on inspiration + expiration
Retractions	None	Mild	Suprasternal, intercostal	Severe, may see sternal retractions
Color	Normal	Normal score = 0	Normal score = 0	Dusky or cyanotic
Breath Sounds	Normal	Mildly decreased	Moderately decreased	Markedly decreased
Level of Consciousness	Normal	Restless when disturbed	Anxious, agitated	Lethargic

SCORING: To quantify the severity of croup, add up the individual scores for each of the sign categories. A score between 0 to 15 is possible. The rating of mild, moderate, and severe is as follows:
  4–5 is mild.
  6–8 is moderate.
  >8 or any sign in the severe category is severe.

Source: Adapted from Davis, H.W., and others, (1981): "Acute upper airway obstruction, croup, and epiglottitis," *Pediatric Clinics of North America*, 28:4.

In the prehospital setting, the croup score is generally not calculated. Rather, it is important to assess each of the individual signs for severity. Medical control will be most interested in the specific findings noted with each sign rather than the total score. Croup is considered severe any time a child has even one sign among the severe findings on this croup scale, which include the following:

- Severe stridor, on inspiration and expiration;
- Severe retractions, which may include sternal retractions;
- Dusky or cyanotic color;
- Markedly decreased breath sounds; and
- Lethargy, altered level of consciousness.

Management

BLS field care for croup is the same as for any respiratory distress:

- Monitor ABCDE's and vital signs.
- Administer high-flow oxygen by face mask if the child will tolerate it, or administer blow-by oxygen.
- If the child is awake and conscious, do not agitate the child with excessive physical examination or handling.

- Do not attempt to visualize the mouth and throat or use instruments in the airway since it is often difficult to distinguish between croup and epiglottitis in the prehospital setting.
- In cases of severe respiratory distress, be prepared for respiratory arrest, with positive pressure ventilation and implementation of CPR as necessary.
- Transport patient and contact medical control. Let the child choose the position of comfort for transport, either sitting up or lying down.

ALS providers may additionally provide the following care according to protocol or medical control:

- Racemic epinephrine by positive pressure ventilation.

Epiglottitis

Epiglottitis is a bacterial infection localized in the epiglottis, usually caused by *Hemophilus influenzae*, type B. Acute swelling occurs above the glottis, creating an airway obstruction (Figure 6.3b). It most commonly affects children between the ages of 3 to 6 years; however, it does occur in young infants, older children, and adults. Because of the sudden onset and rapid progression of respiratory distress and airway obstruction, the child with epiglottitis is a true medical emergency. Often the child will awaken with a sudden-onset high fever, difficulty breathing, sore throat, and difficulty swallowing.

History

Important information to obtain during the history includes the following:

- When did the child first become ill? Is this a recent illness with sudden worsening, or is this an illness with a sudden onset?
- Does the child have a fever? How high is the fever?
- Does the child have a sore throat? Will the child drink and swallow liquids or saliva? Is the child drooling?
- Is the child's voice hoarse or muffled?
- Has the child ever had an illness like this before?
- Has the child been given any medications?

Assessment

When you arrive at the scene, the child with epiglottitis will appear sick, have a high fever (up to 102°–103°F) and experience difficulty breathing. The patient is in acute distress with a severe airway obstruction and will be in a tripod position, in which the child sits upright with his or her neck extended forward and the weight of the body resting on the patient's outstretched arms in front (Figure 6.4). This position maximizes the airway opening around the swollen epiglottis.

The child generally holds the mouth open with the tongue protruding

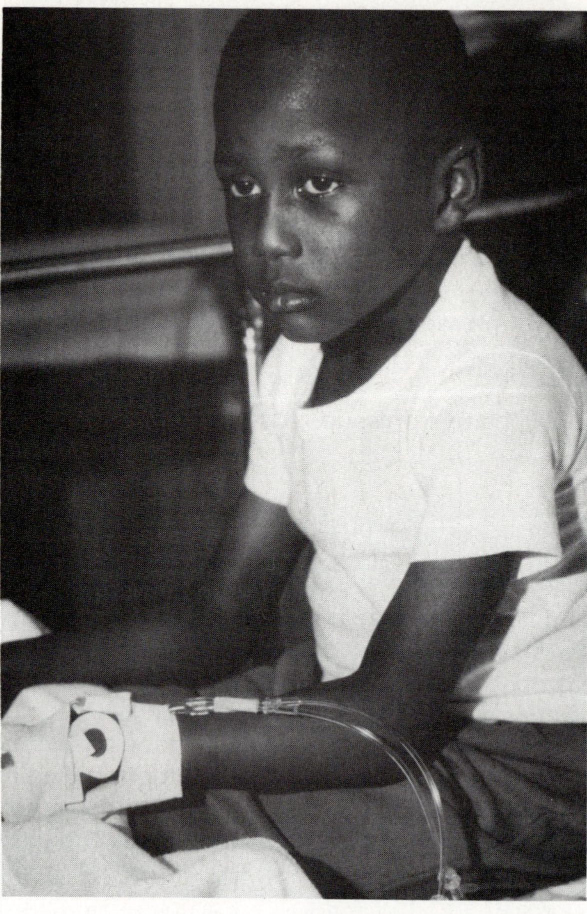

slightly, almost like holding a piece of hot potato on the tongue. The pain from the sore throat is intense, resulting in the refusal to swallow saliva or other liquids. This child looks anxious and is very focused on each slow, deliberate breath. The child will be lethargic and show very little concern for what is happening around him or her (Figure 6.5).

The child will be experiencing hypoxia and respiratory distress. Typical signs of respiratory distress, such as nasal flaring and intercostal and suprasternal retractions, will be present. Occasionally a muffled voice or stridor will be present; however, there is rarely a cough. Respiratory rate will generally not be increased. The child will have tachycardia and cyanosis in cases of progressive hypoxemia.

The child with epiglottitis should be identified immediately from history and initial observation of the patient. Do not attempt to examine the child's mouth.

Management

BLS field care for the child with suspected epiglottitis includes the following:

- Monitor ABCDE's and vital signs.
- Because maintenance of a patent airway is your primary concern, DO NOT MANIPULATE THE AIRWAY IN ANY WAY! *Do not* attempt

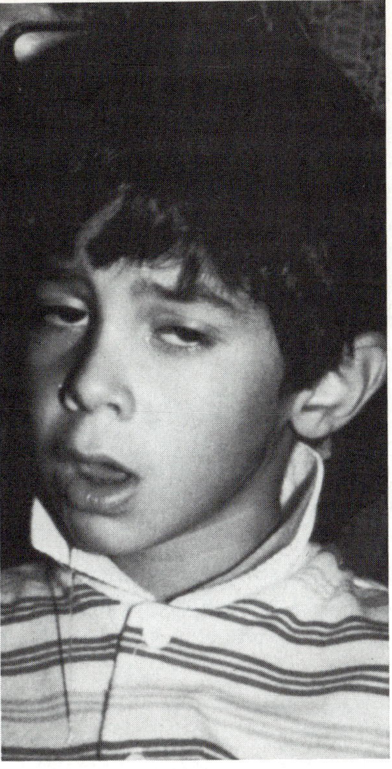

to visualize, insert a tongue blade, or shine a flashlight into the patient's mouth. It may produce a laryngospasm and totally occlude the airway.

- Permit the child to remain sitting. *Do not* attempt to have the child lie down; the swollen epiglottis can fall back into the airway and cause obstruction.
- Minimize handling and examining of the child to prevent agitation and crying.
- Keep child with the parent or primary caretaker at all times.
- Administer high-flow oxygen by face mask. Approach the child very gently with the oxygen mask or give the mask to the parent to hold. If the mask distresses the child, administer oxygen via blow-by.
- Transport immediately. Notify the hospital to be prepared for a child with suspected epiglottitis.
- If an airway obstruction occurs, administer positive pressure ventilation with high-concentration, high-flow oxygen after getting a good seal. Use enough pressure to get beyond the obstruction; however, be prepared for gastric distention. Some oxygen will get beyond the obstruction and buy time until you get the child to the hospital.
- Perform CPR as indicated.

ALS providers will not need to provide any additional care beyond that of BLS providers. Field intubation of the child with epiglottitis is contraindicated. The swollen epiglottis totally obliterates the larynx and other landmarks used for tube insertion. In addition, the manipulation of the mouth and throat with the laryngoscope may trigger a total airway obstruction.

Intubation for epiglottitis is performed by the most skilled physician or anesthesiologist in a controlled setting of the hospital, usually the operating room. An emergency tracheostomy can then be performed if intubation is not successful. If the child experiences a total airway obstruction en route to the hospital, and positive pressure ventilation is not effective, medical control may order a cricothyrotomy to establish an airway. While this procedure may be life-saving, it is difficult to perform in the young child.

Respiratory Emergencies References

BARKIN, R. M., "Pediatric respiratory emergencies," *Emergency Care Quarterly*, 5, no. 1 (May 1989), pp. 71–78.

FIREMAN, P., "The wheezing infant," *Pediatric Review*, 7, no. 247 (1986), pp. 247–254.

GOLDHAGEN, J. L., "Croup: Pathogenesis and management," *Journal of Emergency Medicine*, 1, no. 1 (1983), pp. 3–11.

LEFFERT, F., "The management of acute severe asthma," *Journal of Pediatrics*, 96, no. 1 (January 1980), pp. 1–12.

LULLA, S., and NEWCOMB, R. W., "Emergency management of asthma in children," *Journal of Pediatrics*, 97, no. 3 (September 1980), pp. 346–350.

McCONNOCHIE, K. M., and ROGHMANN, D. J., "Bronchiolitis as a possible cause of wheezing in childhood: New evidence," *Pediatrics*, 74, no. 1 (July 1974), pp. 1–10.

TERCIER, J. A., "Bronchiolitis: A clinical review," *Journal of Emergency Medicine*, 1 (1983), p. 119.

WILLIS, R. J., and ROWLAND, T. W., "The early management of acute epiglottitis: A survey of current practice," *Journal of Emergency Medicine*, 2 (1984), p. 13.

Medical Emergencies

7

OBJECTIVES

When you have completed this chapter you should be able to

* Describe fever and hypothermia, identifying their impact on managing the child with other emergencies.
* Describe field management for the child with a seizure.
* Describe the field management for meningitis and sepsis, including special precautions for both patient and field provider.
* Differentiate among mild, moderate, and severe dehydration.
* Describe the physical signs and field management for diabetic ketoacidosis (hyperglycemia) and hypoglycemia.
* List signs of distress in a child with a congenital heart defect.
* Describe the appropriate prehospital care of children at home with high-technology equipment.

Hyperthermia: Fever

Fever is defined as a core body temperature over 100.5°F or 38°C. A temperature of 101°F or 38.4°C is generally cause for concern. Fever usually results from the body's response to an acute viral or bacterial infection. Bacteria or viruses cause the body's thermostat to set at a higher level, and the body responds by generating and retaining body heat. It is believed that fever is a protective response enabling the body to mobilize and fight the infection.

Fever or hyperthermia may also result from an alteration in the brain's ability to regulate body temperature. Various drugs in toxic doses (aspirin, atropine, and antihistamines) can cause hyperthermia by altering the brain's regulation of temperature. Children frequently have a febrile response to illnesses, with a range of temperature between 101°–105°F. Higher temperatures may be present, but *neurologic damage does not occur until the temperature reaches 107°F.*

Fever from an acute illness is generally not a significant prehospital problem unless the child has a febrile seizure. *Febrile seizures* are most common in children under age 5. A febrile seizure is most often triggered by the rapid rise in temperature, rather than the ultimate high temperature. If you find a child at the scene with a 105°F temperature who has not yet had a febrile seizure, it is unlikely that the child will convulse or have a seizure.

Hyperthermia may also result from exposure during hot weather. The child has less ability to reduce body temperature than to produce heat and raise body temperature. Situations producing hyperthermia are sitting in a closed car or apartment during hot weather, which results in either heat exhaustion or heat stroke. The child's core temperature will rapidly rise to dangerous temperature levels, greater than 106°F. This rapid rise in core body temperature is associated with an increased oxygen demand and metabolic acidosis. This seriously strains the cardiac and respiratory systems, leading to respiratory and ventilatory failure.

History

- How long has the child been ill? What other symptoms are present with this fever (i.e., trouble breathing, vomiting, change in behavior)?
- Has there been any change in level of consciousness?
- Have any medications been given for fever, such as aspirin or Tylenol? How long ago? What was the response to medication?
- Has the child ever had a febrile seizure?
- Does the child have any chronic illnesses or health problems?
- Where was the child found? What was the temperature of the environment?

Assessment

During the primary and secondary survey, look for signs and symptoms associated with a fever. These include:

- Flushed, warm/hot skin;
- Chills and shivering (in some cases); complaints of feeling cold;
- Increased perspiration (less common in infants);
- Tachycardia and tachypnea;
- Malaise, vague aches and pains;
- Signs of dehydration, dry mucous membranes;
- Altered level of consciousness (listless, lethargic, or irritable); and
- Loss of appetite.

In cases of heat stroke, the child may rapidly progress from severe headache to fainting, stiff neck, coma, posturing, and seizures, in addition to the above signs of a fever. Sweating may or may not be present.

The degree of temperature elevation is not necessarily associated with the seriousness of the patient's illness. Observe the child's response to the fever to determine the seriousness of the illness. You should be more concerned with a lethargic child having a 102°F temperature than the child who is alert and playful with a 105°F temp.

You should also be more concerned if the febrile child has a chronic illness such as a congenital heart defect, leukemia or cancer, sickle cell disease, or hydrocephalus controlled with a shunt. These children may have a very serious infection requiring urgent medical care.

Management

BLS care for a febrile infant or child should include the following:

- Monitor ABC's and vital signs.
- Remove heavy clothing.
- Give oral liquids if the child is alert, able to swallow, and not vomiting or having diarrhea (usually not recommended for short transport times).
- Prepare for a possible seizure.
- In cases of exposure hyperthermia, administer high-flow oxygen by face mask and prepare to bag-mask ventilate. Begin rapid cooling by removing patient's clothes, placing patient in a cool environment, and begin sponging.
- Transport patient rapidly in cases of exposure hyperthermia. In cases of acute, non-life-threatening illness, encourage the parent to take the child with a fever to the family physician (if local protocols or medical control permit).

ALS providers may additionally want to provide the following care:

- Start an IV with Ringer's Lactate or Normal Saline at a keep-open rate.
- Orotracheal intubation if the child's level of consciousness begins to deteriorate.

Hypothermia

Hypothermia is a core body temperature of less than 95°F (35°C). In children it most often results from prolonged exposure to cold temperatures. Children have a proportionately larger body surface area for their weight than do adults. Their temperature regulation mechanism is also less well developed, so their heat conservation efforts are less effective. Newborns have even greater risk of hypothermia because they have little subcutaneous fat. Causes of hypothermia include:

- Exposure to cool and cold weather;
- Ingestion of alcohol and drugs such as barbiturates (they dilate the peripheral blood vessels and interfere with the body's ability to conserve heat);
- Metabolic problems such as hypoglycemia;
- Trauma or other brain disorders that interfere with the temperature-regulating system;
- Overwhelming infection (sepsis).

Heat loss is accelerated by wet clothes and high winds through the process of convection and conduction. Submersion in cold water has the most profound effect on heat loss, and is further intensified by any movement. Death can occur in as short a time as 15 minutes. If the diving reflex is triggered during rapid cooling, a young child may be successfully resuscitated after a longer period of time (see "Drowning" in Chapter 5).

The progressive response of the body to lowered core body temperatures is as follows:

- The brain senses blood cooling in the extremities and triggers increased muscle tone and a higher metabolic rate.
- Shivering begins when muscle tone is increased.
- Constriction of blood vessels leads to pooling of cool blood in the extremities.

The body is able to increase heat production at about 4 times its normal rate with these efforts. The core body temperature begins to drop when these functions can no longer compensate for the environmental cold.

History

- How long has the child been exposed? Has the exposure been associated with water (i.e., soaking by rain, submersion in cold water)?
- Were any drugs or alcohol ingested?

Assessment

The child will present with progressively deteriorating signs and symptoms as the core body temperature drops (see Table 7.1). Prolonged vasoconstriction is accompanied by a decrease in tissue temperatures and may result in local cold injury or frostbite. Thickening of the blood may lead to clotting, and ice crystals may form when the tissue temperature nears 0°C. The ears, nose, fingers, toes, hands, and feet are most often affected by frostbite. A superficial injury is indicated by pain and flushed, burning skin. A deeper injury is indicated by blistering and loss of sensation.

Management

BLS care for mild hypothermia includes the following (Figure 7.1):

- Move patient to warm environment.
- Remove wet clothing and wrap patient in blankets to passively rewarm.
- Give warm liquids by mouth if the child is conscious.

BLS field care for moderate to severe hypothermia includes the following steps:

- Maintain the airway.
- Give high-flow oxygen by face mask (humidified and warmed to 40–42°C if possible).
- Use a bag mask with high-flow, high-concentration oxygen to assist ventilations when necessary.

TABLE 7.1 Signs and Symptoms of Hypothermia

Mild (32–35°C)	Moderate (28–32°C)	Severe (<28°C)
Slurred speech	Progressively lowered consciousness	Coma, unresponsive
Mild incoordination	Cyanosis	Dilated and fixed pupils
Shivering	Edema	Ventricular dysrhythmias
Poor judgment	Muscle rigidity, no shivering	Respiratory arrest
	Decreased respiratory rate, bradycardia	

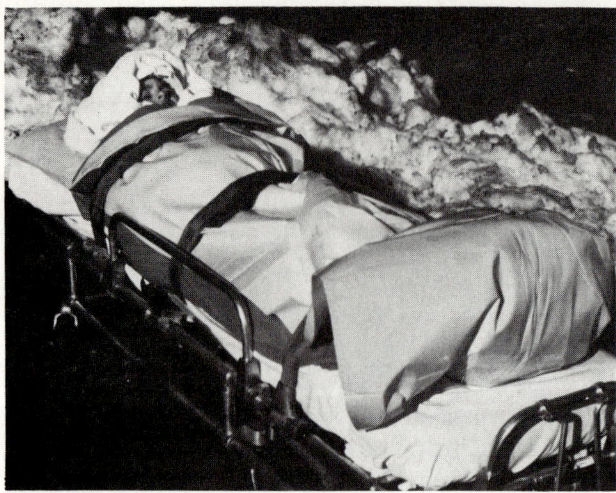

FIGURE 7.1 Passive rewarming for the hypothermic child involves removal of clothing (if wet) and wrapping in blankets. (Reproduced with permission from Grant et al. *Emergency Care*, Fifth Ed., © 1990 Prentice Hall.)

- Perform CPR even if no pulse or respirations are present.
- Avoid active external rewarming of the total body so as to prevent a dilation of blood vessels in the extremities. This will cause a secondary drop in core body temperature, hypovolemia, and a fatal heart dysrhythmia. Heat packs may be placed *around the trunk,* but make certain they are not in direct contact with the skin.
- Prevent injuries to cold extremities; wrap extremities with frostbite in warm, dry material; do not rub them or expose them to dry heat.
- Transport patient immediately.
- *Do not stop resuscitation in the field. No child is declared dead until warm and dead.*

ALS providers should provide the same care as BLS providers. Do not mechanically stimulate the child with orotracheal intubation, CPR, or suctioning when a heart rate is present (even in severe bradycardia). It is important to prevent the development of ventricular fibrillation, which is difficult to manage in the hypothermic child. Providers should also not waste time starting an IV.

Seizures

A seizure is caused by abnormal bursts of electrical discharge from the brain, leading to abnormal body movements and altered mental status. Seizures are caused by a wide variety of disorders, including the following: fever (febrile seizure); epilepsy; inflammation of the brain or its protective lining (encephalitis or meningitis); trauma (birth injury or head trauma); metabolic disorders such as hypoglycemia; poisoning from drugs or lead; and failure to take antiseizure medication. Seizures are not generally life-threatening unless seizure activity is prolonged, as in the case of *status epilepticus.*

History

Important information to obtain during the history from the parent and witness of the seizure event includes the following:

- Has the child ever had a seizure or convulsion? If yes, was that seizure related to a fever, epilepsy, head injury, or other medical illness? Does the child take any seizure medication?
- When did the seizure begin? How long did it last?
- Does the child have a fever or medical illness now?
- How did the child behave when the seizure began (shaking of arms and legs, eyes rolling upward, loss of consciousness, or loss of urinary control)? Has the shaking of arms and legs stopped and started up again?
- Has the child been unconscious the entire time? Has the child seemed to have any difficulty breathing?

Assessment

The seizure activity will usually be over by the time you arrive at the scene. Children for whom EMS is called will usually be experiencing their first seizure or have a medical illness or an acute head injury that has caused the seizure. In cases of a febrile seizure, the child will have a fever that has risen rapidly, triggering the seizure.

The onset of symptoms is very abrupt, and if this is the child's first seizure, the parents will be alarmed. Signs of a seizure may include any of the following: sudden jerking of the entire body followed by tenseness and then relaxation of the body; loss of consciousness; sudden jerking of a part of the body, such as an arm or leg (focal seizure); lip smacking; eye blinking; staring, or confusion. Following the seizure, the child will be lethargic and sleepy.

In cases of status epilepticus, the child has repeated jerking movements alternating with tenseness of the body. These repeated seizures occur so frequently that the child remains unconscious between seizures. This is a true *medical emergency* as the child quickly becomes hypoxemic.

Management

BLS field care for seizures includes the following:

- Monitor the ABC's.
- Maintain the child's airway. Do not insert an oral airway or bite block into the mouth; use the jaw thrust maneuver and suctioning as needed. Children frequently have loose teeth, and one could be knocked out and aspirated.
- Administer high-flow, high-concentration oxygen by mask.
- Protect the child from further injury (Figure 7.2).
- Protect the head and cervical spine if injury to the head or neck could have occurred.
- Transport patient immediately.

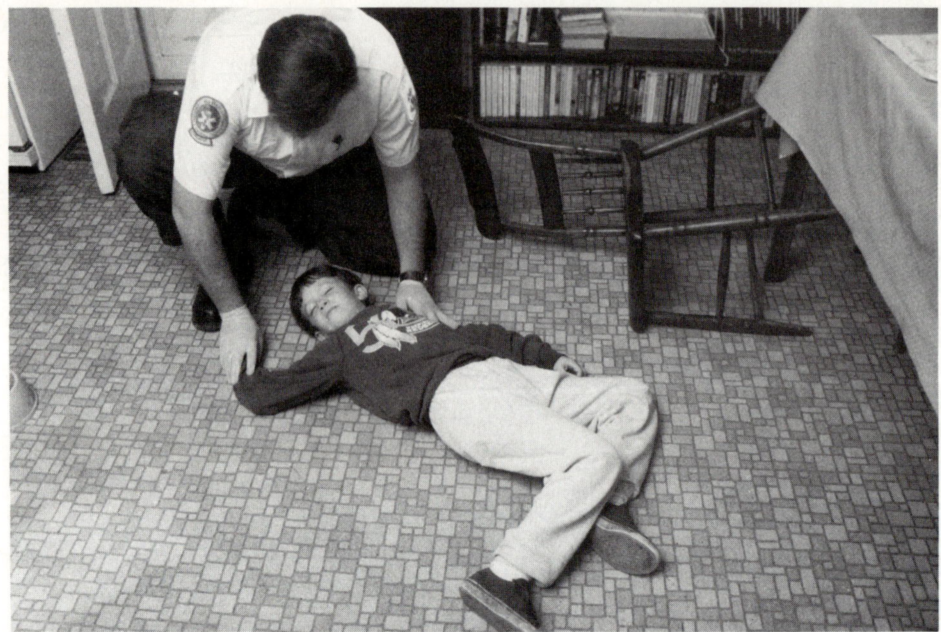

FIGURE 7.2 Protect the child having seizure activity from further injury by moving away furniture or other objects.

ALS providers may provide the following additional care under protocol or as ordered by medical control:

- Orotracheal intubation.
- An IV with Ringer's Lactate at a keep-open rate.
- 2–4 ml/kg of 25% dextrose in water IV, in case seizure is caused by hypoglycemia.
- Diazepam per medical control orders.

Meningitis

Meningitis can be either a bacterial or viral infection of the central nervous system that is localized in the thin layers (meninges) surrounding the brain and spinal cord. The disorder usually follows an upper airway infection such as an ear infection or tonsillitis.

Approximately 38,000 children develop meningitis each year in the United States. While it occurs in all ages, 90% of cases occur in children between 1 month and 5 years of age. The organism causing meningitis differs by age group. Newborns may develop symptoms within a few days of birth, becoming infected with group B streptococcus bacteria acquired from the mother during delivery. *Hemophilus influenzae* is the most common bacteria causing meningitis in infants and young children up to 3 years of age. Meningococcemia (epidemic meningitis) is most common in school-aged children and adolescents.

Bacterial meningitis is life-threatening if antibiotic treatment is delayed. In fact, there is a 5–10% mortality rate in children acquiring bacterial meningitis. Survivors are at high risk for deafness, blindness, retardation, seizure disorders, and learning disabilities.

History

Important questions to ask during the history are:

- Did the baby have any problems in the nursery after birth that you are aware of? (For infants < 1 month old.)
- Has the child had any other illness or fever in the past week? Was the child treated by a physician for that illness?
- How has the child been behaving and eating?

Assessment

Signs and symptoms of meningitis are associated with the age of the child (see Table 7.2). In all cases, the onset of symptoms is abrupt. Some or all of the signs for each age group may be present or develop rapidly as the disease progresses. Any combination of signs should make you more suspicious of meningitis.

The infant or child with meningitis usually has a fever, appears ill, irritable, and does not want to be touched or held. Fever and poor feeding may be the only early signs of meningitis in young infants. Fever and a stiff

TABLE 7.2 Signs and Symptoms of Meningitis in Infants and Children

Signs and Symptoms	Newborns/ Infants	Children/ Adolescents
Fever	± (E)	+, chills (E)
Tachycardia, tachypnea	+	+
Shock	± (L)	± (L)
Unexplained respiratory distress	+ (E)	−
Vomiting	+	+
Diarrhea	±	−
Poor feeding, sucking (may be dehydrated)	+ (E)	−
Seizures	+ (E)	+
Severe headache	−	+ (E)
Irritable, inconsolable	+ (E)	+
Altered level of consciousness (LOC)	+	+ (E) delirium (L) stupor
Stiff neck	± (L)	± (E)
Arching of back and neck	± (L)	−
High-pitched cry	+	−
Bulging fontanelle	±	−
Petechial rash	−	±

KEY: E, early sign; L, late sign;
  +, Present; −, Absent; ±, Not always present.

neck, an altered level of consciousness, or seizures are often clues to meningitis in older children.

Management

BLS field care for meningitis includes the following:

- Monitor ABC's and vital signs (remember that the infant may develop septic shock or be dehydrated from fever, poor intake, vomiting and diarrhea).
- Administer high-flow, high-concentration oxygen.
- Provide ventilatory support with a bag-valve mask if needed.
- Initiate CPR if indicated.
- Prepare for seizures.
- Transport patient immediately. (If meningitis is suspected in an infant or child, be aware that this is considered a true medical emergency. Do not delay transport.)

ALS providers should start an IV of Ringer's Lactate. If the child is in shock, administer a 20 cc/kg bolus IV push. Repeat the bolus if no improvement in vital signs is noted after 15 minutes. A third bolus may be necessary.

CAUTION! 

Meningococcal Meningitis
If meningococcal meningitis is suspected because a petechial rash is present, you should protect yourself with a gown, gloves, and a mask as soon as possible. Disinfect the unit prior to placing it back in service. If meningococcal meningitis is confirmed, antibiotic treatment of exposed prehospital providers may be indicated.

Sepsis and Septic Shock

Sepsis is a bacterial infection of the bloodstream, usually occurring as a complication of another infectious site. It is often associated with meningitis. Toxins released by the bacteria may lead to *septic shock.*

Newborns are particularly susceptible to sepsis because their immune systems are not well developed. They become exposed to bacteria either during delivery or in the nursery. Infants and children with chronic illnesses or impaired immune systems are also highly susceptible to sepsis.

History

Important questions to ask during the history are:

- While in the nursery did the baby have any problems that you know of? (For infants < 1 month.)

- Has the child had any illness or fever in the last week?
- How has the child been behaving and eating?

Assessment

Signs and symptoms of sepsis in the newborn and infant are not related to a specific site of infection. They include:

- Fever (if present in an infant under 2 months of age, sepsis or meningitis is assumed); however, more commonly fever is not present.
- Nonspecific respiratory distress (apnea; irregular, grunting respirations; and retractions).
- Vomiting, diarrhea, abdominal distension.
- Poor sucking and feeding.
- Cyanosis, pallor, or mottled skin; there may be jaundice.
- Neurologic signs (irritability, tremors, seizures, altered LOC).
- Signs of increased intracranial pressure, if meningitis develops.

Signs of sepsis in an older child include: fever, chills, vomiting or diarrhea, pallor, ill appearance, increased lethargy, and tachycardia.

Septic shock is a life-threatening complication of sepsis, with a high mortality rate in children. Toxins produced by the bacteria cause a dilatation of the peripheral blood vessels and pooling of blood in the extremities. The resulting decreased blood flow to the heart leads to decreased tissue perfusion and plasma leakage from the capillaries. The onset of shock is rapid and can lead to death within a few hours. Signs of shock include the following:

- Altered level of consciousness—confusion to coma;
- Cool, or cold and clammy skin;
- Tachycardia;
- Prolonged capillary refill time;
- Hyperventilation to respiratory failure;
- Blood pressure normal or hypotension.

Management

BLS field care for an infant or child with sepsis and septic shock includes the following:

- Administer high-flow high-concentration oxygen.
- Monitor ABC's and vital signs.
- Prepare for respiratory and cardiac arrest.
- Transport patient immediately and notify the receiving hospital. *This is a true medical emergency.* As soon as your assessment leads you to suspect sepsis, transport should begin.

- Obtain further history en route.

The ALS provider should provide the following additional care (Figure 7.3):

- Start an IV en route with Ringer's Lactate or Normal Saline, and give a bolus of fluid, 20 cc/kg IV push. If vital signs do not stabilize, repeat the fluid bolus.
- Perform orotracheal intubation and provide assisted ventilation when the child becomes less responsive.

Dehydration

Dehydration is an acute loss of body fluids resulting from an imbalance between fluid intake and output. Water (body fluid) is normally lost from 4 systems in the body:

1. The skin by sweating;

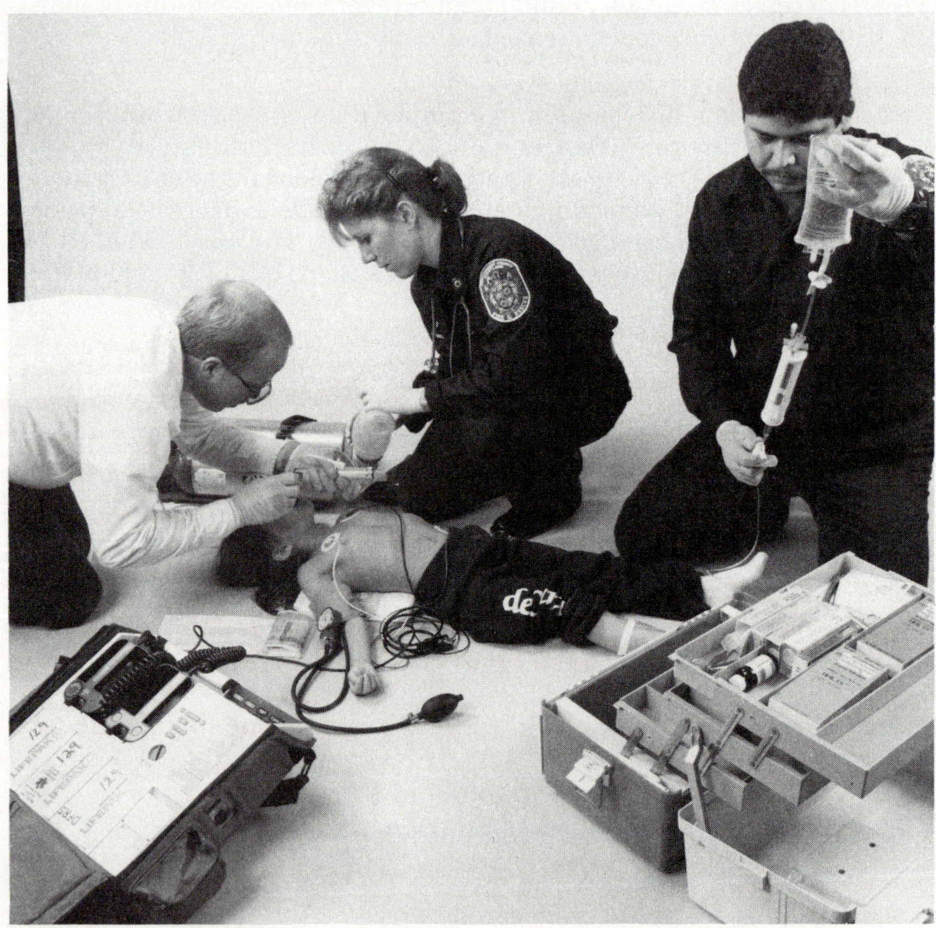

FIGURE 7.3 Advanced life support for the child in septic shock includes intubation, assisted ventilation, and IV fluid administration of Ringer's Lactate in boluses of 20 cc/kg, IV push.

2. The respiratory tract to humidify the air breathed;

3. The gastrointestinal tract in the stool and vomitus; and

4. The kidneys in urine.

Infants are more susceptible to dehydration than adults because a greater proportion of their body is water and their fluid maintenance needs are higher. (See Table 7.3 for distribution of body fluids by age group.)

Infants and children need different amounts of fluid each day to maintain their intake and output balance.

- Infants up to 10 kg need 100 ml/kg of fluid.
- Children between 10 and 20 kg need 1000 ml plus 50 ml for each kg over 10 kg.
- Children over 20 kg need 1500 ml plus 20 ml for each kg over 20 kg.

For example, an infant weighing 9 kg needs 900 ml, an infant weighing 14 kg needs 1200 ml, and a child weighing 26 kg needs 1620 ml of fluid each day.

Acute medical illnesses and sometimes diet interfere with the balance between intake and output in the following ways:

- A fever is associated with increased sweating and tachypnea. At the same time a child may refuse food and fluids, further jeopardizing the balance.
- Viral gastrointestinal disorders, vomiting, and diarrhea may cause rapid dehydration, especially if oral fluids stimulate further vomiting.
- Diabetic ketoacidosis results in dehydration as the kidneys attempt to flush the high concentration of glucose from the blood.
- Errors in infant formula preparation (making it too concentrated) will result in dehydration as fluid is drawn from the cell spaces to dilute the formula in the intestines.

History

Important questions to ask about the child's fluid intake and output include:

- When was the last bottle or drink taken?

TABLE 7.3 Distribution of Body Fluids by Age Group

Fluid Characteristics	Newborn	Infant (1 year)	Adult
Weight: lb (kg)	7.5 (3)	22 (10)	154 (70)
Percent of total weight that is water	78	65	60
Percent of body fluids replaced every 24 hours	45	25	20

Source: Adapted from Hochman, H.I., and others (1979): "Dehydration, diabetic ketoacidosis, and shock in the pediatric patient," *Pediatric Clinics of North America*, 26(4):804.

Dehydration Severity	Percent of Body Weight Lost	
	Infants	Children/Adults
Mild	0–5	0–4
Moderate	5–10	4–8
Severe	10–15	8–13

- How much was consumed? How much was offered (i.e., 4 oz out of 8 oz)? Is this typical for the child?
- When was the infant's last wet diaper? Was the diaper as wet as usual?
- Has the infant had diarrhea or vomiting? How frequently?
- Has the infant had a fever? How long?

Assessment

Dehydration can be a true medical emergency in all age groups, but it tends to strike infants more frequently. Its severity (mild, moderate, and severe) is based upon the percentage of fluid lost (determined from body weight lost), and signs and symptoms exhibited by the child (see Table 7.4).

Signs and symptoms of dehydration are variable, but they progress as dehydration worsens (see Table 7.5). The child with mild dehydration will demonstrate signs and symptoms as moderate dehydration develops. The child with severe dehydration will look very ill and is in hypovolemic shock with impending circulatory collapse.

TABLE 7.5   Signs and Symptoms of Dehydration

Assessment	Dehydration Severity		
	Mild	Moderate	Severe
Vital Signs			
Heart rate	normal	increased	tachycardia, >130/min
Respiratory rate	normal	increased	tachypnea
Blood pressure	normal	normal	hypotensive, systolic <80
Capillary refill	normal	2–3 seconds	>2 seconds
Mental Status	alert	irritable	lethargic
Skin			
Color	pale	ashen	mottled
Turgor	normal	poor	tenting
Temperature	warm	cool	cool, clammy
Texture	normal	dry	doughy
Fontanelle	flat	depressed	sunken
Mucous Membranes	dry	very dry/±tears	parched/no tears
Eyes	normal	darkened/sunken	sunken/soft
Thirst	increased	intense	intense if conscious
Urine Output	normal	decreased/concentrated	minimal/very concentrated

Even though the precise severity of dehydration is difficult to determine, an estimate of severity will be possible with information from the history and assessment of the child. You may be called for a child with moderate to severe dehydration, but mild dehydration may be present when summoned for other medical conditions.

Management

BLS field care for mild to moderate dehydration includes the following:

- No special management is needed.
- Offer clear oral liquids if the infant or child can tolerate them without vomiting.
- Monitor ABC's and vital signs.
- Transport patient and contact medical control.

BLS field care for severe dehydration includes:

- Monitor ABC's and vital signs.
- Administer high-flow, high-concentration oxygen.
- Prepare to administer CPR.
- *Transport patient immediately* and contact medical control.

ALS providers should give the following additional care as directed by medical control or protocol:

- Start an IV and give a bolus of Ringer's Lactate or Normal Saline, at 20 ml/kg IV push. Monitor vital signs for improvement, and repeat the bolus if no change in status is apparent within 5 minutes. A third bolus may be needed.

Diabetic Ketoacidosis

Diabetes mellitus is a chronic disease in which the pancreas does not produce insulin. When insulin is not available, glucose, broken down from foods, is not able to enter muscle or fat cells. Glucose builds up in the bloodstream, causing a high blood sugar or hyperglycemia. The body attempts to compensate for hyperglycemia by diluting the sugar in the blood with water from the cells. The kidneys excrete some of the sugar and excess water, leading to frequent urination (polyuria), dehydration, an electrolyte imbalance, and excessive thirst (polydipsia). Onset of the disease frequently occurs during childhood or adolescence.

Ketoacidosis occurs when cells cannot use glucose for energy and the body attempts to break down fats to use as energy. Organic acids called *ketones* are a by-product of fats. An increase in ketones leads to metabolic acidosis and an acetone or fruity odor to the breath. If this condition is not reversed with insulin therapy and fluid replacement, it becomes life-threatening.

History

Ketoacidosis occurs most often in known diabetics; however, it can also occur in children with disease onset. Questions to ask during the history include:

- Has the insulin been given regularly?
- Does the child have an acute illness?
- Has the child been growing rapidly? When was the last time the insulin dose was checked by the doctor?
- What was the last urine test or blood glucose test result?
- Has the child recently experienced an emotional stress?
- Has the child had recent prolonged physical activity, or a change in thirst or hunger?

The balance between food eaten and insulin dosage is often difficult to maintain in children because they are growing and physically active. Their insulin dose is often changed to adjust to these special requirements.

Assessment

Signs and symptoms of hyperglycemia and ketoacidosis are progressive if the insulin dosage is not adjusted. The development of ketoacidosis takes several days in the case of disease onset or diet and insulin imbalance. However, ketoacidosis may develop rapidly (in several hours) when triggered by an acute illness, especially if fever, vomiting, and diarrhea are present. Specific signs and symptoms associated with each of the stages of diabetic ketoacidosis are listed below.

Early Stage
- Increased thirst;
- Increased urination;
- Weight loss.

Acute Stage (Dehydration and Early Ketoacidosis)
- Weakness, abdominal pain, generalized aches;
- Loss of appetite; nausea and vomiting;
- Signs of dehydration, except frequent urination may continue because of the kidneys' response to hyperglycemia;
- Fruity breath odor;
- Tachypnea, hyperventilation to blow off CO_2, tachycardia.

Precomatose Stage: Ketoacidosis
- Altered level of consciousness (responsive to verbal or pain stimuli);
- Tachypnea, tachycardia;
- Nausea, vomiting, abdominal pain;
- Signs of moderate dehydration.

Comatose Stage
- Deep and slow respirations (Kussmaul);
- Signs of severe dehydration;

- Tachycardia, weak pulse;
- Hypotension;
- Rigid abdomen.

Management

BLS field care for diabetic ketoacidosis includes the following:

- Monitor ABC's and vital signs.
- Protect the airway, preventing aspiration if vomiting occurs.
- Should the child have hypoglycemia rather than early diabetic ketoacidosis, give oral fluids with sugar if the patient is alert and able to swallow (Figure 7.4).
- Administer high-flow oxygen by face mask and assist ventilations as needed.
- Transport patient promptly.

ALS providers may additionally start an IV with Ringer's Lactate or Normal Saline, administering a 20 ml/kg bolus IV push, and repeating the bolus if no change in vital signs is apparent.

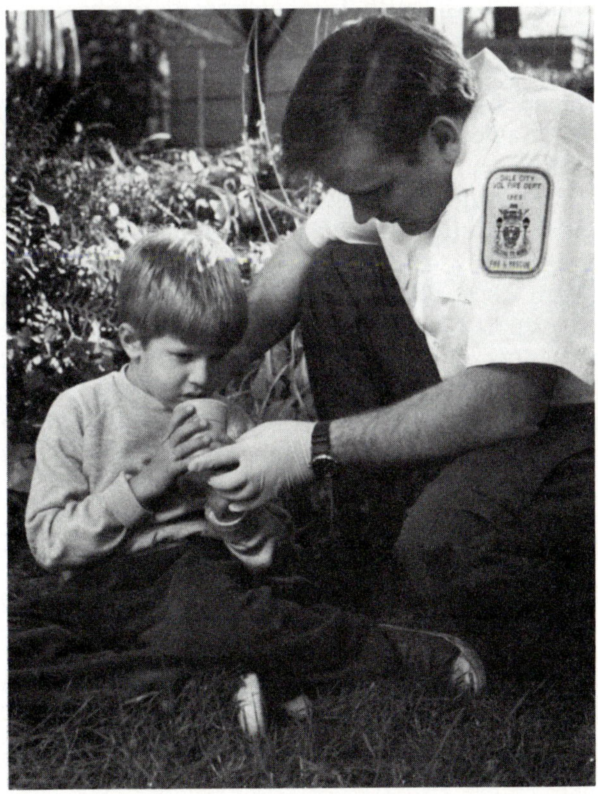

FIGURE 7.4 When a diabetic child develops symptoms of early diabetic ketoacidosis or hypoglycemia and no Dextrostix is available, give oral fluids with sugar. Until the child gets to the hospital, it is more important to manage hypoglycemia, which may become life-threatening, than to worry about increasing the child's blood sugar.

Hypoglycemia

Hypoglycemia, or low blood glucose level, in the prehospital setting is usually a problem associated with known diabetics and newborn infants. It can be as life-threatening as hyperglycemia, and if not promptly treated can result in permanent brain damage.

Causes of hypoglycemia in known diabetics can result from either an:

- Increase in exercise without adequate food support or a reduction in prescribed insulin, or
- An increase in administered insulin, whether accidental or intentional without additional food support.

History

Important questions to ask during the history include:

- Is the child a known diabetic?
- How quickly did symptoms occur? Was any juice or sugar given?
- Has the child recently changed daily exercise routine or sports involvement?
- Was there a change in the amount of insulin administered prior to symptoms?

Assessment

Children with *mild hypoglycemia* generally have feelings of hunger, weakness, as well as a rapid respiratory rate and heart rate.

Children with *moderate hypoglycemia* will have more severe symptoms such as sweating, tremors, irritability, vomiting, and mood swings. They may complain of a stomachache, headache, dizziness, or blurring of vision.

Children with *severe hypoglycemia* have an altered level of consciousness (responsive to verbal or painful stimuli), seizures, tachycardia, and perspiration.

It is very difficult to determine the difference between hypoglycemia and hyperglycemia symptoms in children. Prehospital providers who carry blood glucose test strips should check the blood glucose level prior to initiating management. Because hypoglycemia may be life-threatening if not treated promptly, treatment is initiated (even when blood glucose test strips are not available) when it is strongly suspected.

Management

BLS field care for hypoglycemia includes the following:

- Monitor ABC's and vital signs.
- Assessment may include a blood glucose test when available.
- Give oral fluid with sugar or glucose paste by mouth when child is alert and able to swallow.

- *Transport patient immediately* when there is an altered level of consciousness or when there is no response to sugar or glucose paste.

ALS providers should perform the following additional care as directed by medical control or protocols:

- Start an IV with Ringer's Lactate and then administer a bolus of 25% dextrose 2–4 cc/kg (0.5–1.0 g/kg) IV push. (The 50% dextrose should be diluted with sterile water in a 1:1 concentration. The 25% concentration is less irritating to the child's veins.)
- If IV access is not possible, administer glucagon IM (when available), 0.03–0.1 mg/kg per dose. It may be repeated in 20 minutes as necessary.
- When available, repeat the blood glucose test 10–15 minutes following dextrose infusion to determine a response.

Congenital Heart Defects

The heart has two circulatory pathways—transporting blood requiring oxygen to the lungs (pulmonary circulation) and transporting oxygenated blood to the major organs and extremities (systemic circulation). In the normal heart without defects, these two circulatory pathways do not allow the two bloods to mix.

Congenital defects of the heart or the aorta and pulmonary artery are the primary cause of heart disease in children. These defects are present, but not always detected, at birth. They are usually detected during infancy and early childhood. The cause of most congenital defects is unknown, although heredity and maternal infection or drug use during pregnancy are associated with such defects.

Heart structures that may be defective include:

- A valve that is too small, does not completely close, or is absent.
- The wall between two heart chambers has an opening where none should exist.
- The aorta and pulmonary artery are improperly formed or in the wrong position.
- The channel between the pulmonary artery and aorta (ductus arteriosis, an important feature of fetal circulation) does not close after birth.

Single or multiple defects can occur. Some defects allow blood in the two circulatory pathways to mix, often resulting in cyanosis. Other defects are not associated with cyanosis. *Cyanotic spells* occur when the blood going to the lungs is mixed with the blood going to the rest of the body (i.e., hole in the wall between heart chambers). Cyanotic spells occur when the oxygen demand acutely exceeds the oxygen in the blood supply (hypoxemia), and metabolic acidosis often results. These spells rarely occur prior to 3 months of age, but they tend to increase in frequency and duration once they begin.

History

When the EMS is called for these children, the parents know the child has a heart defect. In these instances, specific information to obtain during the history includes:

- What is the name of the defect? (to share with medical control)
- Does the child take any medications such as digoxin or diuretics? Did the child receive any medication today?
- Does the child use oxygen, and was it used today?
- Does the child use any special feeding devices?
- Has the child had any recent illnesses or stresses?
- Has the child had any heart surgery? If so, how long ago? Was the defect totally corrected?
- What is the child's normal color?
- What kind of spell did the child have? How long did it last? What treatment has been given to the child?

Assessment

A request for assistance and transport will most often occur when the child develops respiratory distress associated with an acute illness, congestive heart failure, or a "cyanotic spell."

Progression of Signs and Symptoms during a Cyanotic Spell

- Uncontrollable crying in the infant, irritability;
- Severe dyspnea, hyperpnea, progressive cyanosis;
- Unconsciousness, seizures, and even cardiac arrest.

Signs and Symptoms of Respiratory Distress Associated with a Congenital Heart Defect

- *Respiratory*—intercostal retractions, dyspnea, tachypnea, crackles or wheezing on auscultation;
- *Circulatory*—tachycardia, cyanosis or duskiness noted in the mucous membranes for some defects;
- *Neurologic*—drowsiness, loss of consciousness during "cyanotic spells," limpness of extremities;
- *Skin*—cool, moist skin; noticeable perspiration; pallor;
- *General*—fatigue and exhaustion in infants; irritable when disturbed; small and poorly developed for stated age.

Management

BLS field care for the infant or child with a cardiac emergency includes:

- Monitor ABC's and vital signs.
- Maintain the airway.
- Administer high-flow, high-concentration oxygen.
- Provide ventilatory support as necessary.

- For a cyanotic spell, place the child in knee-chest position (see Figure 7.5).
- Prepare for cardiopulmonary arrest.
- *Transport patient immediately.*

The ALS provider should initiate the following additional care:

- Start an IV with D5W at a keep-open rate if there is an anticipated lengthy transport time.

Children Dependent on High-Technology Equipment

Children with a wide variety of chronic illnesses are often cared for at home by parents. Some of the conditions that these children have include the following: respiratory and cardiac disabling conditions, feeding disorders, disabilities associated with severe trauma, and terminal illnesses.

These children are at home, primarily because of benefits to the child, family, and the health care system. The home is a more positive environment for the child to grow and develop than is a hospital intensive care unit. However, families take on a tremendous burden to care for the child at home, often disrupting the lives of all family members. Parents are often exhausted caring for the child 24 hours a day. They often have no relief because other family members and babysitters are afraid to care for the child.

The *respiratory disabled* include such children as premature babies who require life-saving, long-term mechanical ventilation. Surviving babies often develop a chronic lung disease characterized by hypoxia, hypercarbia, and oxygen dependence. Advanced cystic fibrosis is another respiratory disorder sometimes requiring high-tech care. Such children will have signs of respiratory distress with crackles, wheezes, abundant secretions, retractions, and cyanosis on exertion. They may be treated at

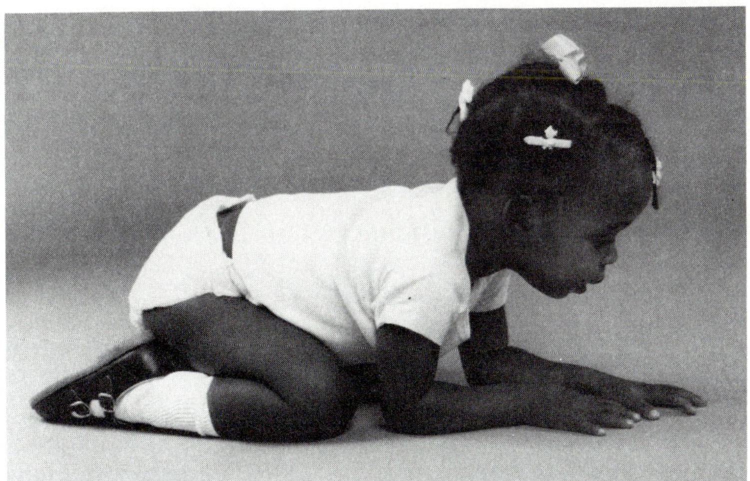

FIGURE 7.5   Place the infant having a ''cyanotic spell'' in knee-chest position. This will decrease the blood flow from the legs to the heart and reduce the heart's workload temporarily.

home with any of the following adjuncts: oxygen, mechanical ventilators, suction, tracheostomies, and apnea monitors.

Cardiac disabled infants and children include those with congenital cardiac defects who are waiting for surgery or have a defect that cannot be surgically corrected. They will have signs of hypoxemia, decreased exercise tolerance, and sometimes congestive heart failure. These children are treated at home with oxygen and feeding pumps.

Children with major *trauma disabilities* that are the result of a head or spinal cord injury, or near drowning, are often treated at home after discharge from a rehabilitation hospital. They may be on life-support equipment such as oxygen, mechanical ventilators, suction, and feeding pumps. Some of these children will have a gastrostomy tube that permits tube-feeding directly into the stomach or a Broviac catheter for IV nutrition.

Some children receive hospice care at home for a terminal illness. Rather than life-support equipment, these children will have equipment necessary for comfort measures, such as IV pumps for drug administration. These families made the decision to permit the child to die at home rather than in the hospital. EMS will not usually be called to administer care to these children, unless the family has not resolved the issue of the child's death. When EMS is called, providers are required to begin resuscitation.

Reasons Why EMS Is Activated

Prehospital care providers are generally called to help these families in times of crisis. EMS providers are often notified about the child in the community by the family or health care providers. In the event of such an occurrence, a higher priority of response will be made when called. While parents have been well trained to manage all types of problems, the child might become acutely ill, equipment might fail, or the parent panics because of fatigue. Examples of some of these problems include the following:

- Severe respiratory distress or respiratory arrest;
- The tracheostomy tube has become obstructed and the parent is unable to clear it or change it; or
- The child has hemorrhaged.

Management

BLS and ALS field care should include the following:

- Assess and manage the ABC's.
- Parents may already be providing emergency care (CPR, manual ventilation, suctioning, etc.), so support their efforts. It is not always necessary to take over for the parents.
- When an equipment malfunction has occurred, attach the child to your equipment, rather than try to determine what is wrong with the child's equipment. Vendors will repair the equipment.
- Provide rapid transport to the hospital, notifying the hospital to contact the child's physician.

ADAMS, F. H., and EMMANOUILIDES, G. C., eds., *Moss' Heart Disease in Infants, Children, and Adolescents.* Baltimore: Williams and Wilkins, 1983.

CHAMEIDES, L., ed., *Textbook of Pediatric Advanced Life Support.* Dallas: American Heart Association, 1988.

DAVIDSON, L., and DIERKING, B., "Medical emergencies in the pediatric patient," *JEMS,* 14, no. 3 (1989), pp. 74–78.

HALLOCK, J. A., "Meningitis—A true medical emergency," *Emergency Medical Services,* 9, no. 1 (1980), pp. 36–37.

HENRY, J. G., "Cardiac emergencies in pediatrics," *Emergency Medical Services,* 9, no. 1 (1980), pp. 53–56.

HOCHMAN, H. I., and others, "Dehydration, diabetic ketoacidosis, and shock in the pediatric patient," *Pediatric Clinics of North America,* 26, no. 4 (1979), pp. 803–825.

LAMB, L. S., "Think you know septic shock—read this," *Nursing 82,* 12, no. 1 (1982), pp. 34–39, 43.

LEVI, M., "On managing the febrile child," *Emergency Medicine,* 16, no. 3 (1984), pp. 166–168, 173–175, 178–180.

LONG, S., and HENRETIG, F., "Fever in children," *Pediatric Consult,* 6, no. 1 (1987), pp. 1–8.

ROBINSON, M., and SEWARD, P. N., "Environmental hypothermia in children," *Pediatric Emergency Care,* 2, no. 4 (1986), pp. 254–257.

SILVERMAN, B. J., ed., *Advanced Pediatric Life Support.* Dallas: American College of Emergency Physicians, 1989.

WHALEY, L. F., and WONG, D. L., *Nursing Care of Infants and Children,* 3rd ed. St. Louis: The C.V. Mosby Co., 1987.

WITTE, M. K., and others, "Shock in the pediatric patient," *Advances in Pediatrics,* 34 (1987), pp. 139–174.

Poisoning Emergencies

8

OBJECTIVES

When you have completed this chapter you should be able to

* Describe the contribution of developmental stage to childhood poisoning.
* List signs of toxins on various body systems.
* List important information to collect at the scene of a poisoning emergency.
* Describe poisoning emergencies in which vomiting should be induced.
* Demonstrate field management of the child with a poisoning emergency.

Developmental Considerations

In 1986 nearly 1.1 million cases of poisonings were reported to U.S. poison control centers nationwide. Children accounted for the majority of these cases. More boys than girls were victims in children under 12 years of age, but this frequency reversed in adolescents. More than 90% of all poisoning events occurred in the home (Table 8.1).

Poisoning is a major cause of preventable death in children under 5 years of age, with a peak incidence in children between 2 and 3 years of age. This age group is at greater risk for poisoning because of certain developmental characteristics (Figure 8.1).

- They explore by putting objects in their mouth.
- Taste is not well developed, so they will drink or eat (ingest) seemingly distasteful liquids and other substances.
- They are becoming more independent, mobile, and curious.
- Their fine motor skills have developed so they can open drawers, closets, and most containers.
- They cannot read labels.

The Poison Prevention Packaging Act of 1970 has helped reduce the incidence of poisoning by requiring child safety caps on all potentially toxic substances and drugs. The caps are designed to *delay* access to the substance by a child under 4 years of age. However, children still get access to toxic substances for the following reasons:

- Child safety caps are not replaced properly on containers.
- A nonsafety cap is requested for a drug at the pharmacy.
- Substances are put in different containers without safety caps, such as paint thinner in a soda bottle.
- Substances are packaged in containers similar to those used for food, such as milk and Clorox both in plastic bottles.

Poisonous substances that young children most often ingest include the following:

- Over-the-counter medications such as aspirin, Tylenol, vitamins with iron, skin care preparations, diaper care products, etc.;
- Prescription drugs—sedatives;

TABLE 8.1 Distribution of Poisonings by Age Group and Percentage of Poisonings Reported for All Age Groups to Poison Control Centers in 1986

Age Groups	Number of Poisonings (%)
< 3 years old	516,476 (47.0)
3–5 years old	171,381 (15.6)
6–12 years old	57,535 (5.2)
13–17 years old	47,335 (4.3)

Source: Adapted from Litovitz, T. L., and others (1987): "1986 Annual Report of the American Association of Poison Control Centers National Data Collection System. *American Journal of Emergency Medicine,* 5(5):405–435.

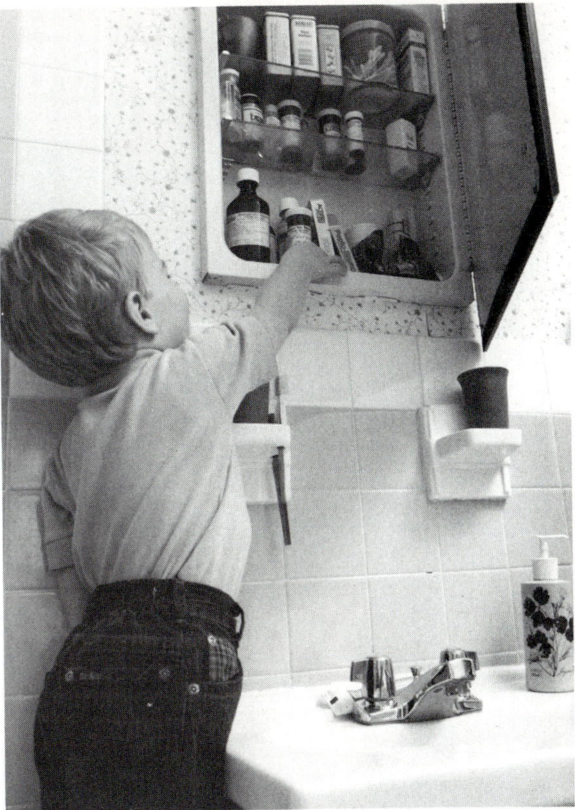

- Plants, such as poinsettias;
- Household cleansers;
- Cosmetics and personal care products;
- Petroleum products or hydrocarbons;
- Alcohol and alcohol-based products.

School-age children and adolescents often experiment with various drugs, and they may unintentionally take an overdose. They are curious about the effect of various drugs and are greatly influenced to use drugs recreationally by their peers. These children use drugs to experience perceptual and sensory sensations. Some children experiment with drugs as part of a social group, sharing the experience and feeling as though they are getting away with something by breaking the rules (Figure 8.2).

Chronic drug use and drug dependence may be the result of children who have other motivations. Such motivations may include seeking

- An escape from reality or their problems;
- An escape from feelings of anger, depression, and disenchantment with the adult world;
- Feelings of power, excitement, and confidence.

Drugs most often used by school-age children and adolescents include:

- Alcohol;
- Organic solvents (hydrocarbons and fluorocarbons are contained in

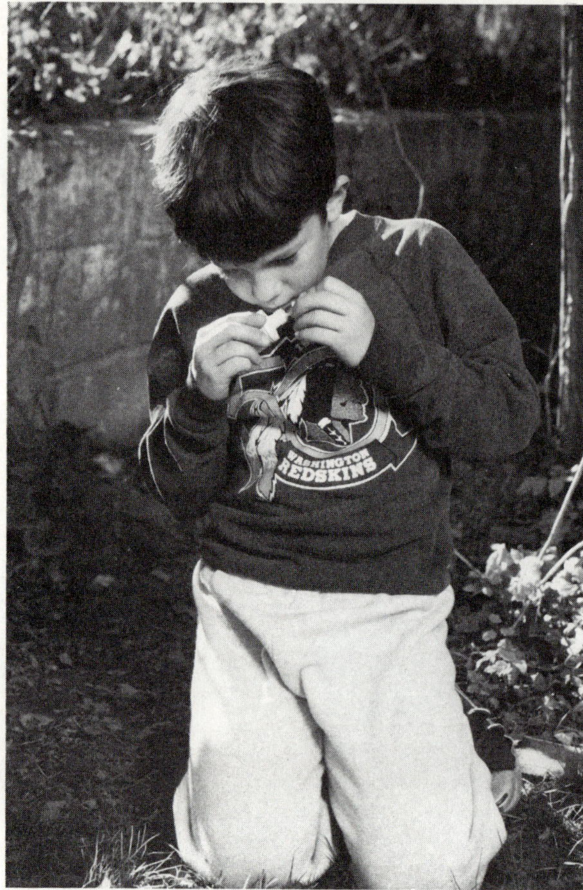

FIGURE 8.2 Older children often experiment to experience the feelings associated with inhaling substances.

such substances as airplane glue, typewriter correction fluid, and gasoline);

- Mind-altering drugs (marijuana, hashish, LSD, PCP, mescaline);
- Narcotics (heroin, morphine);
- Central nervous system depressants (barbiturates);
- Central nervous system stimulants (amphetamines, cocaine, or crack).

Drug overdose may be intentional in school-age children and adolescents who are attempting suicide. (See Chapter 16, "Suicide.")

Effect of Toxins on Body Systems

The initial concern in poisonings is whether the drug will quickly depress the respiratory system, leading to respiratory arrest. Depending upon the type of substance, various systems will be affected directly or through complications caused by the toxic substance. Some poisons cause life-threatening symptoms in the respiratory, circulatory, and central nervous systems. The gastrointestinal system is often burned and irritated by the corrosive substance ingested, such as drain cleaners, dishwasher

140

detergent, toilet bowl cleaners, and other concentrated cleansers (see Table 8.2).

History

The following information should be collected at the scene:

- What was taken, how much, and how long ago?
- Was the substance swallowed, inhaled, injected, or absorbed through the skin?
- What symptoms have developed as time has passed?
- What treatment has been initiated?
- Was vomiting induced or did it occur spontaneously?

TABLE 8.2 Effect of Various Poisonous Substances on Body Systems

Drug/Poison	Respiratory System	Circulatory System	Nervous System	Gastrointestinal System
Alcohol (A) Barbiturates (B) Sedatives (S)	Depressed rate	Tachycardia, first Bradycardia Low blood pressure	Aggression Violence ↓ coordination ↓ perception Slurred speech Loss of inhibitions (A) Constricted pupils (B)	
Amphetamines (A) Cocaine (C) Hallucinogens (H)	↑ rate	Tachycardia ↑ blood pressure Dysrhythmias	Euphoria Agitation Restlessness Dilated pupils (A,H) Seizures	
Digitalis (D) Beta-blockers (B)		Bradycardia (D) Dysrhythmias		
Narcotics	Depressed rate	Bradycardia ↓ blood pressure	Euphoria, first Lethargy Loss of consciousness Constricted pupils	
Anticholinergics (atropine)	↑ rate	Tachycardia ↑ blood pressure		
Aspirin	↑ rate (metabolic acidosis)	Shock (GI bleeding)	Fever	Abdominal pain Nausea, vomiting
Hydrocarbons	↑ rate, distress (with aspiration)			Abdominal pain Nausea, vomiting
Organophosphates	↑ rate, wheezing		Seizures, fever Pinpoint pupils	Vomiting, drooling, ↑ salivation
Corrosive substances	Obstruction	Shock		Drooling ↑ salivation Abdominal pain Nausea, vomiting Burns to mouth
Organic solvents (inhaled)			Loss of coordination ↓ perception Euphoria Lethargy Loss of consciousness	

Assessment

Upon arriving on the scene, conduct the primary survey to identify any life-threatening problems. Corrosive substances may cause swelling in the mouth and throat. Spontaneous vomiting can occur with any substances swallowed.

The actual signs and symptoms present in the child will vary depending upon both the poisoning substance and the time since the child was exposed. Refer to Table 8.2 for common signs and symptoms for various groups of poisons.

Inspect the scene for signs of a mechanism of injury (bottles or containers, plastic bags, traces of substances, injection paraphernalia, plants). Be sure to take any evidence to the hospital for analysis. Any drug paraphernalia at the crime scene indicates the need for police involvement. Note the general condition of the environment and any signs of poison prevention for the young child.

Management

General BLS care for poisonings includes the following:

- Upon arrival at the scene, conduct the primary survey, identifying any immediately life-threatening problems.
- Ensure the airway, and protect the cervical spine if head injury could have occurred.
- Continually reassess the child's ABCDE's and monitor vital signs.
- Call the poison control center or medical control to obtain directions for specific treatment. State the signs and symptoms noted in the child, and give any specific information about the toxin that is known. *In many states, the poison control center has no medical director, and medical control must be consulted prior to initiating management.*
- For substances without a hydrocarbon or corrosive base, follow guidelines to induce vomiting with syrup of ipecac (page 143) when appropriate (see also Caution box, page 143). In cases of corrosives, dilute the toxin with milk or water.
- Administer high-flow oxygen by mask and closely monitor for vomiting.
- Assist ventilations in cases of deteriorating level of consciousness. Prepare to do CPR if the child's level of consciousness begins to deteriorate.
- Transport rapidly and contact medical control.

ALS providers should consider the following additional management procedures for the child who has any altered level of consciousness, seizures, or coma possibly resulting from a poison:

- Perform orotracheal intubation in cases of altered level of consciousness.
- Start an IV with Ringer's Lactate or Normal Saline at a keep-open rate, unless signs of shock are present. If shock is present, adminis-

ter a 20 ml/kg bolus IV push and repeat if no change in vital signs is apparent.

- Charcoal can be ordered because of its binding action with many poisons. Give 1 g/kg mixed in water to the child to drink or by nasogastric tube. It can be given even after the child vomits.
- Administer dextrose 0.5–1.0 g/kg/IV dose (2–4 ml/kg/D25W), if no mechanism of injury is present.
- Administer naloxone 0.1 mg/kg per dose IV initially to a maximum dose of 0.8 mg. If there is no response in 10 minutes, then give 2 mg IV if a narcotic overdose is suspected.
- Administer atropine 0.5–1.0 mg IV, if organophosphate poisoning is suspected.

Guidelines for Use of Ipecac

While there is some controversy, vomiting is often induced in cases of swallowed poisons in an attempt to reduce the amount of poison absorbed through the gastrointestinal tract. For best effect, this should be done as soon after ingestion as possible, before the stomach empties the poison into the intestinal tract (2–3 hours). Syrup of ipecac is often used by pre-hospital care providers to induce vomiting, but it takes approximately 20 minutes to work. The dosage is dependent upon age:

10 ml to infants between 6 and 12 months of age;

15 ml to children between 1 and 12 years of age;

30 ml to children over 12 years of age.

Then give 8 oz of water, which dilutes the poison and stimulates vomiting (Figure 8.3). If the patient does not vomit in 20 minutes and you have a long transport time, the dose can be repeated if the child is still expected to be alert for the next 20 minutes. If the child vomits, take the vomitus to the hospital for analysis.

 **CAUTION!**

Inducing Vomiting

Prior to giving syrup of ipecac, it is important to determine if the child's level of consciousness is expected to deteriorate over the next 20 minutes. There is an increased risk of aspiration with altered levels of consciousness. Do *not* induce vomiting in the child who

- is having seizures
- is lethargic and in danger of further loss of consciousness
- has already vomited
- has ingested a corrosive substance or hydrocarbon compound. 

Vomiting is often induced in the child who ingests a hydrocarbon compound (organophosphate pesticide, camphor, or heavy metals) containing a substance more harmful to the central nervous system than the effects caused by aspirating the hydrocarbon.

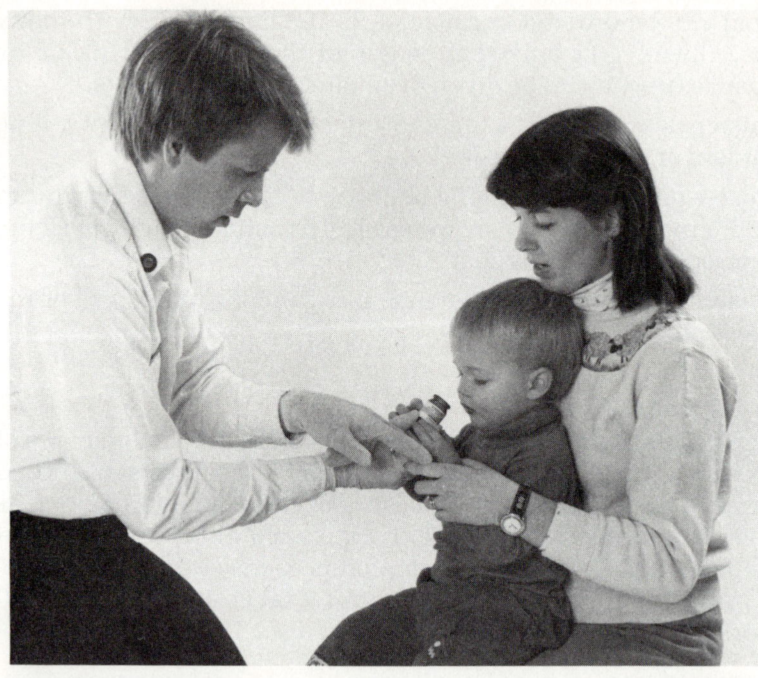

FIGURE 8.3 Administration of syrup of ipecac to stimulate vomiting after ingestion of a poison.

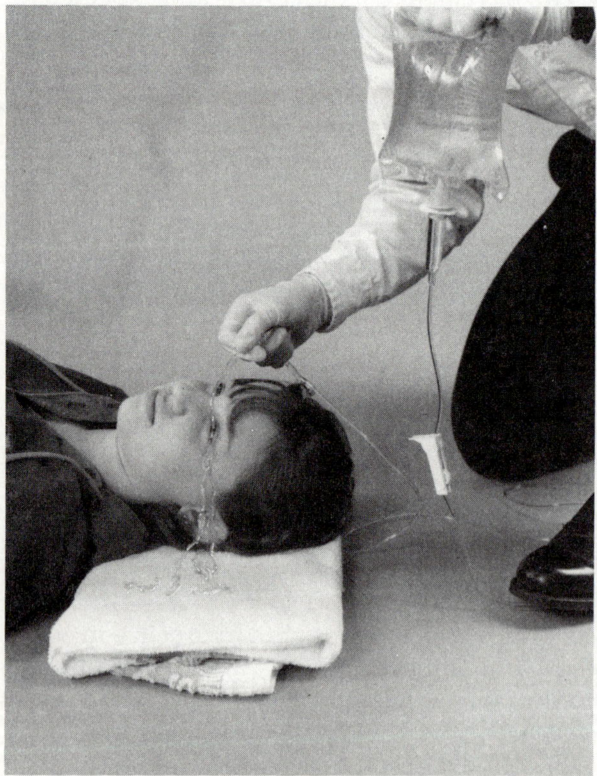

FIGURE 8.4 Flushing the eye to remove any poisons.

144

Poisons on the Skin or in the Eyes

BLS care for the child with poisons *absorbed by the skin* includes the following:

- Clothing should be removed as the child is flushed with copious amounts of water. The prehospital provider should wear gloves and eye protection to avoid exposure.

- Any poisons in direct contact with the eyes should be flushed for 15 to 20 minutes using water or saline. Hold the child's head over the sink or tub and pour the solution directly into the eye. Avoid draining into the unaffected eye (Figure 8.4). During transport, use IV solution with the end of the IV tubing used to direct the solution away from the unaffected eye.

- Refer to the management of chemical burns in Chapter 12.

Poisoning References

BARKIN, R. M., and ROSEN, P., eds., *Emergency Pediatrics*, 3rd ed. St. Louis: The C. V. Mosby Co., 1990.

DYMOWSKI, J. J., and UEHARA, D. T., "Common household poisonings," *Pediatric Emergency Care*, 3, no. 4 (1987), pp. 261–265.

KUNKEL, D. B., "Plant poisoning in children," *Pediatric Annals*, 16, no. 11 (November 1987), pp. 927–932.

LITOVITZ, T. L., and others, "1986 Annual Report of the American Association of Poison Control Centers National Data Collection System," *American Journal of Emergency Medicine*, 5, no. 5 (May 1987), pp. 405–435.

VICTORIA, M. S., and NANGIA, B. S., "Hydrocarbon poisoning: A review," *Pediatric Emergency Care*, 3, no. 3 (March 1987), pp. 184–186.

WHALEY, L. F., and WONG, D. L., *Nursing Care of Infants and Children*, 3rd ed. St. Louis: The C. V. Mosby Co., 1987.

9

Pediatric Trauma Assessment

OBJECTIVES

When you have completed this chapter you should be able to

* List the most common causes of trauma to the child and the most frequent injuries to the child with multiple trauma.
* Describe the steps of the primary survey.
* Describe effective airway management and ventilation in an injured child.
* List signs that may indicate shock in the child.
* Describe management of the injured child in shock.
* Describe the essential components of a secondary trauma assessment.

Introduction

Trauma is the leading cause of death in children in the United States today. Statistics show that half of all childhood fatalities, approximately 8000 children under 15 years of age, occur each year as a result of injury. Motor vehicle crashes are the mechanism of injury in 40% of cases; this is followed by drowning, burns, falls, and firearms. Pediatric patients make up 10% to 15% of trauma seen in the emergency setting and are nearly twice as likely as adults to die in transport to the hospital or during resuscitation in the emergency department.

Mechanism of Injury

The most common childhood injuries seen in multiple trauma—resulting from a motor vehicle crash—affect the head, trunk, and extremity (triad of injury). It is not unusual to have a child hit by a vehicle and sustain a head injury, lung contusion, spleen laceration, and femur fracture (Figure 9.1). Most of pediatric trauma is blunt trauma, although the incidence of penetrating trauma in children is increasing.

When standing or sitting on a bike a child is lower to the ground than is an adult. When a child is involved in a motor vehicle collision, the car bumper strikes the child's femur, the car's hood hits the child's chest and abdomen, and the child is thrown to the ground with impact to the head. Young children are particularly vulnerable on a "big wheel" tricycle, sitting low to the ground, because their head is at the bumper level of the oncoming vehicle.

The sequence of pediatric assessment and management at the scene is similar to care of the injured adult. Use the ABCDE's of the primary assessment and immediately treat the life-threatening conditions. Pediatric trauma care differs from adult care because of the child's unique physiologic response to the injury. Rapid deterioration may occur in the young patient who is not managed efficiently and effectively. Most children die from lack of oxygen (hypoxemia) due to poor airway and ventilation control, or from ineffective circulation (shock).

Primary Survey

The primary survey is performed to detect and correct life-threatening conditions. The priority areas assessed during the primary survey are: air-

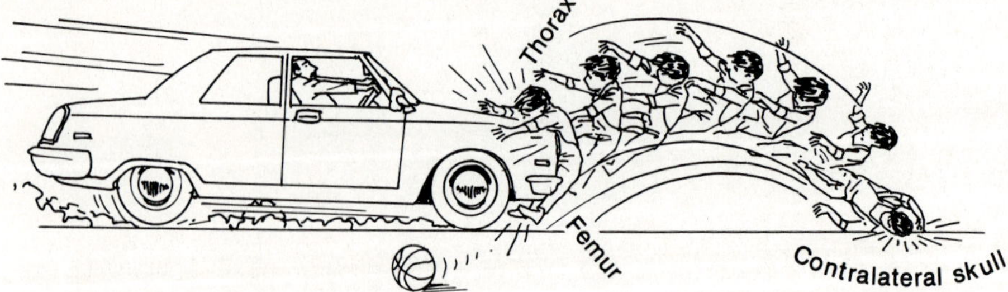

FIGURE 9.1   The triad of injury associated with a child pedestrian–motor vehicle crash includes injury to the head, chest, and femur.

way, cervical spine stabilization, breathing, circulation, neurological disability, and exposure.

Airway

Assessment

When approaching the child, first check the airway. If the child is talking, crying, or answering questions, the child's airway is adequate and patent *at this time.* Because the child's airway is smaller in diameter than an adult's, it can be easily obstructed by blood, vomitus, tongue, and broken teeth. During the primary and secondary assessment, the airway is frequently reevaluated because respiratory compromise can occur, especially if there is an underlying head injury. Repeated assessment will alert you to the need for any supplemental action to maintain the airway. *Caution!* With any head injury or other major injury, assume an injury to the cervical spine. A fracture can only be ruled out by X ray at the receiving hospital.

Look for spontaneous chest motion and listen for spontaneous breath sounds or other sounds such as stridor, bubbling, or gurgling (Figure 9.2).

Management

BLS providers should provide the following care in cases of an obstructed airway:

- Control and stabilize the C-spine in neutral alignment.
- Open the airway if it is not patent or adequate. Use the most simple and least invasive maneuver to open and secure the airway.
- Place the child in neutral or sniffing position. This brings the tongue

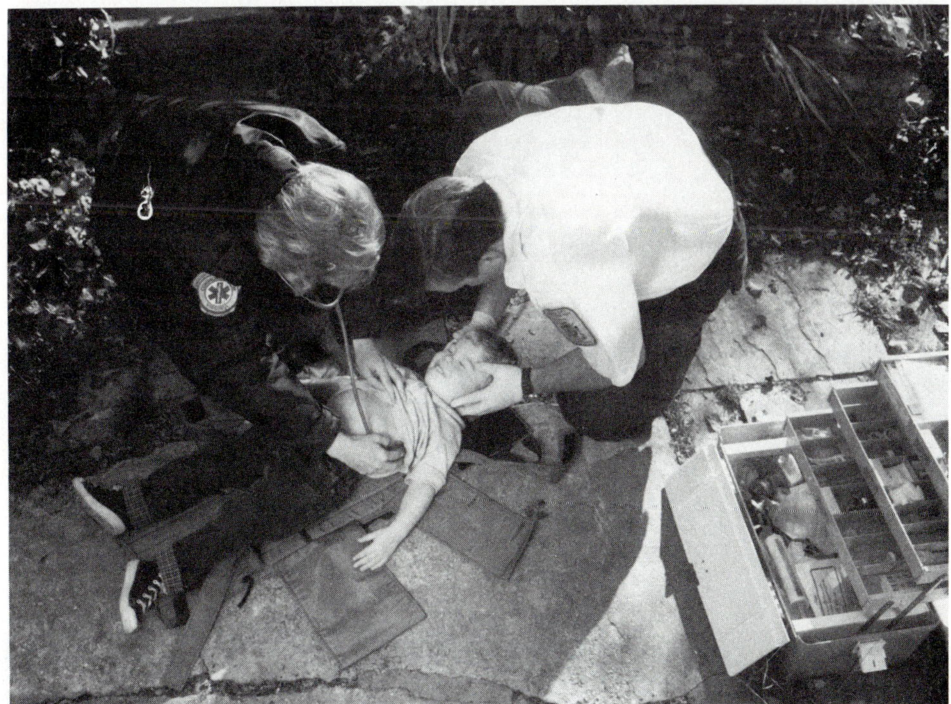

FIGURE 9.2　Reassessment of airway, ventilation, and breath sounds while maintaining cervical spine stabilization.

forward and straightens the trachea, thus giving patency to the full diameter of the airway.

- Perform the jaw-thrust maneuver if further manipulation is necessary to bring the tongue even further forward in the mouth.
- Suction with a DeLee or Yankauer apparatus to remove mucous, blood, or vomitus. Head-injured children are at risk for posttraumatic seizures and vomiting.
- Insert an oral airway in the unconscious child if necessary; use with extreme care. (See Chapter 4, "Equipment and Procedures.")
- Administer high-flow, high-concentration oxygen when the airway is secured.

ALS providers should consider the following additional care for airway management:

- Orotracheal intubation should be performed when the airway remains inadequate or airway control must be secured to free the provider for other tasks. Recheck the placement of the tube frequently because minimal movement may displace it (Figure 9.3).
- Needle cricothyrotomy is indicated only in the rare instance of severe facial trauma or unresolved upper airway obstruction. It is a last-ditch effort to establish an airway.

Breathing

Because of the pliability of the child's rib cage, a very severe blow to the rib is required to produce a rib fracture or flail chest. Blunt trauma to the chest may cause pulmonary contusion or a spontaneous pneumothorax because the energy from the blow must be dissipated and is absorbed by the lung

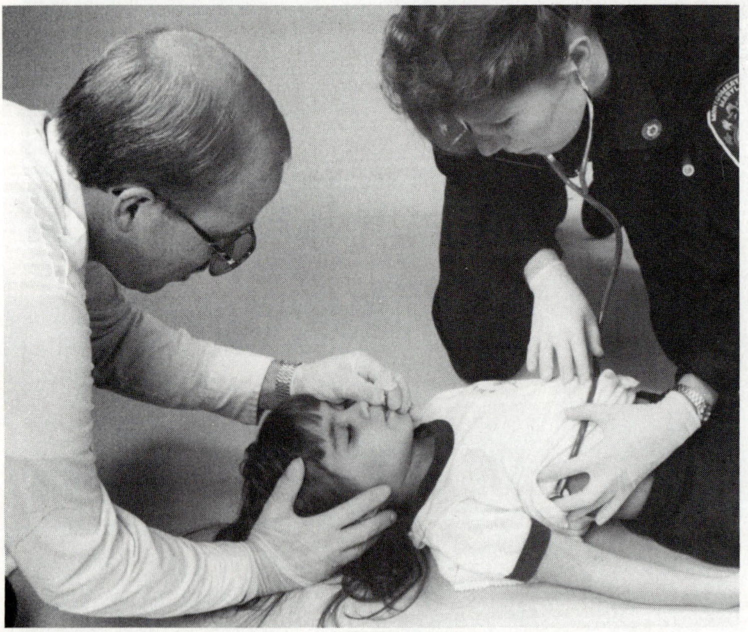

FIGURE 9.3 Checking ET tube placement prior to taping.

tissue. Because of the mobility of organs within the mediastinum, tension pneumothorax is a potential life-threatening disorder (see Chapter 11).

Assessment

Observe the child's color. Check for pallor, mottling or cyanosis of the lips, tongue, mucous membranes of the mouth, and nail beds.

Assess breathing with the chest and abdomen exposed. To count the respiratory rate in young children, observe the rise and fall of the abdomen. Remember the expected respiratory rate of the child. Rates lower than 20 breaths/min in a small child may indicate ventilatory failure due to chest muscle fatigue. Rates greater than 60/min indicate oxygen hunger, reflective of ineffective breathing.

Inspect the chest, noting any swelling or bruising or penetrating chest wounds. Look for other irregularities such as retractions, unequal rise and fall of the chest, paradoxical breathing or "see-sawing" of the chest and abdomen. Note other signs of respiratory distress such as nasal flaring, apprehension, noisy breathing, or hoarseness.

Using a stethoscope listen for bilateral breath sounds under each clavicle and at the mid-axillary line halfway between the axilla and the lower margin of the rib cage. Note any wheezing or other abnormalities such as unequal breath sounds.

Palpate for tracheal deviation, which is a sign of tension pneumothorax. This is especially difficult to evaluate in young children owing to their short, chubby necks; thus, do NOT rely on this as the only sign of a tension pneumothorax. Other signs of tension pneumothorax development include increasing respiratory distress, crepitus, subcutaneous emphysema, and any guarding during the palpation of the neck.

Management

BLS providers should administer the following intervention for ineffective ventilation:

- Monitor ABC's and vital signs.
- Administer high-concentration, high-flow oxygen by bag-valve mask to all children with major trauma.
- Perform mouth-to-mask ventilation until positive pressure ventilation can be implemented.
- Provide positive pressure ventilation when the respiratory rate is less than 20 breaths/min or the child is not breathing.
- Treat open chest wounds immediately with a petroleum gauze dressing or cellophane taped on four sides. Monitor the ABC's and burp the dressing to release pressure if a tension pneumothorax develops (Figure 9.4).
- Administer CPR if necessary.
- Transport patient *immediately.*

ALS providers should additionally provide the following management for life-threatening ventilation problems:

- Orotracheal intubation.
- If tension pneumothorax develops, perform needle thoracostomy to relieve the intrathoracic pressure.

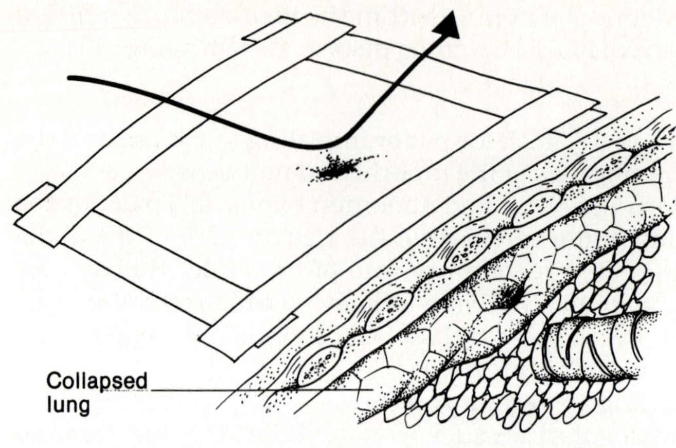

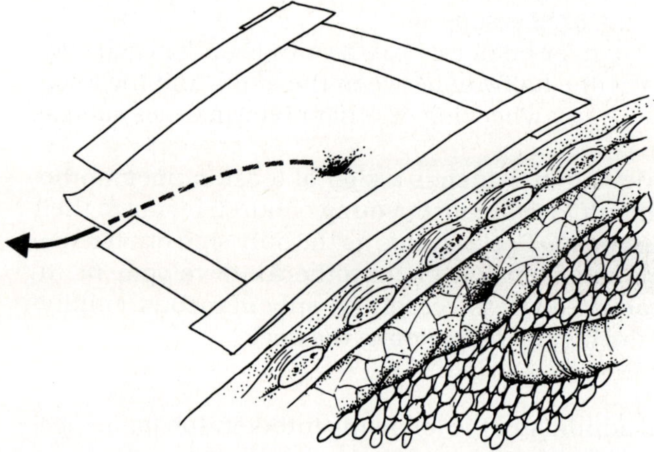

FIGURE 9.4 Management of sucking chest wound. Cover an open chest wound with cellophane or petroleum gauze dressing taped on all four sides to prevent air entry on inspiration. Peel back a corner of the dressing if tension pneumothorax occurs to permit air escape on expiration.

Circulation

The child's blood volume is proportional to weight (see Table 3.2). A 3-year-old with a total blood volume of 1275 ml will be in shock with a loss of 255 ml of blood (about 1 cup!). Young children may develop significant hypovolemic shock from a scalp laceration (Figure 9.5).

Identification of *early hypovolemic shock* is extremely important in children because of their physiologic ability to compensate for shock. As shock develops, they will constrict their arteries and veins, actually shunting blood to the central circulation. As blood loss increases, this compensatory mechanism becomes less effective. Once the blood pressure begins dropping, usually after 20–25% blood loss, the child is in *late* shock. Resuscitation of the child in late shock is more difficult because the condition will deteriorate very rapidly.

Assessment

Assess the patient's circulation by observing the child's color. Look for any obvious bleeding and investigate any dark stains on clothing. Apply

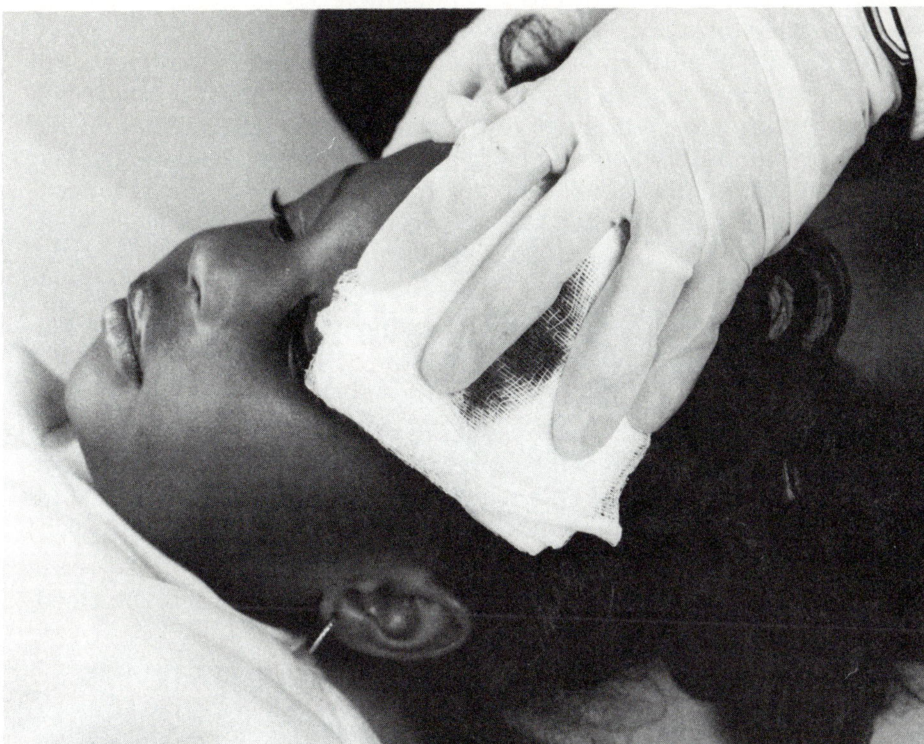

FIGURE 9.5 Applying manual pressure to scalp laceration to control bleeding.

manual pressure to control bleeding. Check the capillary refill time. Because of the child's tendency to become hypothermic, perform this test in an area of central circulation, such as over the forehead or sternum. A capillary refill time longer than 2 seconds indicates poor perfusion.

Auscultate the chest, listening for the apical heart rate below and medial to the left nipple. Because of the child's thin chest wall, the heart sounds should be clear and distinct. Note any muffling or indistinctive sounds of the heart that might indicate cardiac tamponade. Palpate the pulse rate and check for weak or absent brachial or femoral pulses. Take the blood pressure.

The best indicators of *early shock* in children are:

- Sustained tachycardia (greater than 130 beats/min) in a quiet child;
- Increased capillary refill time greater than 2 seconds;
- Cool, pale skin.

Altered mental status is also associated with hypovolemic shock; however, this sign may be difficult to evaluate when head trauma is suspected.

A drop in the systolic blood pressure is a late indicator of hypovolemic shock. The child will have lost at least 20% of the total blood volume before a decrease in systolic blood pressure is noted. The child with a systolic blood pressure less than 70 mm Hg is in late shock. If a child shows signs and symptoms of shock without obvious hemorrhage be suspicious of internal bleeding. The body spaces of the chest, abdomen, and pelvis can harbor large enough quantities of blood to put a child into shock. Except for small infants, bleeding into the skull alone does not cause shock; it causes increased intracranial pressure.

Children with hypothermia also have a delayed capillary refill time and cool, mottled, or pale extremities. Their pulse rate and blood pressure will usually be within normal limits or low. The child with altered mental status and cool, pale skin who has a capillary refill time of 2 seconds or less and a systolic blood pressure of 100 may have a head injury or other central nervous system dysfunction rather than hypovolemic shock.

Management

BLS providers should provide the following care to children with life-threatening circulatory problems:

- Control external bleeding by placing a dressing with pressure over the site and elevation of the extremity, if indicated. Use your entire hand to place pressure on a scalp laceration, in case there is a skull fracture underneath. Manual pressure is better than a "pressure dressing."
- Place pressure over a pulse point between the heart and the bleeding site to control a bleeding artery.
- Administer high-flow, high-concentration oxygen by bag mask.
- Keep the child warm.
- Apply PASG if protocols so direct and an appropriate size is available. See Chapter 4 and Figure 4.23 (page 72) for indications and application directions.
- Transport patient *immediately*.

ALS providers should additionally perform the following management as directed by medical control or protocols:

- Start an IV with Ringer's Lactate or Normal Saline. Do NOT delay transport to start the IV. Limit your attempts to two sticks en route to the hospital. If the extrication is lengthy, attempt IV start at the scene.
- If the child is unconscious and in severe hypovolemic shock, and attempts at a peripheral line are unsuccessful, insert an IO line if local protocols permit.
- Administer a fluid bolus (20 ml/kg), as rapidly as possible, IV push with a syringe or pressure bag.
- Recheck the child's vital signs and capillary refill for signs of improved circulatory perfusion. If signs of shock do not improve after 5 minutes, repeat the fluid bolus. Up to three boluses may be needed in severe shock.

Disability: Neurologic Exam

An altered level of consciousness commonly results from hypoxemia or a head injury. No improvement with oxygenation, or progressive deterioration, indicates either a massive injury or that complications of the injury have occurred.

Assessment

The Glasgow Coma Scale (GCS) provides a standardized, quantifiable evaluation of mental status. It can be repeated over time by prehospital and hospital personnel to determine whether the child is improving or deteriorating. See Table 3.3 for GCS criteria.

Management

The BLS provider should provide the following care if altered mental status is present and head injury is suspected:

- Administer high-concentration, high-flow oxygen by bag-valve mask.
- Hyperventilate at a rate 5 to 10 breaths faster than the child's normal respiratory rate.
- Elevate the head and upper body as a unit, unless contraindicated, maintaining immobilization of the spine.
- Observe and prepare for posttraumatic seizure.

Exposure

Before removing all of the child's clothes to begin the rapid body scan for injuries that may have been overlooked during the ABCDE's, remember the tendency for children to develop hypothermia. Children cool more quickly than do adults, even in mild weather, because of their greater body surface area to mass ratio. Children with hypothermia (core body temperature less than 98°F) do not respond as well to resuscitation efforts. Drug absorption will also be delayed.

Assessment

Expose only that body part being assessed to reduce heat loss. Once assessment of that body part is completed, recover it and move on to another body part. Observe the child for signs of mild hypothermia, such as cool, pale or mottled extremities, and an increased capillary refill time greater than 2 seconds in the extremities.

Management

All prehospital providers should provide the following care to the child with potential for heat loss:

- Cover the child to retain body heat during further assessment, management, and transport.
- Use warmed oxygen and IV fluids, if possible, during cold weather. Turn the ambulance heater on.

Secondary Survey

When the ABCDE's of the primary survey are under control, proceed to the secondary survey. Transport immediately if your primary assessment reveals life-threatening injuries or respiratory distress or shock. In this circumstance the secondary survey is done in the back of the ambulance. Do not delay transport for treating wounds or applying traction at the scene if the child's survival is in danger. Remember to reassess the ABCDE's frequently during care.

Minimal time should be spent in the field with the secondary survey. In many cases, the secondary survey is performed during transport. A rapid head-to-toe exam is performed in a systematic order to find additional injuries and plan management strategies during transport. For example, bruises on the abdomen will alert you to the possibility of internal bleeding and the potential for the child to develop shock.

While pieces of the child's history have been obtained during the primary assessment, additional information must be obtained to complete the history. Full information about the child's medical history, allergies, and mechanism of injury should be obtained from parents or care providers. In addition, gather further information from family members or bystanders.

Head and Neck

- Palpate the head for any lacerations, swelling, deformities, or depressions.

- Check eye movement for coordination in following objects and note if the eyes are focusing. Use a penlight to check pupils for size, shape, and reaction to light.

- Look for any blood or fluid drainage in the ears, nose, and mouth. Any bruising around the eyes (raccoon sign) or behind the ears (Battle's sign) are both late signs of basilar skull fracture. Clear fluid draining from the nose may indicate a basilar fracture in the cribiform plate of the nose.

- Palpate the facial structure and neck for any swelling, deformity, or depression (Figure 9.6). Check for proper alignment of the mandible and any missing teeth. Complaint of pain on palpation of the neck is an important sign of neck injury in children.

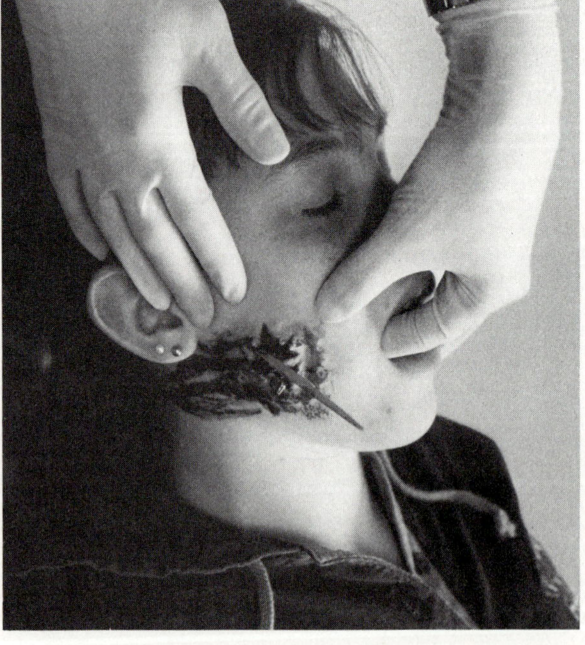

FIGURE 9.6 Palpate for facial deformity.

- Palpate the infant's fontanelle for tense bulging (may indicate increased intracranial pressure). A depressed fontanelle indicates hypovolemia.

Back

As you log-roll the child to place him or her on the backboard, quickly inspect and palpate the patient's back and spine. Note any lacerations, bruising, or deformities (Figure 9.7).

Chest

This exam should have been completed during the primary survey.

Abdomen

- Lightly palpate the abdomen noting any guarding, tenderness, pain, or rigidity (Figure 9.8).
- Inspect for bruising, ecchymosis, abrasions, lacerations, or distension.
- Check the femoral area, noting any swelling or hematomas and presence of pulses.
- Palpate pelvic girdle for tenderness or deformity. Carefully compress the pelvis by pushing the two wings of the ilium toward the symphysis pubis to determine if this maneuver is painful, indicating a pelvic fracture.
- Inspect genitalia and perineal areas for hematoma. Blood at the urethra and ecchymosis of the perineum may indicate bladder rupture or pelvic fracture.

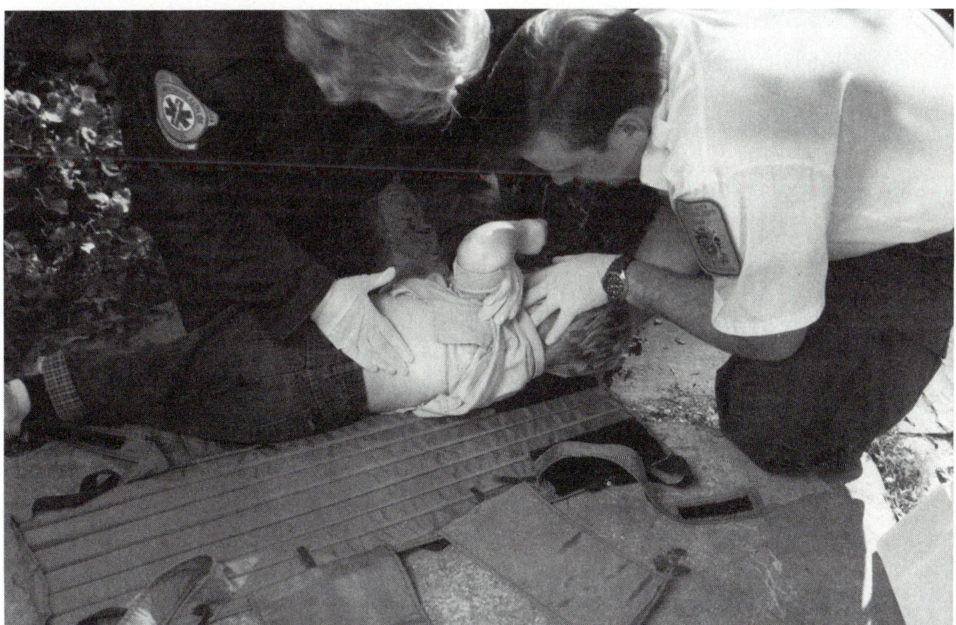

FIGURE 9.7   As you log roll the child onto a backboard, quickly inspect and palpate the back and spine.

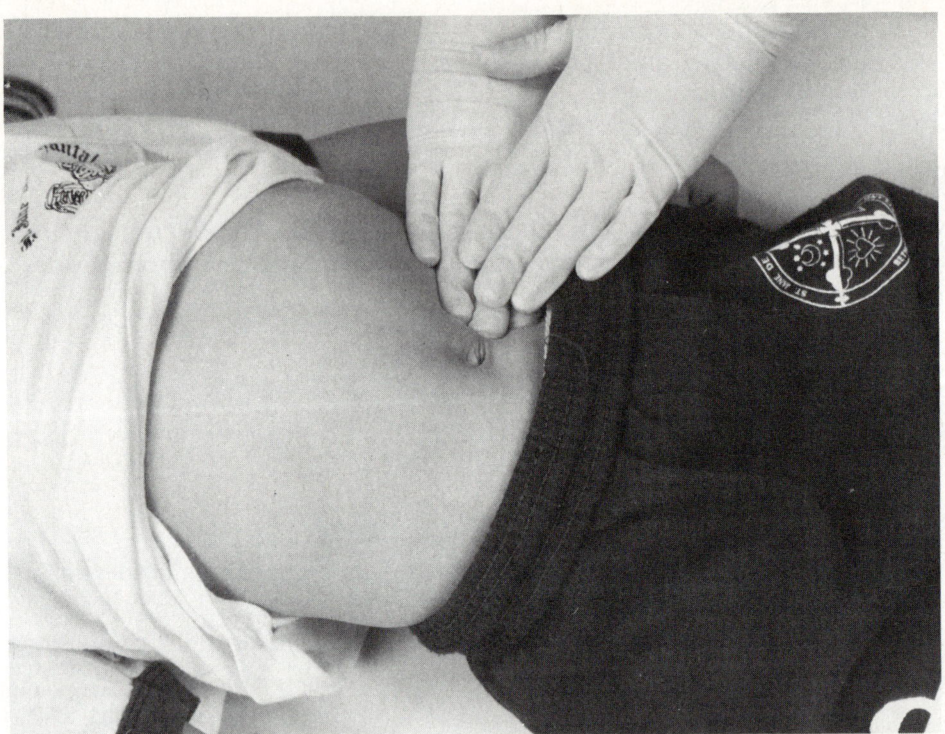

FIGURE 9.8 Palpate the abdomen for pain, tenderness, and rigidity.

Extremities

- Manually examine the arms and legs, noting obvious deformity, swelling, and open wounds with or without exposed bone.

- Assess vascular status distal to the injury by checking for the presence of a pulse, color, and temperature of the extremity, and capillary refill time.

- Note any loss of sensation, pain or tenderness on palpation or motion; inability to move the extremity; asymmetry of extremities or improper alignment. Note excessive pain that persists after immobilization. This could indicate *compartment syndrome*, a condition in which the pressure within the closed space of a muscle increases to the point where the blood supply is inadequate to oxygenate tissue. The pressure might be caused by hemorrhage, swelling of tissues, or a tight tourniquet-like dressing. It is extremely painful and requires emergency surgical intervention at the hospital.

- Palpate all major joints and long bones. Significant swelling can arise from displacement, which can also lead to nerve and blood vessel damage.

- Periodically check and recheck pulse and capillary refill distal to the injured extremity (Figure 9.9).

Management

All prehospital providers should continue assessment and management of the ABCDE's and transport the child.

- For orthopedic injuries to the upper extremities, splint the extrem-

     Pediatric Trauma Assessment

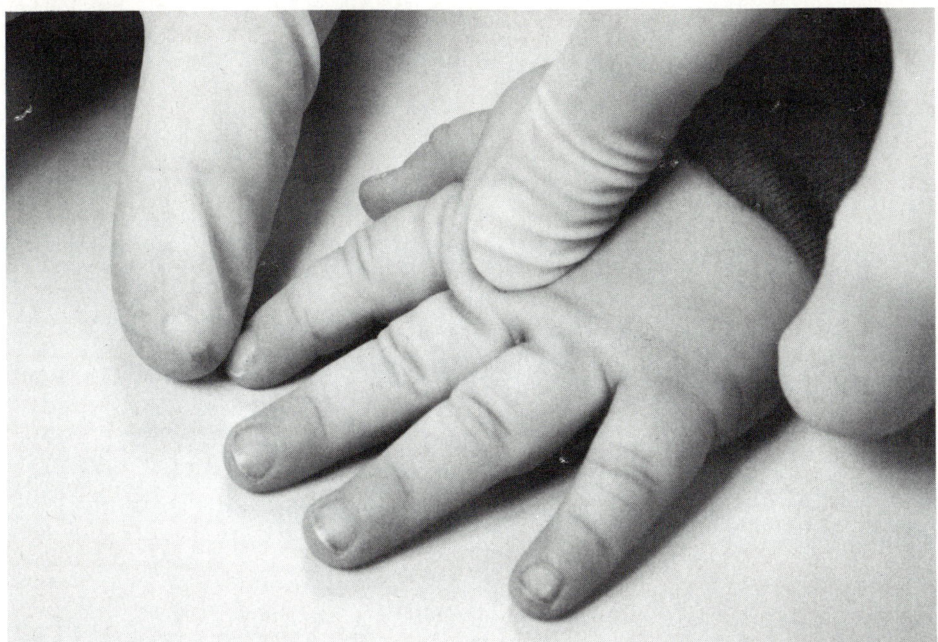

FIGURE 9.9   Assessing capillary refill time.

ity in the position in which it was found. If there is no pulse present, realign and splint.

- For injury to the lower extremities between the hip and knee, apply gentle traction in the line of the extremity and splint. Palpate for the presence of a distal pulse before and after realignment, and after splinting.

- Cover any open wounds near a fracture site with a sterile dressing. Be sure to report any suspicion of an open fracture to the emergency department.

For more information about specific chest, abdominal, and extremity injuries, refer to Chapter 11.

Primary and Secondary Trauma Assessment References

EICHELBERGER, M. R., and ANDERSON, K. D., "Sequelae of thoracic injury in children." In Hix, W.R., and Aaron B. L., eds., *Residua of Thoracic Trauma.* Mount Kisco, N.Y.: Futura Publishing Co., 1987, pp. 247–264.

HOLMES, M. J., and REYES, H. M., "A critical review of urban pediatric trauma," *Journal of Trauma,* 24, no. 3 (March 1984), pp. 253–255.

RIMAR, J. M., "Shock in infants and children: Assessment and treatment," *Maternal and Child Nursing,* 13 (March/April 1988), pp. 98–105.

SEIDEL, J. S., HOENBEIN, M., YOSHIYAMAK, and others, "Emergency medical services and the pediatric patient: Are the needs being met?" *Pediatrics,* 73, no. 6 (June 1984), pp. 769–772.

10

Head and Spinal Cord Injury

OBJECTIVES

When you have completed this chapter you should be able to

* List and describe the types of skull fractures.
* List and describe the types of injuries to the brain.
* List the characteristics of head injury with varying severity.
* Describe the assessment and management of the head-injured child.
* Describe the assessment and management of the spinal cord injury.

Head Injury

Head injury claims the lives of 10 out of every 100,000 American children between 1 and 14 years of age annually. Death or disability from head injury affects the lives of 25,000 children each year. Up to 75% of all children sustaining multiple trauma suffer head injury, and nearly 80% of all trauma deaths in children are associated with significant neurologic injury.

The mechanism of head trauma varies by age and developmental abilities of the child and their environmental exposure to these mechanisms.

- Infants and small children most commonly fall, either off the bed, out of the crib, down a flight of stairs, or out of windows.
- Children frequently sustain head injuries from bicycle and skateboard accidents, horseback riding, climbing trees, etc.
- Older children and adolescents sustain head injuries from sport injuries, such as soccer, football, and diving.
- Motor vehicle crashes involving unrestrained passengers and pedestrians also account for many serious head injuries.
- Penetrating trauma is seen in suicide or homicide cases primarily in the adolescent.
- Child abuse occurs at any age. Shaken-baby syndrome is a frequent cause of head injury in abused infants. The infant is shaken so hard that the bridging veins in the head rupture and cause a subdural hematoma. (See Chapter 13, ''Child Abuse.'')

Physiology

Children are particularly susceptible to head injury because their heads are proportionately larger and heavier in comparison to the rest of their body. In addition, the musculoskeletal structures of the neck are not as strong as an adult's, making the child more susceptible to high cervical spine injuries. Because a child's head is so large, a significantly larger blood flow goes to the head and brain, and the scalp is highly vascular. Children can bleed enough from a scalp laceration to develop shock if not properly treated.

The brain of infants and young children is less myelinated, and the tissue is thinner, more fragile, and easily bruised. With an acceleration–deceleration injury, the brain receives a *coup and contrecoup injury.* For example, if the child falls and hits the back of the head, the back part of the brain impacts the skull at the injury site and then the frontal lobes of the brain hit the skull opposite the injury site. This brain movement within the skull results in shearing and tearing of small blood vessels as the brain is jolted back and forth. The cranial bones are also thinner and less developed, thus being more susceptible to brain injury (Figure 10.1).

The skull is an enclosed space containing brain tissue, cerebrospinal fluid, and blood, all of which function in balance. When the brain swells or hemorrhage occurs within this confined space, it places pressure on brain tissue, compressing arteries and veins, which cuts off the oxygen supply

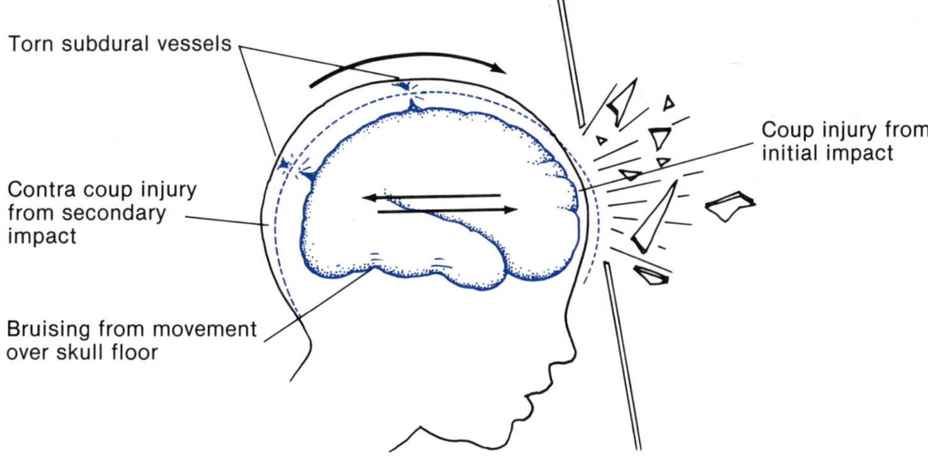

FIGURE 10.1 Coup contrecoup injury: note movement and bruising of the frontal area of the brain at time of initial impact—stretching brain tissue, tearing subdural vessels, and bruising as the brain moves over the floor of the skull. The occipital (posterior) area of the brain is bruised as the brain bounces back to strike the back of the skull.

and other nutrients to the brain. The brain's protective response is to call for more blood, which is one cause of diffuse cerebral edema.

Increased intracranial pressure due to diffuse cerebral edema is common in children. It generally occurs slowly over several hours or days following the initial injury. Seizures and vomiting may occur after the intracranial pressure level has begun to increase.

Increased intracranial pressure, if untreated, is fatal. However, intracranial pressure is better tolerated for a short time in infants than adults because the skull sutures are not fused and the anterior fontanelle allows expansion of the skull to accommodate the bleeding or swollen tissue.

Because of the rapid maturation of the brain, which occurs between 2 and 8 years of age, the skull and brain of children over 8 years of age respond to trauma similar to that of an adult.

Types of Head Injury

Fractures

A *linear* skull fracture occurs along one of the skull's suture lines. A fracture across the temporal bone may tear the middle meningeal artery resulting in an epidural hemorrhage.

A *depressed* skull fracture is palpable on physical examination, usually 5 mm below the contour of the skull. The brain tissue underneath may be contused or lacerated.

A *compound* skull fracture is an open fracture, either linear or depressed under a scalp laceration (Figure 10.2).

A *basilar* skull fracture is a fracture on the floor of the skull. Leakage of clear or amber-colored cerebrospinal fluid from the nose or ear indicates a cribiform plate fracture inside the skull. Other signs of a basilar skull fracture include bruising under the eyes (raccoon eyes) or behind the ear (Battle's sign).

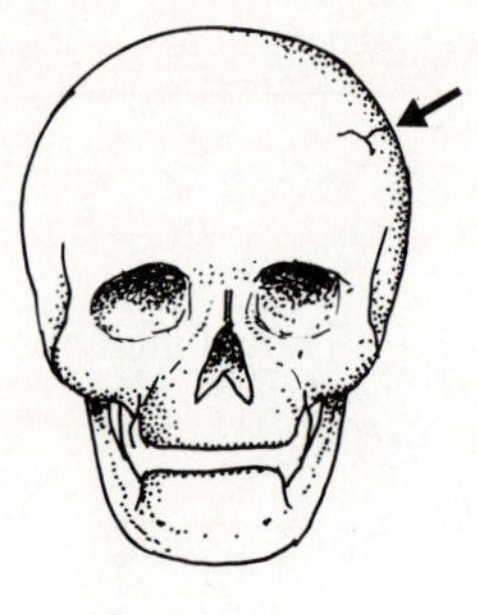

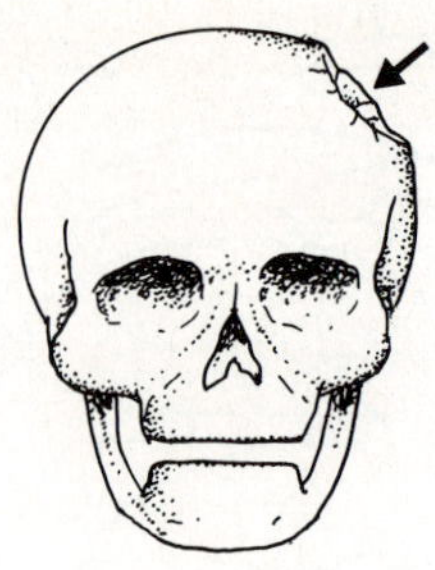

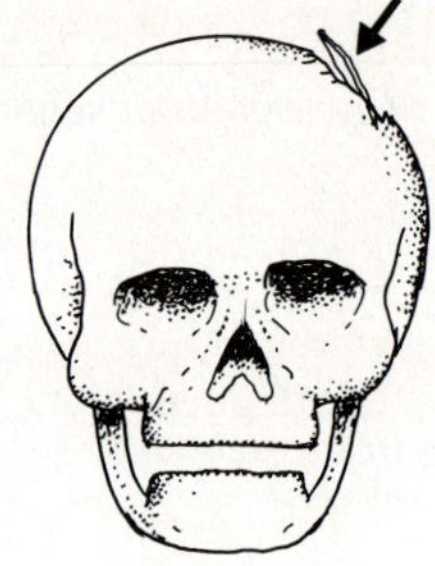

FIGURE 10.2   Skull fractures.

Concussion

This is a violent shaking or jarring of the brain that results in transient loss of consciousness disappearing within either minutes or days. There is no permanent neurologic damage. Other symptoms may include headache, vomiting, and memory loss or confusion. The child is usually not hospitalized unless loss of consciousness lasts longer than 5 minutes or persistent vomiting is present (Figure 10.3).

Contusion

Scalp, forehead, or facial contusions are associated with local swelling and tenderness with variable bruising. There is usually no neurological deficit.

Brain contusions represent a severe injury with hemorrhage and swelling in the brain tissue, usually resulting in marked alterations in level of consciousness (Figure 10.3).

Hemorrhage

An *epidural* hemorrhage occurs with a skull fracture and meningeal artery bleed located between the skull and the dura. A *subdural* hematoma results from a laceration of the vein network between the dura and the surface of the brain. These hematomas can occur hours to days after the injury. An *intracerebral* hemorrhage results from a brain laceration (Figure 10.4).

Patient Care

History

During assessment it is important to note the mechanism of injury and establish by history the circumstances surrounding the injury. The information should be obtained from the parents, teachers, or bystanders.

- What happened? Was the child struck on the head or did the child

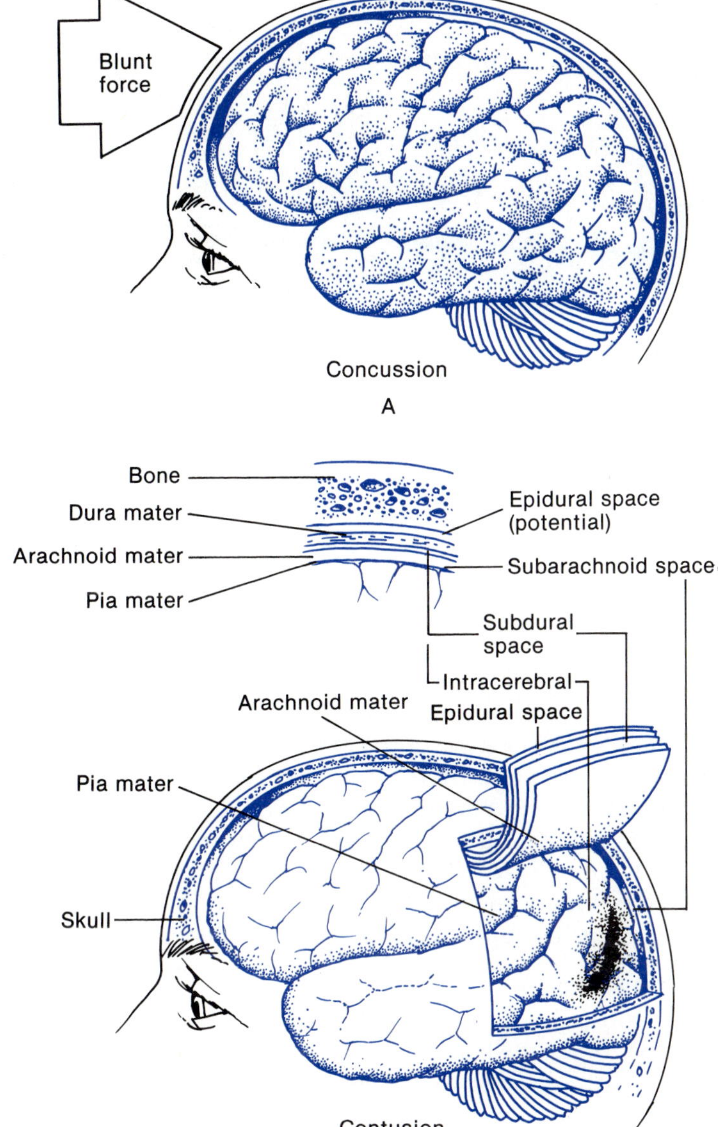

FIGURE 10.3 (A) Concussion vs. (B) contusion. Closed head injuries: (A) In a concussion there is no detectable brain damage. (B) In a contusion there is bruising or rupturing of the brain tissue and vessels at any of the identified levels.

fall? What was the approximate force of the injury? When did the injury occur?

- Did the child lose consciousness immediately or at a later time? Was the child ever disoriented after the head injury? How long did the loss of consciousness or disorientation last?

- Did the child vomit? If so, how long after the head injury?

- Did the child have a seizure before or after the head injury?

- If the child can respond, ask about any visual disturbance, severe headache, tingling or numbness in the extremities.

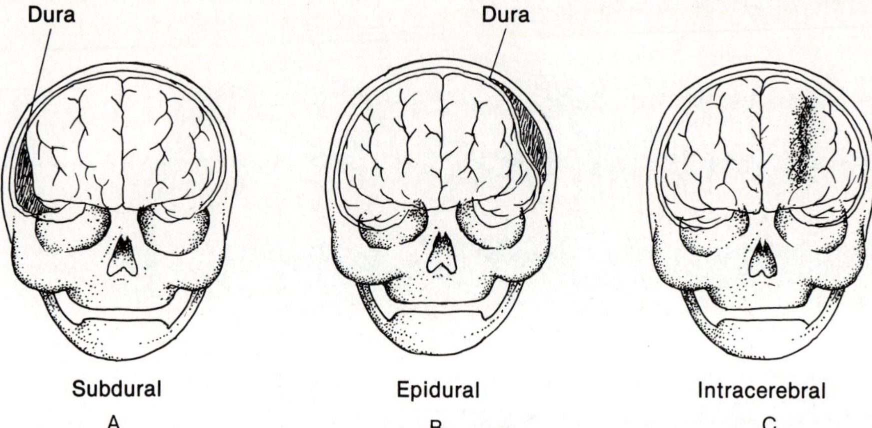

FIGURE 10.4 Hematomas within the skull: (A) subdural, (B) epidural, (C) intracerebral.

Assessment

Expect any child with a head injury to have an associated cervical spine injury. Some children will have a maxillofacial injury, so carefully inspect the airway for teeth, blood, mucous, and loss of continuity of the jaw when performing the primary trauma assessment.

After assessment and management of the ABC's, assess the level of consciousness with the Glasgow Coma Scale (see Table 3.3). Ask older children questions to test their orientation to time, place, and person. Altered mental status is present when a child asks the same question over and over, even when it has already been answered.

The child with a head injury may be alert or have any level of alteration in level of consciousness: lethargy, stupor, or coma. Note any decorticate, decerebrate, or other abnormal posturing in the comatose child.

Secondary Survey

Inspect and palpate the skull for fractures or depressions. Note any clear or amber drainage from the nose or ears, which is indicative of a basilar skull fracture. Check for bruising behind the ear (Battle's sign) or around the eyes (raccoon eyes), signaling a basilar skull fracture.

Check pupillary response, noting size of the pupils and their reactivity to bright light. Asymmetry of the pupil size, abnormal lateral gaze, and roving eye movements are indications of head trauma (Figure 10.5). See Table 10.1 for characteristics associated with mild, moderate, and severe head injuries.

CAUTION! 

Shock in Children with Head Injury
Children with signs of hypovolemic shock generally have other associated injuries. Only infants who have an open fontanelle and open sutures can hold enough blood in the head to cause hypovolemic shock. If there is an associated cervical spine injury, the child may be in *neurogenic* shock. Signs of hypovolemic shock include tachycardia and cool, clammy skin. In contrast, signs of neurogenic shock include bradycardia and warm, dry extremities.

Head and Spinal Cord Injury

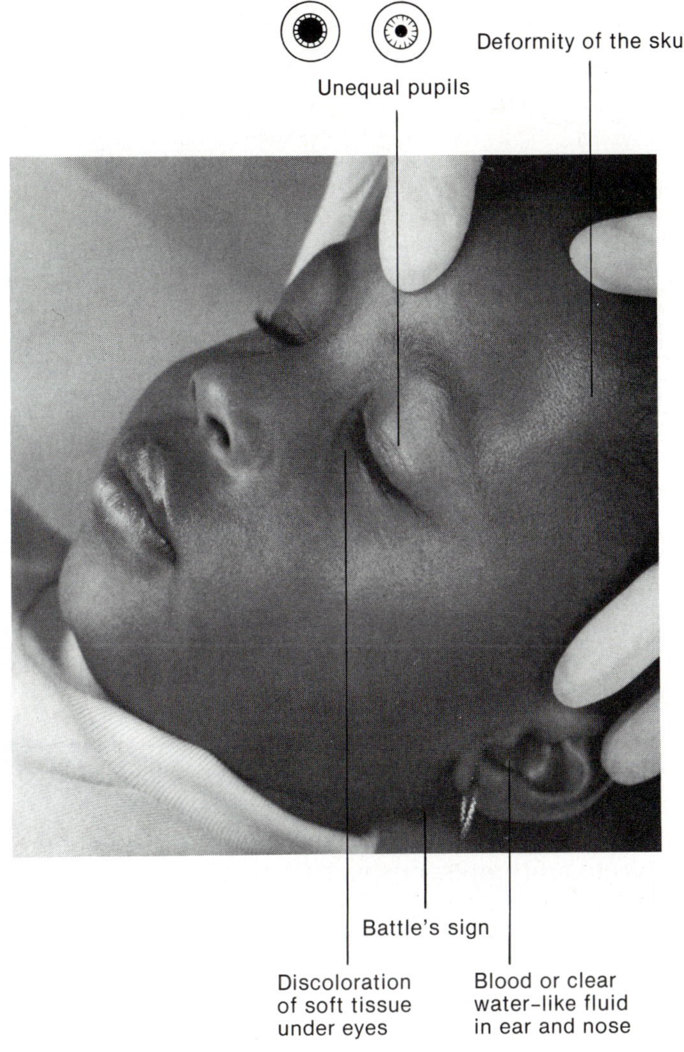

FIGURE 10.5 Inspect the skull and head for signs of a skull fracture.

Increased Intracranial Pressure

In the early stages of rising intracranial pressure (ICP), the blood pressure may be elevated, the heart rate is slow, and breathing is slow and deep, alternating with rapid deep breaths (Cheyne-Stokes respiration). The child is responsive to pain and might demonstrate decorticate posturing. Typical decorticate posturing includes adduction of the arms at the shoulders; the arms are flexed on the chest with the wrists flexed and the hands fisted; and the lower extremities are extended and adducted.

The infant with ICP has a bulging fontanelle, irritability, and listlessness. The child usually exhibits altered mental status along with the three signs of the Cushing's reflex (widening pulse pressure, decreasing heart rate, and abnormal respirations). As the intracranial pressure continues to rise, the systolic blood pressure increases while the heart and respiratory

Characteristic	Mild	Moderate	Severe
Consciousness	Transient loss Altered mental status	Loss of consciousness	Coma
Glasgow Coma Score	14–15	9–13	<9
Behavior	Crying, agitated, easily consoled	Agitated, combative, not easily consoled	Quiet, unresponsive
Signs	Local tissue swelling Redness over injury site	Moves spontaneously May have CSF leak Pupils reactive	Bulging fontanelle Pupils unresponsive Posturing Increased intracranial pressure (ICP)
Type of Injury	Simple skull fracture Concussion	Hemorrhage (subdural, epidural, intraventricular)	Brain laceration Acute subdural and intracerebral hematoma

Source: Developed by author.

rates decrease. Pupils become fixed and dilated, and the child becomes flaccid and unresponsive to pain. This child needs immediate transport and efficient prehospital management.

The findings at the scene, on reassessment during transport, and how they change over time are essential to detect signs of deterioration or improvement in the child. This information is important for the receiving hospital to plan definitive treatment of the head-injured child.

Management

Effective recognition of the head-injured child with hypoxemia and hypovolemia along with aggressive intervention can save a child's life and prevent long-term disability.

BLS field care of the child with a head injury should include the following:

- Assess and monitor ABC's and neurologic status.
- In the case of a facial injury, suction blood, mucous, and vomitus from patient's airway. Remove broken teeth. *Do NOT insert a nasogastric tube or suction catheter in the nose if a cerebrospinal fluid leak, raccoon eyes, or Battle's sign are present.*
- Maintain the airway in the unconscious child by jaw thrust, or insert an oral airway using extreme care. The nasopharyngeal airway should not be used in the head-injured patient.
- Stabilize and immobilize the cervical spine.
- Using a bag-valve mask, hyperventilate the child with high-concentration, high-flow oxygen at a rate at least 5 breaths/min faster than the child's usual respiratory rate. This will increase the blood oxy-

gen level and decrease the blood carbon dioxide level, causing constriction of the blood vessels. This is the most effective method for temporarily lowering increased intracranial pressure.

- Manage shock with PASG application, if protocols permit. Hypovolemia must be managed even when increased intracranial pressure is present to allow adequate perfusion of brain tissue.
- Cover any scalp lacerations and apply pressure to stop the bleeding (see Chapter 9, "Trauma"). Use your entire hand to apply pressure over an area of suspected skull fracture.
- Apply normal saline-soaked gauze to open fractures.
- Do NOT remove impaled foreign bodies.
- Cover injured eyes with sterile gauze patch.
- Immediately transport patient.

ALS providers should also initiate the following additional care:

- Intubation to maintain the airway, only if necessary, such as in cases of long transport time or deteriorating respiratory status (see "Intubation Risks" box).
- Insert an IV of Ringer's Lactate or Normal Saline to run at a keep-open rate. In cases of hypovolemic shock, treat the child with boluses of Ringer's Lactate at 20 ml/kg IV push.

Intubation Risks
Intubation of the head-injured child is often difficult because of the need to keep the patient's neck stabilized. It also creates more risk for the child with facial or basilar skull fractures or increased intracranial pressure. In the case of the head-injured child, intubation in the controlled hospital setting is preferable to attempts in the field. Children can usually be adequately ventilated by bag-mask ventilation. 

Spinal Cord Injury

Spinal cord injuries are fortunately not as common in children as they are in adults; however, the types of injuries that do occur in children are potentially life-threatening or may cause permanent disabilities. Major causes of spinal cord injuries in children are falls, motor vehicle crashes, and sports injuries. Cervical spine injuries occur in approximately 1% of all injured children; however, about 18% of children injured in a motor vehicle crash have an injury to the cervical spine.

Cervical Spine

By 8 years of age the bony structure of the child's cervical spine has achieved an adult appearance on X ray. In the younger child, significant physiologic differences exist in the development of the spinal column that contribute to significant injuries.

- There is much greater mobility in the cervical spine of a young child because the vertebrae are wedge-shaped. Subluxation can occur with relatively little force.
- The fulcrum of neck motion occurs much higher in children (C2–3 level) than in adults (C5–6 level), leading to higher cervical spine injuries. The most common sites of cervical spine injury in young children are at C1, C2, and C3.
- Because the head is heavier, greater stress is placed on the spinal cord with flexion-extension injuries. The spinal cord is also less elastic than the ligaments and cartilage that protect it.
- The neck muscles of the infant are not well developed; some of the forces involved in injury are not reduced. Infants who have not yet achieved head control are at great risk for cervical spine injury.

Assessment

As with adults, assume there has been a cervical spine injury every time a head injury is suspected in the pediatric patient. During the secondary survey, assess for spontaneous and purposeful movement and sensation in the extremities. Pain on palpation of the neck is another sign of neck injury.

Management

All prehospital care providers should institute immediate stabilization of the cervical spine while performing the primary survey. Immobilize the child on a backboard with a small towel or pad at the shoulders to maintain the cervical spine in straight alignment. This will compensate for the large occiput of the child's head, which would normally result in a flexion of the cervical spine.

Lumbar Spine

The increased emphasis and use of car safety belts for children has led to occasional lumbar spine injury. Lap belts in cars are not designed for the child with a small, bony pelvis. This frequently results in an elevated position of the lap belt across the abdomen. Approximately 10% of all children who wear safety belts at the time of a motor vehicle crash will have the "lap belt syndrome" of abdominal and lumbar spine injuries. The spinal injury (dislocation, fracture, subluxation, or rupture of the spinal ligaments) is caused by hyperflexion of the spine around the lap belt. See Chapter 11 for a description of abdominal injuries. Children should ride in vehicles equipped with safety seats or lap/shoulder strap combination (Figure 10.6).

Assessment

During the secondary survey of any child passenger in a motor vehicle crash, ask the parent if the lap belt was fastened, and then inspect the abdomen for the classic sign of abdominal bruising and abrasion in the shape of the lap belt.

Management

All prehospital care providers should provide the following care to the child with a suspected lumbar spine injury from the lap belt syndrome.

- Place the child on a backboard and immobilize the entire spine.
- Assess and manage any potential shock from the abdominal injuries as outlined in the sections in Chapter 9 dealing with primary and secondary trauma assessment.

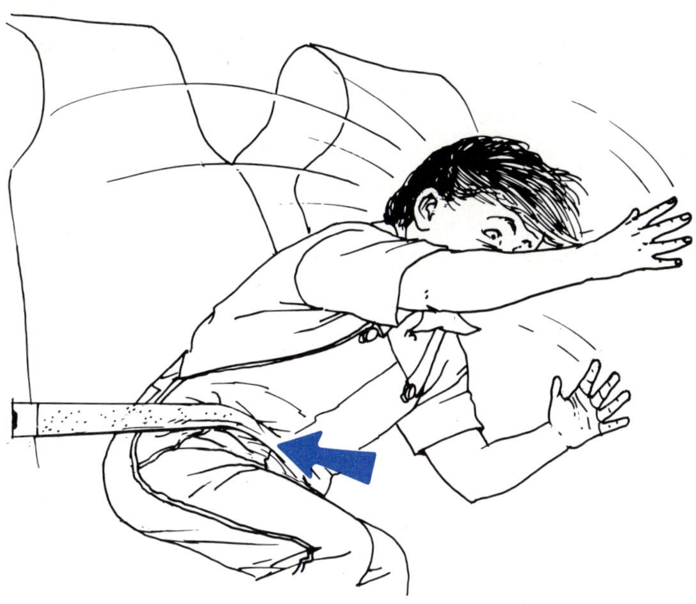

FIGURE 10.6 Forces on the abdomen and lumbar spine from a lapbelt in cases of an accelerating–decelerating injury.

Head and Spinal Cord Injury References

AMACHER, A. L., "Pediatric head injury: A national tragedy." In Chapman, P. H., ed., *Concepts of Pediatric Neurosurgery.* New York: Karger, 1985, pp. 76–83.

FUCHS, S., and others, "Cervical spine fractures sustained by young children in forward-facing car seats," *Pediatrics,* 84, no. 2 (August 1989), pp. 348–354.

GILMORE, H. E., "Emergency management of head trauma in children," *Emergency Care Quarterly,* 3, no. 1 (1987), pp. 37–44.

HERZENBERG, J. E., and HENSINGER, R. N., "Pediatric cervical spine injuries," *Trauma Quarterly,* 5, no. 2 (1989), p. 73.

JOHNSON, D. L., "Head Injury." In Eichelberger, M. R., and Pratsch, G. L., eds., *Pediatric Trauma Care.* Rockville, Md.: Aspen Publishing Co., 1988, pp. 87–99.

LARSON, L., and others, *Trauma Nurse Core Course Manual,* 2nd ed. Chicago: Emergency Nurses Association, 1988.

MAYER, T., and others, "The modified injury severity scale in pediatric multiple trauma patients," *Journal of Pediatric Surgery,* 15, no. 6 (December 1980), pp. 719–726.

MAYER, T., and others, "Causes of morbidity and mortality in severe pediatric trauma," *Journal of the American Medical Association,* 245, no. 7 (Feb. 20, 1981), pp. 719–721.

NEWMAN, K. D., and others, "The lap belt complex: Intestinal and lumbar spine injury in children," *Journal of Trauma,* 30 (1990), pp. 1133–1140.

REEVES, K., "Assessment of pediatric head injury: The basics," *Journal of Emergency Nursing,* 15, no. 4 (July/August 1989), pp. 329–332.

REYNOLDS, E., DIERKING, B., and RAMENOFSKY, M. L., "Head care for kids," *Emergency,* 20, no. 10 (October 1988), pp. 43–48.

RUGE, J. R., and others, "Pediatric spinal injury: The very young," *Journal of Neurosurgery,* 68, no. 1 (January 1988), pp. 25–30.

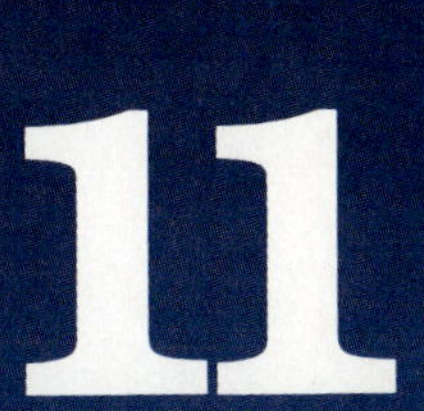

Chest, Abdominal, and Extremity Injuries

OBJECTIVES

When you have completed this chapter you should be able to

✴ Describe the unique characteristics of the child's anatomy pertaining to chest injuries.

✴ Describe the assessment and management of the life-threatening chest injuries in children.

✴ List the two abdominal organs most commonly injured in children.

✴ List and describe the most common fractures in children.

Chest Injuries

Chest injury is second to head injury as the leading cause of death from accidental injury in the United States. Thoracic trauma in children is usually blunt, with a wide range of mechanisms of injury that include motor vehicle crashes, either as a pedestrian or as an unrestrained passenger, and bicycle crashes, again as a pedestrian struck or from a handlebar injury to the chest wall. Falls from heights also produce chest injuries. Penetrating injury to the chest comes from plate glass, stones, guns, and knives.

Several unique characteristics of the child's anatomy pertain to chest injuries. The bone and cartilage of the chest are extremely resilient, accounting for the low incidence of rib fractures, but contusion to the lung can occur. The mediastinum in a child, and particularly in infants, is capable of wide shifts, with dislocation of the heart, compression of the lung, and angulation of the great vessels and of the trachea. The upper airway is much smaller and prone to obstruction from blood and mucous. Children who sustain major injury swallow air, which results in gastric distention that impinges on the movement of the diaphragm, further compromising the already limited lung volume. Children under 9 years of age are abdominal breathers. If the abdomen fails to move with respiration, a serious abdominal problem may be indicated.

Assessment and management of chest injuries are part of the primary survey. Several chest injuries are life-threatening, and prompt recognition and response can affect the mortality rate.

Pneumothorax / Hemothorax

Pneumothorax is spontaneous collapse of the lung from blunt or penetrating trauma. It is the most common life-threatening chest injury in children. *Hemothorax* is the accumulation of blood in the pleural space caused by a tear in a blood vessel or lacerated lung. The accumulation of blood in the pleural space causes the lung to collapse. The key symptom is decreased breath sounds on the side of the injury and respiratory distress. If shock is present without an apparent bleeding site consider the possibility of a hemothorax (Figure 11.1).

Tension Pneumothorax

Tension pneumothorax is the progressive entry of air from the lung or through the chest wall into the pleural space that results in lung collapse. It may result from an open chest wound or blunt trauma in which the trachea or bronchi are torn. This produces a shift of the trachea, heart, and esophagus toward the unaffected lung, resulting in angulation of the major blood vessels of the heart and decreased cardiac output. Signs of a tension pneumothorax are decreased breath sounds and paradoxical chest motion. This is a *true medical emergency.* A child with these signs should be transported immediately to the hospital. Administer high flow, high concentration oxygen and cover any open chest wound. This injury can be exacerbated by positive pressure ventilation. ALS management is needle thoracostomy (Figure 11.2).

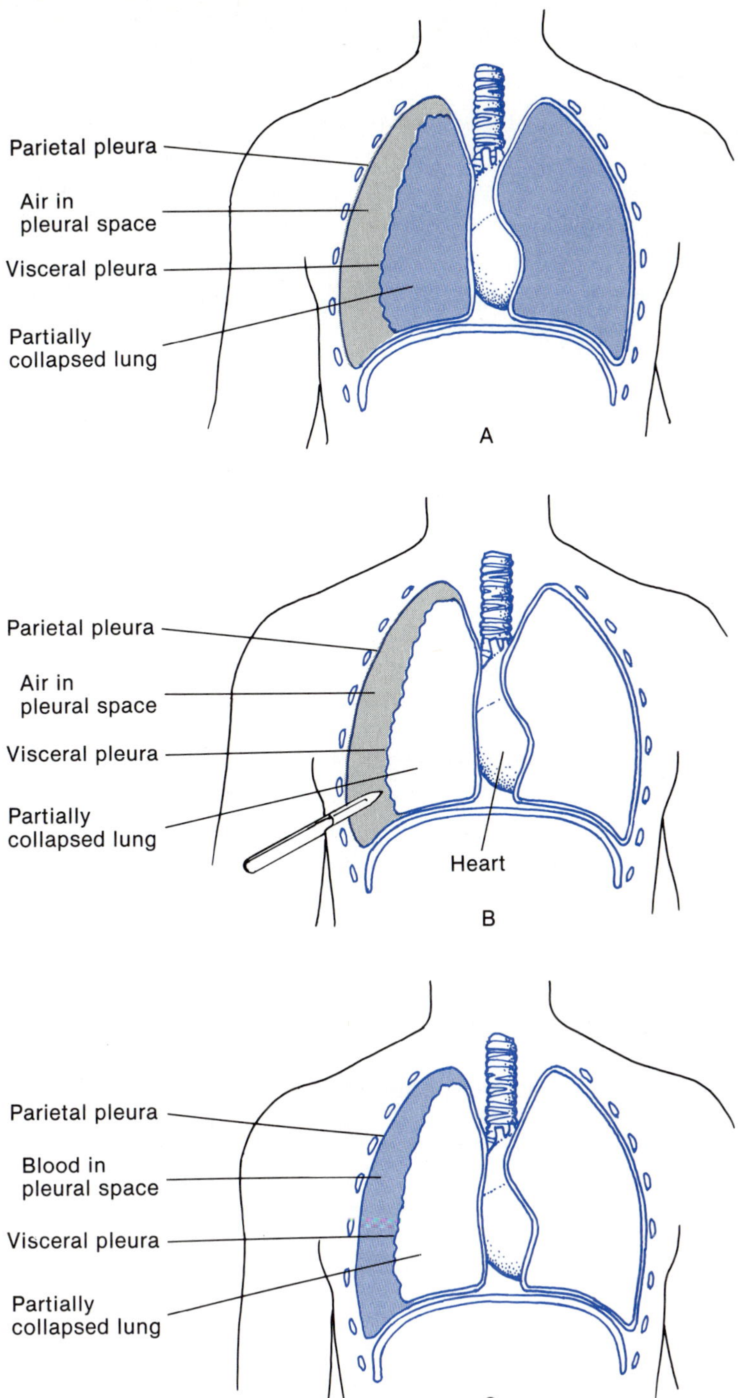

FIGURE 11.1   Injuries to the chest: (A) closed pneumothorax, (B) pneumothorax from a penetrating injury, (C) hemothorax.

Cardiac Tamponade

Trauma to the heart and major blood vessels in the chest is uncommon in children. It does occur with penetrating injuries, however. This injury causes bleeding into the pericardial space around the heart, resulting in impairment of the efficient pumping of the heart. Symptoms are distended

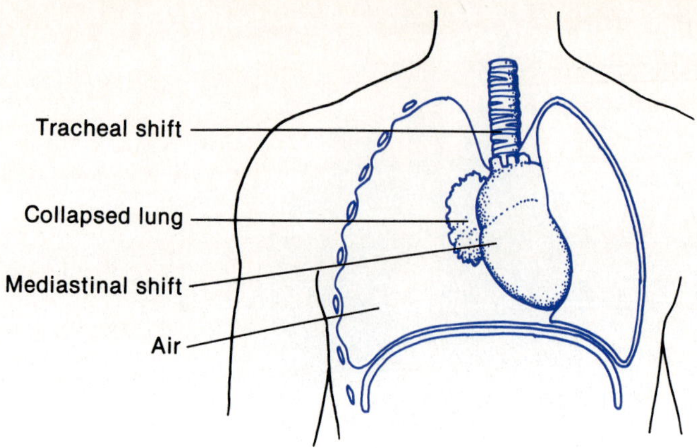

FIGURE 11.2 Tension pneumothorax.

neck veins, weak pulse, muffled heart sounds, and narrowing pulse pressure. Narrow pulse pressure is the difference between systolic and diastolic pressure observed at a specified interval. A pulse pressure below 15 mm Hg is critical, indicating an immediate life-threatening emergency. Cardiac arrest is the end result if these symptoms go untreated. This situation requires immediate transport. Treatment is performed at the hospital by inserting a needle into the pericardial space to aspirate the accumulated blood.

Flail Chest

Flail chest results from multiple rib fractures in sequence, where three or more ribs are each broken in at least two places, creating an unstable chest wall, or the detachment of the sternum. This results in a shifting back-and-forth movement of the major structures—lung, trachea, heart—with every respiration. Symptoms are palpable rib fracture, dyspnea, and the flail segment being unstable that it moves independently of the chest wall (paradoxical movement). (See Figure 11.3.)

Abdominal Injury

Blunt trauma is the most common cause of injury, and the spleen and liver are the organs most often affected. These injuries result from motor vehicle crashes, falls, child abuse, play, or sport-related injuries. Penetrating injuries are from guns, knives, or impalement on sharp objects.

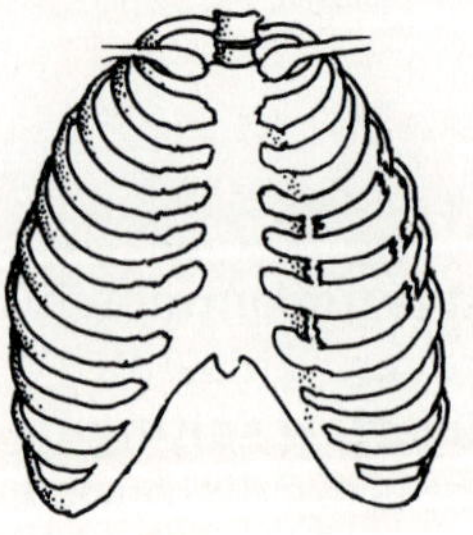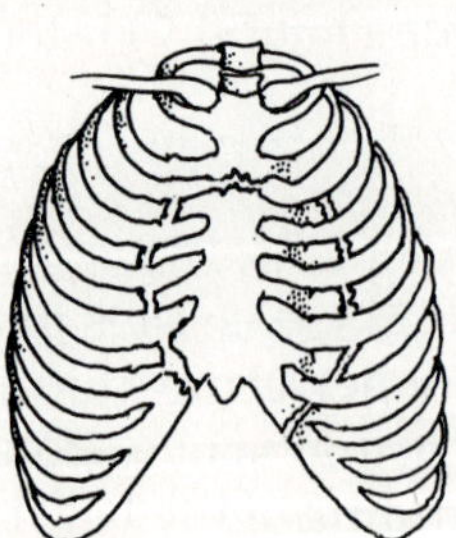

FIGURE 11.3 Flail chest.

The unique features of the child's abdominal cavity are that the abdominal organs are slightly large in relation to the abdominal cavity, the undeveloped abdominal muscles offer little protection, and the liver, spleen, and other organs are more exposed to direct trauma because of the broad costal arch (Figure 3.1).

The main concern with abdominal injuries for the prehospital provider is that major abdominal trauma may result in life-threatening shock. After the primary survey is completed, the abdominal assessment, part of the secondary survey, is performed keeping the following in mind: Observe the abdomen anteriorly, laterally, and posteriorly for any lacerations, contusions, and distention; palpate for pain and tenderness.

Spleen

This is the most commonly injured organ in children. Injury to the spleen most often occurs after blunt trauma from a motor vehicle crash, fall, or blow to the flank or torso. Abrasions, ecchymosis, and tenderness suggest the possibility of this injury.

Liver

Injury to the liver occurs as frequently as spleen injury. A common mechanism of injury is a blow to the right upper quadrant or chest. Severe hemorrhage can result from vascular injuries inside the liver, or injuries to the vena cava and hepatic veins. Symptoms include right upper quadrant pain that may be referred to the shoulder. Rupture of the liver has a high mortality rate with the child presenting in shock, and a tense, distended abdomen.

Pelvis and Perineal Areas

Pelvic trauma usually occurs after trauma from a fall or a motor vehicle accident. Assess femoral pulses (note swelling or hematomas). Palpate pelvic girdle for tenderness or deformity. Inspect genitalia and perineal areas for hematoma (blood at the urethra and ecchymosis of the perineum may indicate bladder rupture or pelvic fracture).

Extremity Injuries

Children are very active and grow at a rapid rate. At times their coordination cannot keep up with the physical demands placed on their bodies; cuts, bruises, and fractures are the result. The types of fractures in children are determined by the child's age, developmental skills, and the season of the year (Table 11.1).

Fractures are not life-threatening, except for amputation or major arterial hemorrhage from a bone fragment severing the vessel. However, skeletal fractures have the potential for producing permanent disability, especially when there is associated nerve and blood vessel damage. When approaching a child with multiple injuries including fractures, the pri-

TABLE 11.1 Orthopedic Injuries According to Children's Developmental Level

Age Group	Mechanism of Injury	Types of Injury
6–12 months Rolls over Creeps Crawls	MVC*: passenger Falls: high chair, crib, tables, stairs	Brain injury Fractures: skull extremity
Toddler 1–3 years Walking Climbing	MVC: passenger, pedestrian Falls: stairs, tables, playgrounds, windows Held up, pulled, or lifted up by one arm	Brain injury Fractures: skull extremity Soft tissue injury Nursemaid's elbow
Preschooler 3–6 years Growth spurts Very Active Very curious	MVC: Pedestrian, passenger bike and big wheel Falls: playground, windows Lawnmower	Brain injury Fractures: skull, pelvis, extremity
School Age 6–12 years Growth spurts Peer pressure Accepts dares	MVC: Pedestrian, passenger bike Falls: bike, skateboard Sports	Brain injury C-spine injury Fractures: skull, pelvis, extremity Subluxation L1-2, dislocation Soft tissue injuries

*MVC, motor vehicle crash.

mary survey priorities of airway, breathing, circulatory assessment, neurologic exam, and keeping exposure to a minimum always remain.

Children's bones are unique compared to the adult; they are more porous and more flexible, resulting in different patterns of injury. This results in bone that bends and splinters during the stress of an injury, increasing the risk for soft tissue damage, as well as vascular and nerve damage. Bone healing occurs faster in children; the younger the child the faster the healing process.

Long bones of children grow from a narrow strip of preosseous material called the *epiphyseal plate* at the ends of the bone. Significant injuries to this area of bone result in growth deformities and discrepancies of bone length and joint deformities (Figure 11.4).

Types of Fractures

- *Bend* fracture: A child's flexible bone can be bent 45° or more before breaking. The bone will straighten slowly, but not completely, to produce some deformity but without the angulation seen when the bone breaks.

- *Buckle* fracture: This appears as a raised or bulging projection at the fracture site.

Chest, Abdominal, and Extremity Injuries

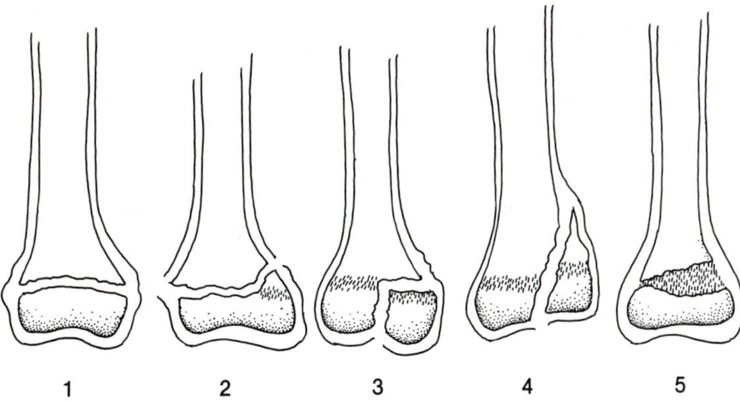

FIGURE 11.4   Types of epiphyseal fractures (Salter classification).

- A *green-stick* fracture is an incomplete fracture similar to the break observed when a green stick is bent and partially breaks.
- A *complete* fracture is one that divides the bone fragments. They often remain attached by a periosteal hinge (Figure 11.5).
- *Epiphyseal* fractures are classified as Salter I through Salter V, with the type of growth disruption increasing from type I through type V.

Potential for Disability

Even though a skeletal injury is not life-threatening, there is the potential for great disability if evaluation of the extremities does not include a neurovascular assessment (see Chapter 9).

FIGURE 11.5   Types of fractures in children.

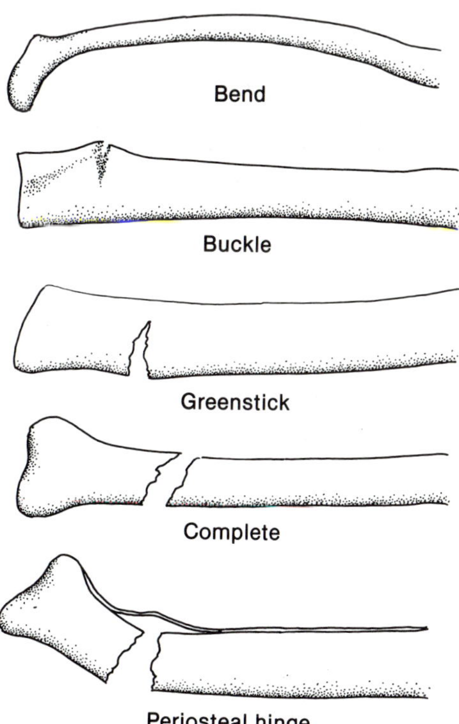

Compartment Syndrome

Compartment syndrome is a true emergency in a child. It is a condition whereby the pressure within the closed space of the muscle increases to the point where the blood supply to the muscle fibers is occluded. The pressure is usually caused by hemorrhage, swelling of tissues, or a tight tourniquet-like dressing. It is extremely painful and requires emergency surgical intervention at the hospital.

The primary symptom of compartment syndrome is severe pain. If your assessment does not reveal major extremity injury perform a neurovascular assessment, looking for changes such as diminished pulses, poor capillary refill, and decreased sensation in the affected extremity to alert you to the possibility of compartment syndrome.

Open Fracture

Children's bones splinter and may cause pinpoint open wounds (Figure 11.6). Treat any open lesion over a fracture as an open fracture. Do not reduce an open fracture but notify the receiving hospital of the fracture. Treatment of potential infection in the bone must be initiated quickly.

Management of open wounds requires the reduction of contamination and control of bleeding. Flush generously with Normal Saline or Ringer's Lactate. Cover with a sterile gauze roll bandage. Open bleeding wounds require a pressure dressing. Because of the possibility of causing a tourniquet effect resulting in compartment syndrome, do not use elastic bandages for additional pressure.

Splinting Management

Splinting an extremity fracture lessens the possibility of further damage to the nerve, blood vessel, muscle, and skin that may occur with movement of the extremity. Perform the following steps:

- Remove the clothing from around the fracture site.
- Check pulse, capillary refill, and sensation in the extremity before and after application of the splint.

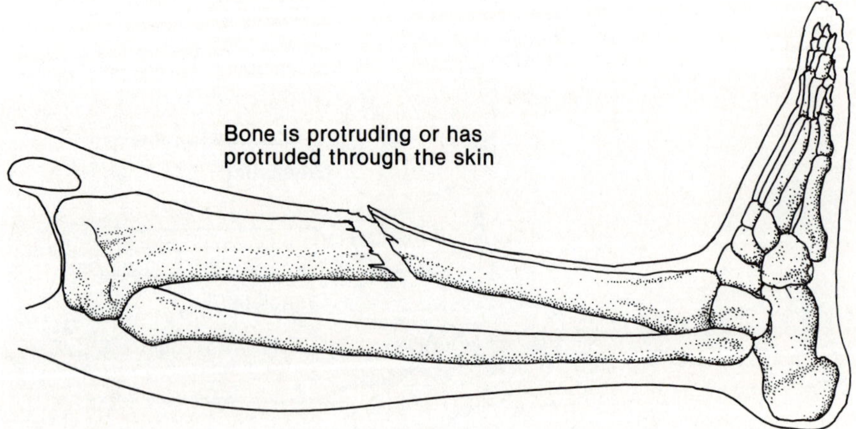

FIGURE 11.6   Open fracture—the bone may have splintered, protruding through the skin and then withdrawing.

- Apply sterile dressings to any open wounds before splinting.
- Immobilize the fracture site above and below the fracture site.
- Splint in the position found; do not try to correct the deformity.
- Take caution when the application of the PASG is needed. Assess the lower extremities carefully to detect any fracture of the long bones, deformity, instability, ecchymosis, weak or absent pulses. Any extended length of time in the PASG may result in vascular compromise producing compartment syndrome.

Chest, Abdominal, and Extremity Injuries References

BUDASSI, S., and BARBER J., *Emergency Nursing Principles and Practice*, St. Louis: The C. V. Mosby, Co., 1981, p. 506.

EICHELBERGER, M. R., and RANDOLPH, J. G., "Chest trauma in children." In Brook, B. F., ed., *The Injured Child.* Austin: University of Texas Press, 1985, pp. 44–52.

EICHELBERGER, M. R., "Trauma of the airway and thorax," *Pediatric Annals,* 16, no. 4 (April 1987), pp. 307–316.

EICHELBERGER, M. R., and RANDOLPH, J. G., "Abdominal trauma." In Welch, K. G., and others, eds., *Pediatric Surgery.* Chicago: Yearbook Medical Publishers, 1986, pp. 154–174.

NEWMAN, K. D., EICHELBERGER, M. R., and RANDOLPH, J. G., "Abdominal injury." In Eichelberger, M. R., and Pratsch, G. L., eds., *Pediatric Trauma Care.* Rockville, Md.: Aspen Publishing Co., 1988, pp. 101–104.

Burns

OBJECTIVES

When you have completed this chapter you should be able to

* Describe common mechanisms of burn injury to children of each developmental age.
* Describe the application of the "rule of nines" to children of different ages or sizes.
* List the signs indicating the possibility of airway burns.
* Identify the burned child needing care in a burn center.
* Describe the field management for each of the following types of burns:
  * Thermal
  * Inhalation
  * Chemical
  * Electrical

Epidemiology of Burn Injuries

Burns, the second leading cause of death, claim the lives of 1200 children annually in the United States, accounting for approximately 15% of all accidental deaths. The death rate from flame injuries in the United States is the second highest in the world and by far the highest among industrialized nations.

Burns also leave 60,000 children hospitalized, many of whom suffer significantly from the physical and psychological scars of being a burn victim. The average age of burned children is 32 months. Child abuse is suspected in approximately 16% of these cases (Table 12.1).

Types of Burns

Thermal Burns

Thermal burns are the result of contact with direct flame, or with hot liquids such as water, tea, coffee, or grease.

Scald burns are the most common type of burns in children. Toddlers like to explore and can easily pull a cup of hot liquid onto their face, neck, arms, and chest. Fortunately, liquids cool quickly and run off, minimizing contact time. Hot grease and thick soup stay in contact with the skin longer, transmitting more heat and resulting in a full-thickness or third degree burn.

Immersion into hot water will result in a full-thickness burn after short exposure, depending upon the temperature of the water. The range of exposure time is as follows:

- *2 seconds* when the water temperature is 150°F or higher, hardly enough time to respond and withdraw the extremity, and
- 10 minutes at 120°F in the adult and even less time in the child.

Both the Federal Consumer Product Safety Commission and the plumbing industry have proposed voluntary standards requiring installation of a device that would limit new bathtub and shower hot water heaters to 120°F (50°C), unlikely to cause third degree burns, except in neonates.

Flame burns follow scalds in frequency (13%). Older children are most likely to sustain flame burns from playing with matches. Infants sustain

TABLE 12.1 Distribution of Common Burn Injuries in Children

Type of Burn Injury	Percentage of All Pediatric Burns
Scald	85
Flame	13
Electrical	1
Chemical	1

Source: Adapted from Herndon, D., and Thompson, P., (1985): "Treatment of burns in children," *Pediatric Clinics of North America,* 32(5):1311–1332.

the most severe burns from house fires. The most common early cause of death (within the first hour) from flame burns is respiratory failure from smoke inhalation.

Fireworks injuries are seasonal and may cause full-thickness burns. Fireworks commonly cause injuries to three body areas:

- The hand, when the firecracker explodes while being held;
- The foot, when the firecracker is dropped; and
- The trunk, when the firecracker explodes in the pocket.

Chemical Burns

Chemical burns can result from contact with a variety of solids, liquids, powders, or gases that irritate or burn the skin surface, mucous membranes, or internal organs. They cause variable tissue damage. Lye is especially damaging to the skin, leaving a full-thickness burn as it runs along the skin. Chemical burns also result from ingesting harmful agents such as household products or caustic chemicals. See Chapter 8, "Poisoning Emergencies," for more information.

Electrical Burns

Electrical burns result from contact with low-voltage electrical cords or high-voltage tension wires. There are about 1300 fatalities annually in the United States from electrical injury with pediatric patients accounting for about a third of the victims.

Toddlers can be injured while playing with electrical appliances, sucking on an electrical cord, or, more infrequently, playing with wall sockets. There have also been a significant number of incidents involving the use of blow dryers and curling irons, especially in association with bathtub electrocutions. Older children can sustain electrical injuries when struck by lightning or when playing on high voltage structures.

The degree of tissue damage in electrical burns is related to the length of exposure to the voltage and the resistance of the tissues. A high-voltage injury can be compared to a crush injury. In addition, the child may be thrown when coming into contact with the electrical current. The injury occurs to large areas of the body and body organs as the current passes through. The heart and central nervous system are especially vulnerable to injury, with a lethal ventricular dysrhythmia resulting if the current crosses the heart at a critical time. Respiratory distress is common, and hypovolemic shock can result from internal bleeding. Moist skin in the antecubital, axillary, and popliteal spaces has a far lower resistance to electrical current, sometimes enough to ignite clothing and resulting in thermal burns.

Electrical injuries leave an entrance and exit wound. The entrance wound often appears dry, charred, and depressed in the center. Exit wounds often have a "blow-out" appearance. Oral burns in toddlers from chewing on electrical cords have a blown-out appearance. These burns may be significantly deeper, with more tissue destruction than their initial appearance would indicate, and require hospitalization. The eschar (dead

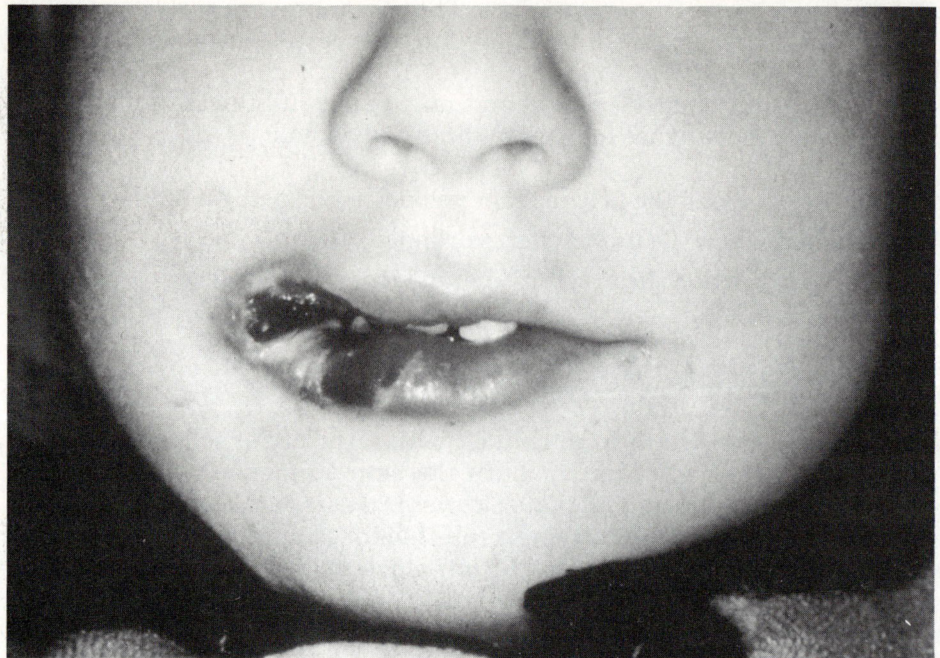

FIGURE 12.1   Burn from biting electrical cord.

tissue) begins to separate between 10 to 14 days, and hemorrhage can occur owing to sloughing of an artery near the wound (Figure 12.1).

Care for the Burn Injury

History

On arrival at the scene it is important to collect the following information about the child and mechanism of injury:

- How long ago did the injury occur?
- How did the injury occur?
- Was the child confined in an area with intense heat or smoke?
- Did the child have any other injury in addition to burn (i.e., fall, struck by falling objects, etc.)?
- Has there been any loss of consciousness?
- Does the child have any chronic diseases?

Assessment

Depth of Injury

The depth of burns are generally classified as *partial thickness* and *full thickness.* Another form of classification consists of first, second, and third degree burns (Figure 12.2 and Table 12.2).

Partial-thickness burns include both first degree and second degree

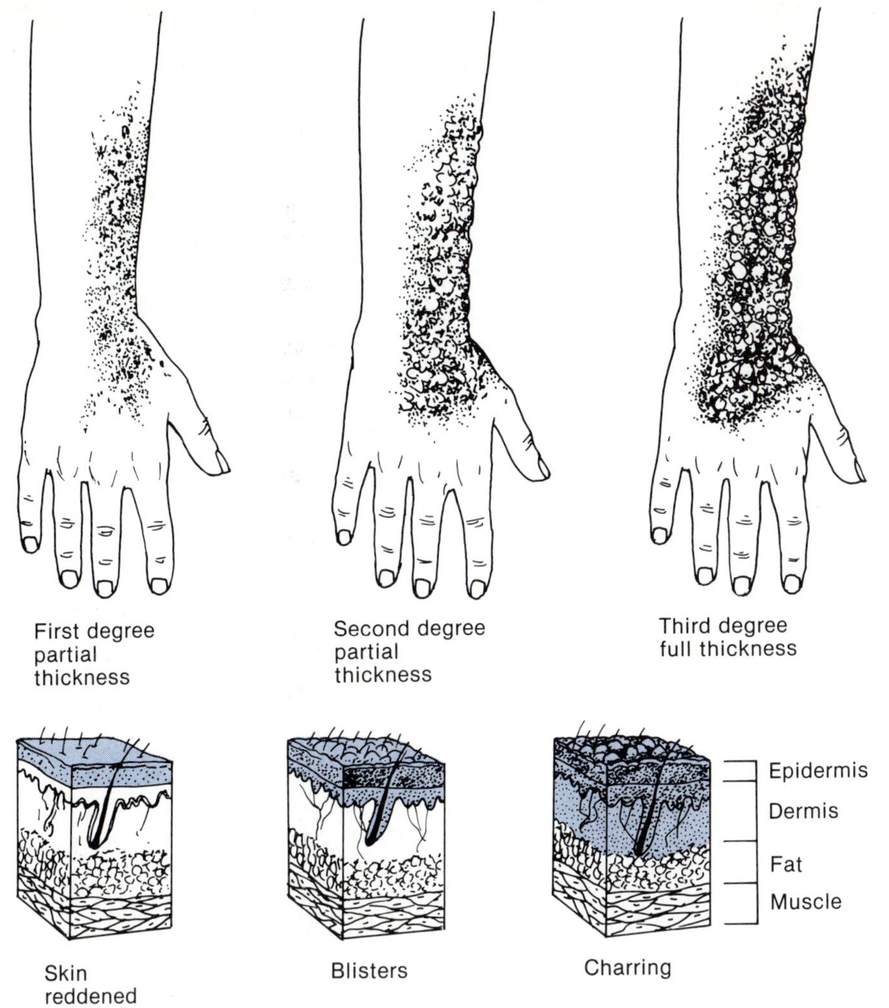

FIGURE 12.2 Severity by burn depth classification.

burns. A first degree burn is superficial, affecting the epidermis of the skin. It is very painful, and blanches readily with pressure. These result from a brief contact with a hot liquid or object, flame, or prolonged exposure to sunlight.

A second degree burn affects the dermis; however, the hair follicles, epidermis, sebaceous glands, and sweat glands are not injured. The burn is red and painful with blisters. These burns result from an intense contact

TABLE 12.2   Classification of Burn Severity in Children

Major Burns
Partial thickness—20% body surface area (BSA)
Full thickness >10% BSA
Burns to hands, face, eyes, ears, feet, perineum
Airway burn or smoke inhalation suspected
Electrical burns
Additional injuries, signs of shock
Children with chronic health conditions

Moderate Burns
Partial thickness—10–20% BSA
Full thickness—3–10% BSA

Minor Burns
Partial thickness <2% BSA
Full thickness <2% BSA

with a hot liquid or object, flame, or prolonged overexposure to sunlight.

A *full-thickness* burn (third degree) damages the epidermis, dermis, and the hair follicles, and the sebaceous glands and sweat glands. These burns are commonly painless, white or charred, and leathery in appearance. They result from contact with live steam, chemicals, and prolonged contact with flame or electric current.

Determination of Burn Surface Area

In adults, the "rule of nines" is used to determine the body surface area (BSA) involved. In children, body proportions and body surface area vary by age. The modified rule of nines for infants and children offers a method to calculate burn percentage (Figure 12.3).

An alternate method to assess BSA is to use the child's palm, or clenched fist, which equals 1% of the BSA. The child's palm serves as a guide for quick estimation of the body surface area burned. Remember to use the child's hand and not your own for the BSA calculation.

Assessment of Physiologic Status

Perform the primary and secondary survey, looking for signs of an airway injury and other major trauma (see Table 12.3). Blunt trauma to the chest may have occurred from a fall or explosion, resulting in a spontane-

FIGURE 12.3 Rule of nines: (A) adult; (B) adaptation for children.

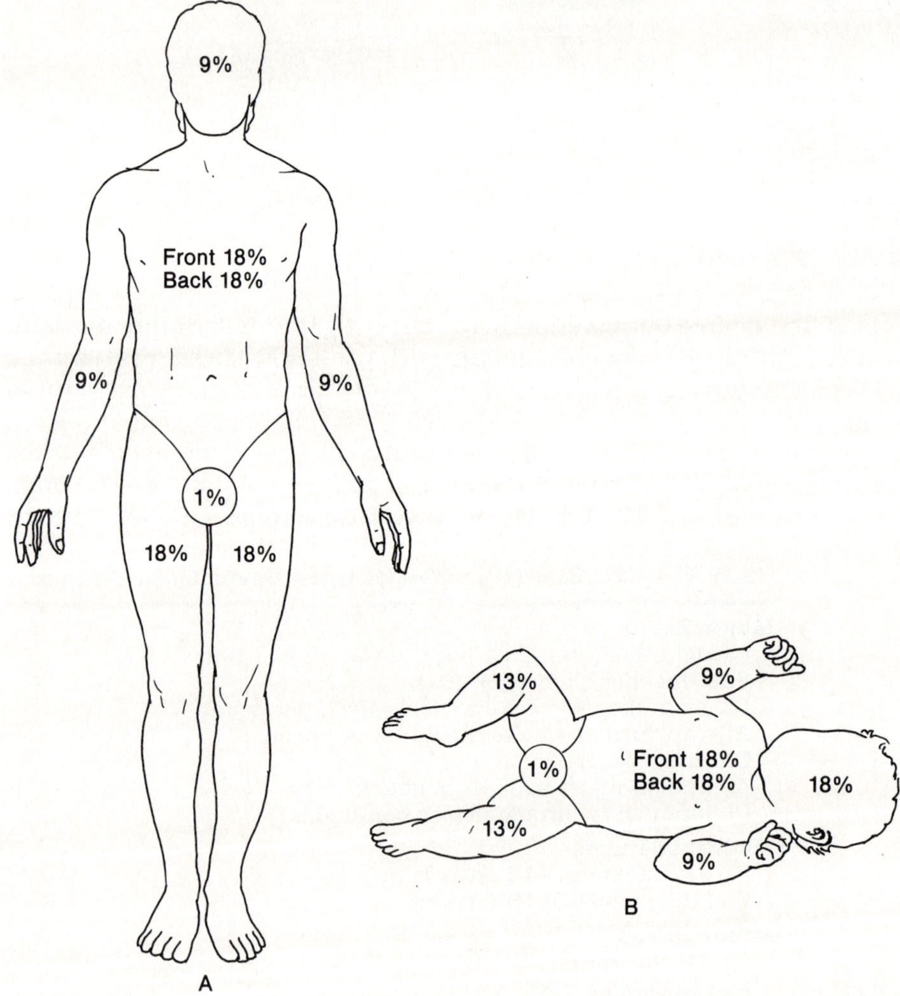

Burns

Child found in a confined space of a smoke-filled environment.
Child found unconscious in a smoke-filled environment.
Singed nasal hair.
Soot in septum, or around the nose and mouth.
Brassy cough, persistent cough.
Sore throat, stridor.
Agitation.
Respiratory distress—cyanosis.

ous pneumothorax or myocardial contusion. Assess the extent of burn injury and note any circumferential burns, those completely circling the chest or an extremity. Full-thickness circumferential burns around the chest or abdomen may interfere with the child's ability to ventilate.

Signs of shock occurring within 30 minutes of injury suggest an internal hemorrhage. Altered level of consciousness may result from a head injury or hypoxemia from smoke inhalation (Figure 12.4).

CAUTION!

Airway Injury

Any child found in a heavy smoke-filled environment is considered to have an inhalation injury. Exposure to the hot air and toxic fumes, including carbon monoxide, will cause the child's airway to swell and occlude up to 50% of the total airway. Because the swelling process is continuous and rapid, the decision to intubate needs to be determined early, especially if there is a long transport time. BLS providers should rapidly transport this child for airway management.

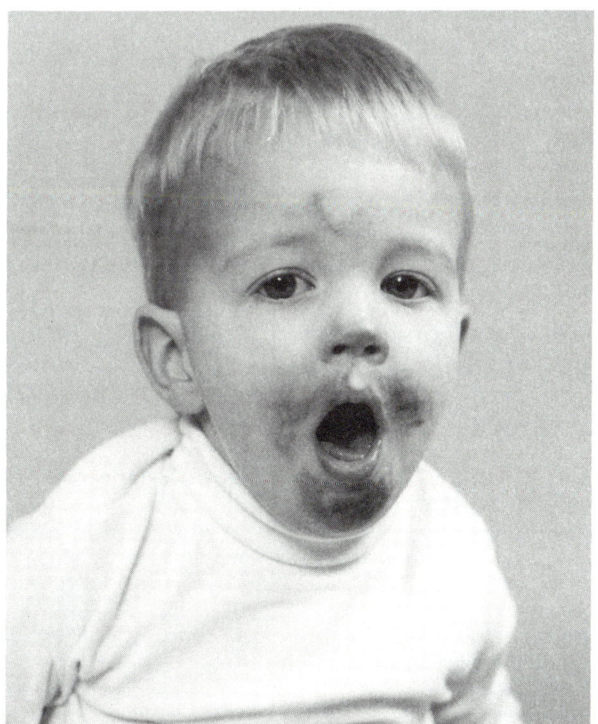

FIGURE 12.4 Suspect an inhalation injury in a child with soot around the nose and mouth and carbonaceous sputum, regardless of level of consciousness. The child's status could change rapidly.

Management of Thermal Burns

BLS care should include the following:

- Remove the child from the source of burn injury and stop the burning process.
- Assess and monitor ABCDE's, especially the airway.
- Administer high-flow oxygen, humidified if possible, by mask.
- When there is suspicion of inhalation injury, administer high-concentration, high-flow oxygen.
- Be prepared to bag-mask ventilate and to initiate CPR.
- Remove clothing over and around the burn, but do NOT remove clothing stuck to the burn. Remove jewelry, belt buckles, rings, boots, etc., which may retain heat and hide burns.
- Cover the child with a sterile or clean sheet. Keep the patient warm. Burned children are particularly susceptible to hypothermia. When the skin is damaged it loses its ability to retain body heat.
- For partial-thickness burns, apply cool, wet compresses to small areas for pain control, if within 2 hours of the injury. Cover no more than 15% of the body surface area at any time with cool, wet compresses to reduce the chance of hypothermia.
- For full-thickness burns, DO NOT wash or apply greasy substances or cool, wet compresses. Cover the child with a sterile sheet and blanket.
- DO NOT apply ice, or rupture blisters.
- Elevate head 30° to assist breathing if no head injury is suspected. Elevate the burned extremity.
- Rapidly transport the child with a major injury to a burn center, if available. DO NOT delay, especially with inhalation injury (Table 12.4).

ALS providers may initiate the following additional care:

- If performing orotracheal intubation, choose an endotracheal tube two sizes smaller than what is usually used for the child. Remember the mucous membranes of the airway are swollen and highly vulnerable to injury from intubation.
- If the burn covers more than 15% BSA, or there is other trauma,

TABLE 12.4   Characteristics of Burns that Should Be Evaluated at the Hospital

Burns greater than 10% body surface area (BSA).
Burns that involve the face, hands, feet, or genitalia even if the burn is less than 10% BSA.
All electrical and chemical burns, especially if the chemical was ingested.
Burns with smoke-inhalation injury.
Burns associated with other injury.

start an IV of Ringer's Lactate at a rate of 10 ml/kg/per hour or as specified in local protocols. Use an extremity without burns, if available, to avoid contamination to the wound.

- If signs of shock are present, give Ringer's Lactate, 20 ml/kg IV push. If vital signs do not improve after 5 minutes, repeat the bolus of Ringer's Lactate. Up to three boluses may be needed in severe shock.

Management of Chemical Burns

All prehospital providers should administer the following care for *chemical burns to the skin:*

- Protect yourself by using protective devices such as disposable rubber gloves and goggles as a precaution.
- For water-soluble chemicals, place the child in the shower, or otherwise flush the burned surface with copious amounts of water. Remove the child's clothing while in the shower, taking care to brush off powder and solid chunks prior to the flushing. Continue flushing until all the chemical has been removed.
- For chemicals that are not water soluble, take the following alternate actions. *Phenol* is poorly soluble in water, so remove clothing, flush with water, and apply baby oil or other oily substance. *Sodium metal* reacts to water by burning, so brush off and apply petroleum jelly to affected skin. For *sulfuric acid,* use soap and water and rinse with copious amounts of water.
- Cover burns with a clean sheet and keep the child warm.
- Transport patient rapidly to the hospital.

All emergency personnel should provide the following care for *chemical burns to the eyes:*

- Flush with large amounts of saline or water for 20 minutes.
- Cover eyes with patches.
- Transport rapidly.

Refer to Chapter 8, "Poisoning Emergencies," for management of chemical ingestions.

Management of Electrical Burns

BLS field care for *low-voltage electrical burns* includes the following:

- Protect yourself. Attempt to disconnect the power source and remove the child from contact.
- Assess and monitor ABCDE's.
- Administer high-flow oxygen by blow-by or mask if tolerated.
- Place a clean dressing over entrance and exit burn sites.
- Assess and manage other injuries.
- Transport patient to hospital.

BLS field care for *high-voltage electrical injuries* includes:

- Protect your own safety. Attempts to remove with ropes or wooden poles high-voltage electrical wires from the child can be very dangerous. Notify the power company immediately to turn off the power prior to extrication. If the child is thrown clear, remove child to an area of greater safety.
- Perform the primary trauma assessment and monitor ABC's.
- Stabilize the cervical spine and maintain the airway.
- Ventilate with high-flow, high-concentration oxygen.
- Perform CPR if indicated.
- Perform secondary trauma assessment.
- Cover burn sites with sterile dressing.
- Keep the child warm.
- Immediately transport to hospital.

ALS personnel should additionally provide the following care according to local protocols:

- Intubate the child if airway control is inadequate.
- Attach a cardiac monitor and record a rhythm strip.
- Initiate defibrillation if the child is in ventricular fibrillation or asystole.
- Start an IV of Ringer's Lactate at a keep-open rate.

Child Abuse and Burn Injury

Children less than 5 years of age represent the age group most often found with burns resulting from child abuse. There are characteristic burns that should make you suspicious of the possibility of child abuse. The child presenting with burns to the back, buttocks, and posterior neck should alert your suspicion of abuse. The child who unintentionally knocks over a cup of hot liquid onto himself has an arrowhead-shaped spill pattern over the anterior shoulder, chest, and possibly the face (Figure 12.5).

Circumferential scald burns of hands or feet that are clearly demarcated and uniform with no splash marks are tell-tale signs of abuse. When the hands or feet are held forcibly under hot running water, there are characteristic burns to the back of the hands or top of the feet. Burns limited to the genitalia and buttocks, with skin folds unburned, occur when children are dipped and held in a tub of hot water. This commonly occurs when parents are frustrated with toilet training. See Chapter 13, "Child Abuse," for more details.

Burns References

BARKIN, R., and ROSEN P., eds, *Emergency Pediatrics*, 3rd ed. St. Louis: The C.V. Mosby Co., 1990, pp. 256–260.

BOURNE, M. K., "Fire and smoke: Managing skin and inhalation burns," *JEMS*, 14, no. 9 (September 1989), pp. 62–82.

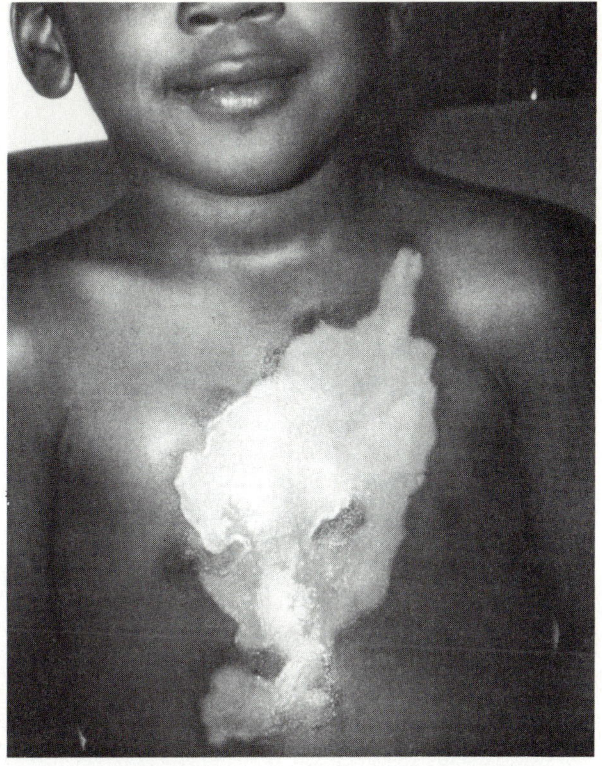

BUDNICK L., "Bathtub-related electrocutions in the United States, 1979–1982," *Journal of the American Medical Association*, 252, no. 7 (Aug. 17, 1984), pp. 918–920.

CLARK, J. R., "Managing burns in children," *JEMS*, 15, no. 4 (April 1990), pp. 90–94.

FELDMAN, K. W., "Child abuse by burning." In Kempe, C., and Helfer, R. E., eds., *The Battered Child*, 3rd ed. Chicago: University of Chicago Press, 1980, pp. 147–162.

FELLE, I., and KEITH, J. C., "National burn information exchange," *Surgical Clinics of North America*, 50, no. 6 (December 1970), pp. 1423–1436.

HERNDON, D. N., CARVAJAL, H. F., and CURRERI, P. W., "The management of burns in children." In Winters, R. W., ed., *The Body Fluids in Pediatrics.* Boston: Little, Brown, 1983.

HERNDON, D., and THOMPSON, P., "Treatment of Burns in Children," *Pediatric Clinics of North America*, 32, no. 5 (October 1985), pp. 1311–1332.

MCLOUGHLIN, E., JOSEPH, M. P., and CRAWFORD, J. D., "Epidemiology of high tension electrical injuries in children," *Journal of Pediatrics*, 89, no. 1 (July 1976), pp. 62–65.

ROBINSON, M. D., and SEWARD, P. N., "Thermal injury in children," *Pediatric Emergency Care*, 3, no. 4 (1987), pp. 266–270.

ROBINSON, M. D., and SEWARD, P. N., "Electrical and lightning injuries in children," *Pediatric Emergency Care*, 2, no. 3 (1986), pp. 186–190.

SURVEYER, J. A., and HALPERN, J., "Age-related burn injuries and their prevention," *Pediatric Nursing*, 7, no. 5 (September/October 1981), pp. 29–34.

13

Child Abuse

OBJECTIVES

When you have completed this chapter you should be able to

✱ Distinguish between physical abuse, sexual abuse, emotional abuse, and neglect.

✱ Describe the range of injuries seen in physically and sexually abused children.

✱ Demonstrate the appropriate method for handling a parent or care provider in a suspected abuse situation.

✱ Describe the procedure by state law for reporting suspected child abuse.

✱ Demonstrate appropriate documentation of findings in suspected child-abuse cases.

Child abuse is a complex health and social problem that is on the rise in today's society; it knows no socioeconomic boundaries. The major difference between child abuse and unintentional injury is that in the former the child is injured or allowed to be injured by his or her parent, guardian, or custodian.

Personal feelings are the greatest obstacle to the successful management of child abuse and neglect. You and your co-workers are often the first individuals in a position to gather information that will later determine whether the hospital care providers are dealing with child abuse or an accidental injury.

> Since repeat abuse occurs in more than 20% of all children, often leading to permanent injury and death, only early recognition of child abuse will allow the interruption of the vicious cycle which may not only kill the involved child but siblings as well. (Kottmeier, 1987, p. 343)

The child may suffer or become at higher risk if you don't follow standard assessment and reporting guidelines. If the parents perceive that you are blaming them, they may not allow you to treat or transport the child to the hospital. If you document in a *subjective* manner your information will be disregarded and the child will most likely continue to be abused.

Epidemiology

- In infants less than 6 months of age, child abuse is second only to SIDS as the leading cause of death.
- Up to 20% of all traumatic injuries seen in children 3 years or younger are caused by maltreatment; however, a third of all child-abuse cases are reported in children over 3 years of age.
- Between 2000 to 5000 children die each year as a result of child-abuse injuries.

Psychosocial Contributors to Child Abuse

A large number of abused and neglected children suffer permanent physical and emotional disabilities, and a large number of these go unreported yearly.

The abusive situation is often precipitated by a crisis, which might be a minor problem that sets off the abuser. It is usually associated with a long series of frustrations or the abuser's inability to cope with problems, such as poverty, unemployment, or too many children. Additionally, factors that can contribute to the abuse of a child include marital disharmony or social isolation, a single parent who is isolated or lacking social support, and drug and/or alcohol abuse.

In some cases the child has certain characteristics that place him or her at higher risk for abuse. The child may be singled out for abuse because he or she is viewed as "different"—such as having a chronic illness, premature birth, or a physical deformity. Hyperactive or difficult-to-manage children are also at high risk for abuse. Sometimes the child may simply resemble a relative or ex-spouse disliked by the abuser.

Classifications of Child Abuse

Physical Abuse

Physical abuse results in trauma to the soft tissue, skeleton, central nervous system, abdominal organs, or teeth. The injuries may be inflicted by beatings, burns, shaking, throwing the child against a wall or on the ground, binding, gagging, twisting extremities, poisoning, or starvation. Overly harsh discipline that results in injury is also considered physical abuse.

Signs of physical abuse include the following characteristic patterns of soft tissue and skeletal injuries:

- Small round burns or scars, often from cigarettes (Figure 13.1).
- Glove or stocking burns from immersion of the hands or feet in hot water. These burns have a characteristic lack of splash marks. Refer to Chapter 12, "Burn Management" (Figure 13.2).
- Burns to buttocks, legs, and feet, often with creases behind the knees and upper thighs spared. These burns occur most commonly in infants and toddlers who soil themselves during toilet training (Figure 13.3).
- Demarcated burns in shape of object used, such as an iron, stove burner, oven rack, or radiator (Figure 13.4).
- Slap marks resembling the shape of a hand.
- Welts showing shape of tool used—belts, buckles, hangers, electrical cords (loop marks), or chains (Figure 13.5).
- Suspicious bruises in various stages of healing (see Table 13.1). Ac-

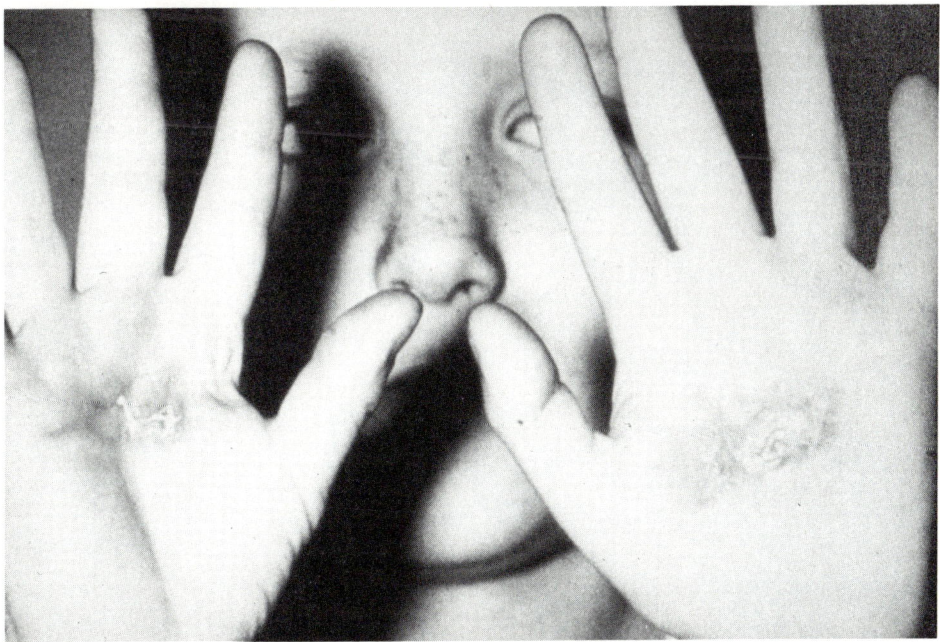

FIGURE 13.1   Small round burns caused by a cigarette held to the skin.

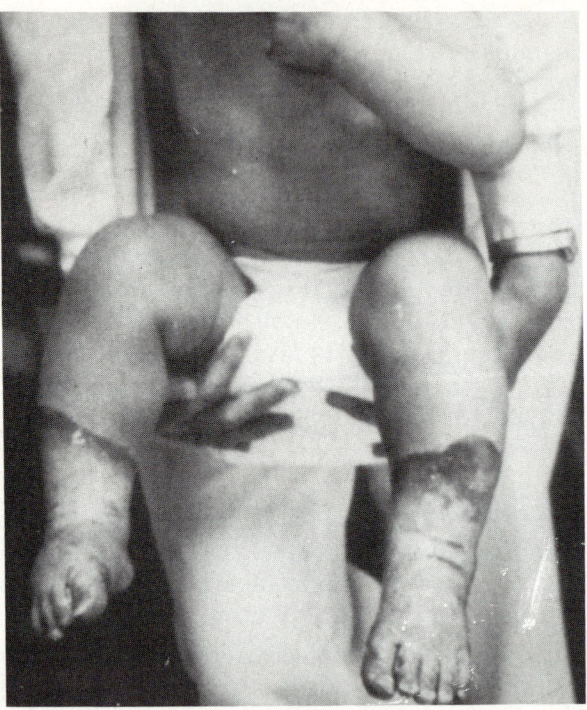

FIGURE 13.2 "Stocking" burns caused by immersion of the feet into hot water. Note the distinct line of the burn on the legs. The lack of splash marks indicates the child was restrained in the hot water and could not escape.

tive children often have bruises over bony prominences (shins, hips, spine, lower arms, forehead, and under the chin) caused by falls and bumping into objects during play. Suspicious sites for bruises are on the upper arms, trunk, upper anterior legs, sides of the face, ears and neck, genitalia, and buttocks (Figure 13.6).

- Human bite marks indicating the pattern of teeth and size of an adult's mouth. Pay particular attention to the characteristics of teeth marks (chips and space between teeth).

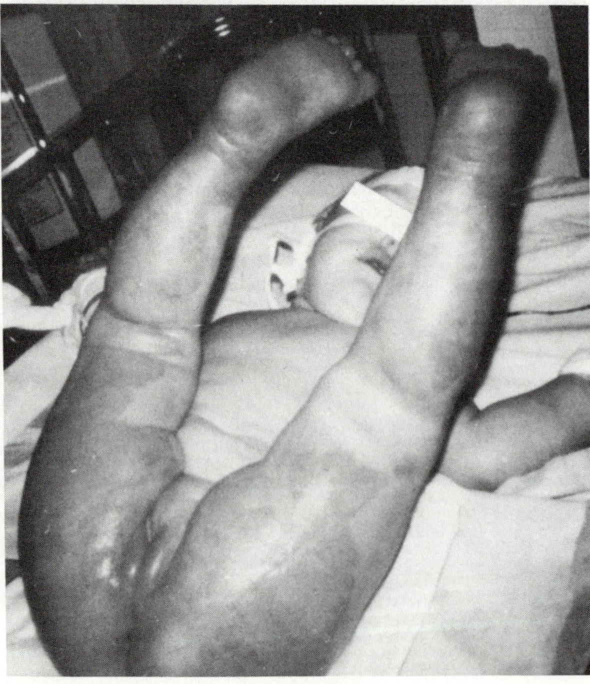

FIGURE 13.3 Burns to buttocks, legs, and feet with creases behind the knees and in upper thighs spared. This immersion burn often occurs as punishment for soiling underclothes during toilet training.

Child Abuse

FIGURE 13.4 Demarcated burns in shape of object used, in this case an iron (from *Atlas of Pediatric Physical Diagnosis*, courtesy of Gower Medical Publishing, New York).

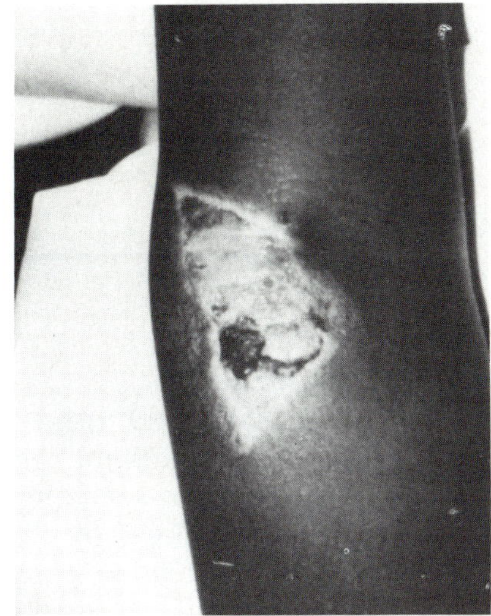

- Marks indicating the child has been bound or gagged.
- Fractures may be detected by poor alignment or the child's sudden unwillingness to use an extremity. X rays of long bones taken at the hospital may reveal numerous fractures in various stages of healing (Figure 13.7).

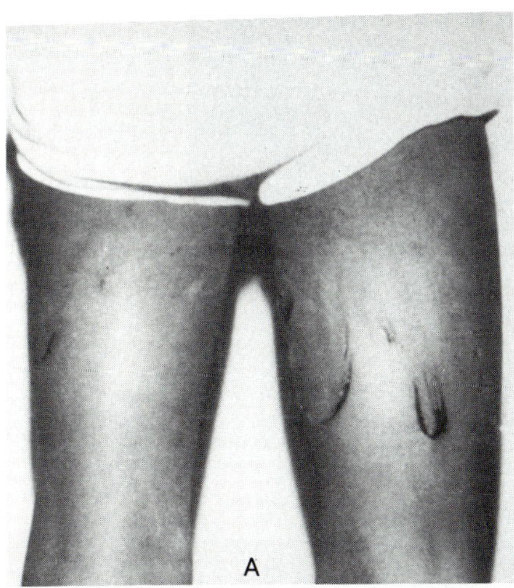
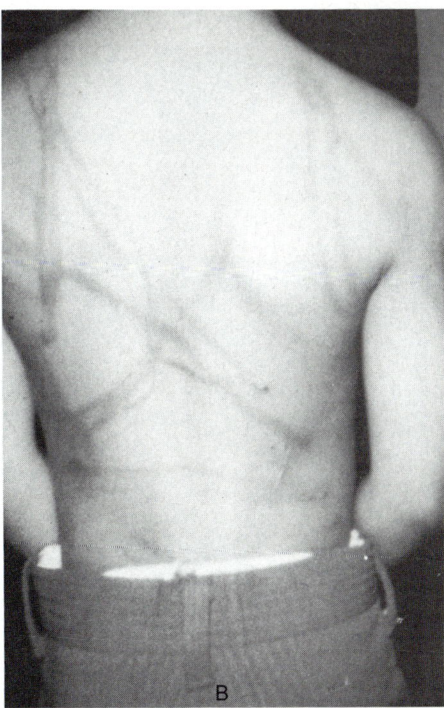

FIGURE 13.5 Welt in the shape of the item used for beating. (A) Welt is caused by a looped electrical cord; (B) welt is caused by a willow branch.

TABLE 13.1   Using Skin Color to Estimate the Age of Bruises

Color	Age of Bruise
Reddish blue	Immediately and up to 48 hours after impact
Brownish blue	2 to 3 days
Brownish green	4 to 7 days
Greenish yellow	7 to 10 days
Yellow-brown	More than 8 days
Normal skin color	2 to 4 weeks

Source: Adapted from Reece, R. M., and Grodin, M. A., (1985): "Recognition of nonaccidental injury," *Pediatric Clinics of North America,* 32(1): 46; Wilson, E. F., (1977): "Estimation of the age of cutaneous contusions in child abuse, *Pediatrics,* 60(5):750.

Shaken Baby Syndrome

Sometimes caretakers become so frustrated with an infant that they shake the baby, not realizing that this action can cause serious injury. After the shaking, the baby often is thrown down on the crib mattress. The blood vessels in the baby's brain are torn as the brain strikes the skull, resulting in bruising and intracranial bleeding. There may be no physical marks on the infant, but the baby will have signs of increased intracranial pressure. If the infant is dead at the scene, you may suspect sudden infant death syndrome (SIDS). However, the true cause of death will be determined by autopsy.

Sexual Abuse

Sexual abuse is defined as sexual contact between a child, 16 years of age or younger, and another person in a position of authority, no matter the age, where the child's participation was obtained through threats, bribery, coercion, or similar tactics. These sexual contacts can include sexual assault or physical force, but they are not limited only to inter-

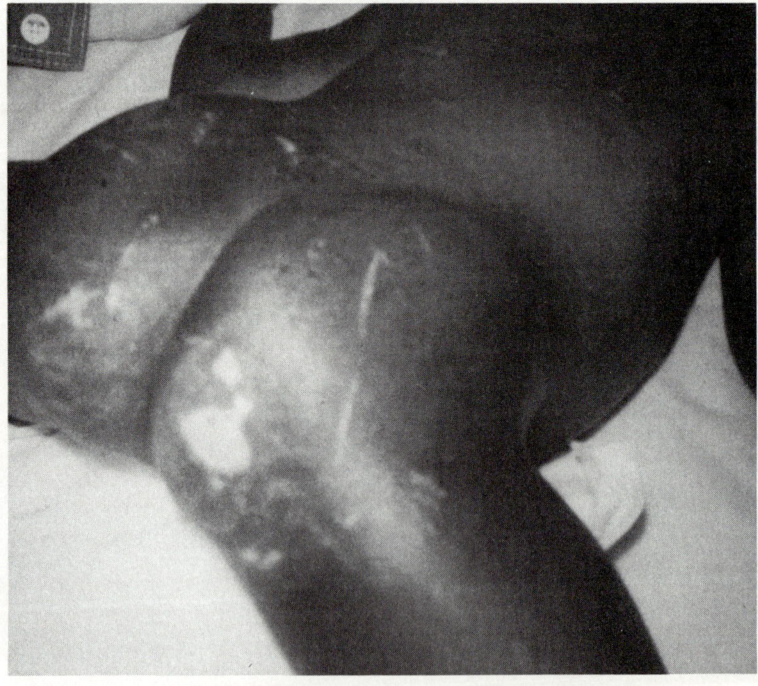

FIGURE 13.6   Bruising on the buttocks from repeated spankings.

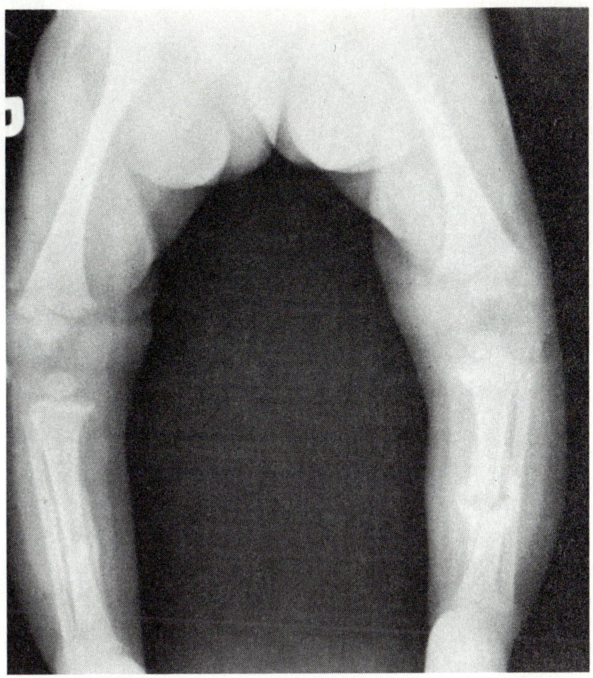

FIGURE 13.7 X-ray of the legs. Note fresh fractures on right tibia and fibula as well as healing fracture on left tibia.

course. Fondling, sodomy, exhibitionism, pornography, and prostitution are also considered forms of sexual abuse.

Often the signs of sexual abuse in young children are subtle because fondling may not result in apparent injury. Some of the more overt signs of sexual abuse include the following:

- Bruising on the genitalia.
- Lacerations indicating vaginal and/or anal penetration.
- Semen on clothes or body.
- Discharge from the vagina or penis, perhaps associated with a sexually transmitted disease.

Neglect

Neglect involves the willful or unintentional absence of care for a child's basic life necessities, which places the child's life or health in jeopardy. These include lack of adequate nutrition, leading to poor growth and development; lack of medical care, lack of psychosocial support, or lack of education. Abandonment and/or lack of committed and consistent daily care is also considered neglect. Signs of neglect include the following:

- The child is unbathed and wearing unusually dirty clothing or has poor hygiene.
- The child is poorly nourished, small, and underweight for age (Figure 13.8).
- The child is inappropriately dressed for the season or weather.
- There seems to be an inappropriate delay in seeking medical care.

Emotional Abuse

Emotional abuse is the most difficult of the four classifications to identify and often goes unreported. It involves the failure of care givers to pro-

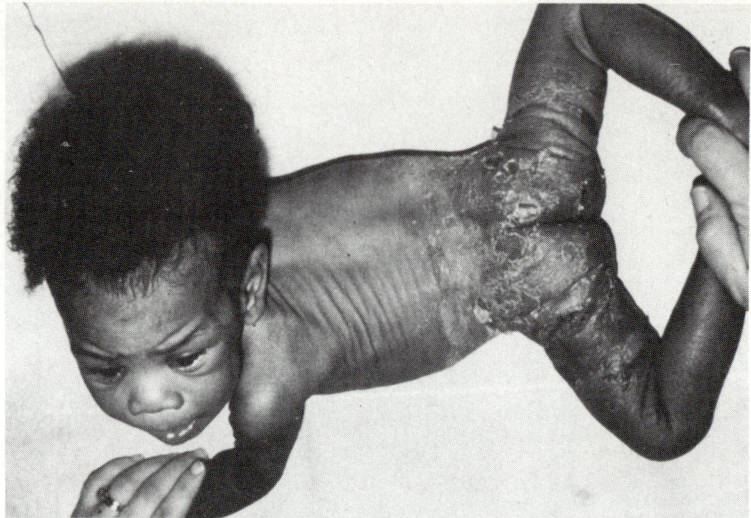

FIGURE 13.8 The neglected infant often appears poorly nourished, small, and underweight for the reported age (from *Atlas of Pediatric Physical Diagnosis*, courtesy of Gower Medical Publishing, New York).

vide a child with the support necessary for the development of a sound personality. This may occur by intimidation, subtle or overt rejection, threats, or excessive criticism.

Care of the Suspected Child-Abuse Victim

It is vitally important that you remember the following important steps when managing a suspected abuse victim:

- Your primary responsibility is to manage the injuries rather than place blame.
- Document history and observations in an *objective* rather than a subjective manner.
- Remain nonjudgmental in the presence of the child's care givers at all times.

History

In addition to the routine history you would obtain for any child with an injury, some additional questions should be asked. Questions should be phrased to obtain facts about the incident so that no apparent blame can be perceived by the care giver.

- How did the injury occur? How long ago did it happen?
- Who was with the child or found the child at the time of injury? Did anyone witness the incident?
- Has the child been moved from the site of the injury?

Assessment

Indications of abuse may be severe or deceptively mild, making your assessment difficult. Remember that many clues to child abuse lie in the assessment of the home; inappropriate attitude of the care giver toward the child's injuries, or of the child's reaction to the injury; and changes in the history or account of the injury given by the care giver over time.

Parental Behavior

Uneasy, unsure, or uncertain behavior on the part of the family member reporting the history of the injury is sometimes your first clue to a child-abuse case. Though the abusive parent or care giver usually has requested your assistance, this individual may react with anger, fear, withdrawal, hostility, or silence to questions about the history of the injury. Overreaction or unusual lack of concern to the injury is sometimes noted as well, but this is difficult to document without seeming subjective. Pay close attention to the behavior the parent or care giver shows toward the child. These individuals may become angry, indifferent, fault the child, or provide little, if any, support or consolation.

Child's Behavior

The child may also show unusual behavior such as the following:

- Demonstrating no expectation of being comforted by the parent or care giver;
- Being overly friendly toward strangers, or less afraid of strangers when compared to other children their own age;
- Having a withdrawn or diminished response to pain.

There may also be some evidence of developmental delay, overt anger and hostility, mistrust, or sexual acting out. Abused children typically will not betray their parents by describing the abuse.

Environmental Clues

Clues of abuse may be found in the environment, and because you may be the only health care provider to see the environment before it is "cleaned up," it is important to document in a factual manner what you observe in the home.

- Are there signs of a struggle or destruction?
- Are family members and/or neighbors discussing who or how the child was injured?
- Is there evidence of drugs or alcohol?
- Is there evidence of the reported accident and does it seem probable for the environment and developmental skills of the child?

Abuse may be suspected if the following items or combination of items is noted:

- A child has noticeable injuries that the parent or care provider doesn't mention.
- The child's injuries and/or age indicates a better explanation than is being offered.

- Your physical findings do not match the history given.
- Information about the injury changes with further questioning.

Management

- Assess and monitor ABC's.
- Treat any major injuries.
- Remove child from situation and transport to hospital.
- Keep the following communication guidelines in mind when at the scene:
    1. *Do not* approach the parent or care provider in an accusatory manner.
    2. *Do not* judge the parents; someone else may be the perpetrator.
    3. *Do not* separate the child from the parents unless the child is in immediate danger. The child is still fearful of separation, even if the parent is the abuser.
- Appropriately document in a factual manner everything heard or observed. See guidelines for documentation below.
- Report suspected abuse to hospital personnel upon arrival at the hospital. *Do not* convey sensitive information over the radio. Hospital personnel can set appropriate social services into motion to protect the child and support the family.
- Report suspected abuse to those authorities required by your state's law. You could be sued for negligence if you do not.

Documentation

Record the child's condition and physical injuries as you would for any other case; however, recognize that this record may well wind up in court. As already stated, it is particularly important in cases of suspected child abuse to record your observations in an objective manner. Here are some guidelines:

- Describe injuries by appearance, shape, color, size, location, and stage of healing, rather than stating your impression of the object that caused the injury. For example: A burn that you suspect was caused by a cigarette should be described by its appearance—a circular burn, approximately ½ inch in diameter, red and weeping.
- Draw pictures of shapes of injuries (burns, bruises, lacerations, etc.) and their location on the body. These drawings do not have to be of artist's quality to convey information.
- Record statements of all persons at the scene as direct quotations, not your summary of what was said. Include any apparent discrepancies in history among those present.
- Describe the setting in which you found the child, as well as the setting of the incident if the child has been moved. You and your coworkers are likely to be the only health care providers to see the environment before all evidence has been cleaned up. You alone can provide a window to the environment for medical and social services personnel to better recognize the case as true abuse.

- Record both the parents' and child's behavior and their interaction with each other.

Reactions of the EMS Provider

It is common for the prehospital care provider to have strong emotional reactions to child-abuse situations. It can be difficult to contain your feelings of anger, frustration, and disbelief at the horror of the situation, and these feelings may get in the way of your physical assessment, reaction toward the family or care provider, and documentation of the situation.

Remember that you are the child's advocate. If you act or appear judgmental toward the parents, they may not let you take the child to the hospital. Difficult as the situation may be, remember that the only way you can help the child, other than providing care for the injuries, is to remove the child from the scene, and transport the child to the hospital and to safety. Remain nonjudgmental, document the facts, and report your suspicions to the receiving hospital personnel.

Once you have delivered the child to the receiving hospital personnel, your feelings may intensify. If so, you need to deal with them for your own emotional well-being. This is an appropriate time to discuss those feelings with personnel at the hospital, such as a physician, nurse, social worker, your partner, or other members of your support group. *Be careful to discuss only your feelings rather than the actual information you have collected about the scene.* Remember that confidentiality is important in the work you do and the patients you manage, regardless of the nature of the call. See Chapter 17, "Crisis and Stress Management," for suggestions to help with managing such an emotionally charged case.

Child Abuse References

"Child abuse: The EMS response," *Emergency Medical Services,* 15, no. 3 (April 1986), pp. 11–42.

CUPOLI, J. M., "Piecing together the pattern of child abuse," *Contemporary Pediatrics,* 4, no. 12 (December 1987), pp. 12–30.

"The darkest side of child abuse," *Emergency Medicine,* 18, no. 4 (Feb. 28, 1986), pp. 117–132.

DERNOCOEUR, K., "Maltreatment of children," *JEMS,* 8, no. 2 (February 1983), pp. 22–27.

EMANS, S. J., WOODS, E. R., FLAGG, N. T., and FREEMAN, A., "Genital findings in sexually abused, symptomatic, and asymptomatic girls," *Pediatrics,* 79, no. 5 (May 1987), pp. 778–785.

GILLESPIE, R. W., "Burns and child abuse," *Emergency Medical Services,* 15, no. 3 (April 1986), p. 26.

HOSCH, I. A., "Munchausen syndrome by proxy," *Maternal Child Nursing,* 12, no. 1 (January/February 1987), pp. 48–52.

KOTTMEIER, P. K., "The battered child," *Pediatric Annals,* 16, no. 4 (April 1987), pp. 343–351.

LEVIN, A. V., "Child Abuse: Challenges and controversies," *Pediatric Emergency Care,* 3, no. 3 (Fall 1987), pp. 211–217.

LUDWIG, S., "Physical and sexual abuse of infants and children," *Pediatric Consult,* 6, no. 2 (1987), pp. 8–12.

McKITTRICK, C. A., "Child abuse: Recognition and reporting by health professionals," *Nursing Clinics of North America,* 16, no. 1 (March 1981), pp. 103–115.

MITTLEMAN, R. E., MITTLEMAN, H. S., and WETLI, C. V., "What child abuse really looks like," *American Journal of Nursing,* 87, no. 9 (September 1987), pp. 1185–1188.

REECE, R. M., and GRODIN, M. A., "Recognition of nonaccidental injury," *Pediatric Clinics of North America,* 32, no. 1 (1985), p. 41.

SAULSBURY, F. T., and HAYDEN, G. F., "Skin conditions simulating child abuse," *Pediatric Emergency Care,* 1, no. 3 (Fall 1985), pp. 147–150.

SWITZER J. V., "Reporting child abuse," *Emergency,* 18, no. 1 (January 1986), pp. 44–47.

WILSON, E. F., "Estimation of the age of cutaneous contusions in child abuse," *Pediatrics,* 60, no. 5 (November 1977), p. 750.

WOODLING, B. A., "Sexual abuse and the child," *Emergency Medical Services,* 15, no. 3 (April 1986), pp. 17–20, 23–25.

Newborn Management

14

OBJECTIVES

When you have completed this chapter you should be able to

* Describe the important parameters for assessment of the newborn.
* Describe the four mechanism of heat loss in a newborn infant and ways to manage each.
* List causes of respiratory distress in the newborn.
* Describe airway management of the newborn.
* Describe appropriate oxygen administration to the newborn.

Physiologic Adaptations at Birth

Newborns must rapidly make a transition to the outside world from a temperature-controlled, protected environment in utero. Newborns must make three major physiologic adaptations necessary for survival:

- Changing their circulatory pattern;
- Emptying fluid from their lungs and beginning ventilation;
- Maintaining body temperature.

Most newborns make this transition with minimal support. Only 10–20% of newborns need some resuscitation.

The newborn's chest is usually compressed during a vaginal delivery, which forces some of the fluid in the lungs out through the mouth and nose. The chest wall recoils after delivery and draws air into the lungs. The initial breath is stimulated by the newborn's response to hypoxia, acidosis, and temperature.

When the umbilical cord is cut, fetal circulation that by-passed the lungs is abruptly ended. As the lungs expand with the initial breaths, resistance to blood flow in the lungs' blood vessels is decreased, making it easier for blood to flow through them. At the same time, the resistance to blood flow in the extremities is increased. This sets the stage for the newborn's blood to be oxygenated by the lungs rather than through the placenta. See Table 14.1 for causes of hypoxemia in newborns.

Newborns have a large body surface area (BSA) for their weight, decreased tissue insulation, and a poorly developed temperature regulation mechanism. Their head is proportionately larger and accounts for 20% of BSA. In addition, newborns enter the world wet, which promotes rapid heat loss. Delivery into a cool environment only increases the heat loss suffered by the infant. See Table 14.2 for mechanisms of heat loss by newborns.

Newborns attempt to conserve heat by maintaining a flexed position and vasoconstriction. Hypothermia develops rapidly in the newborn if not quickly managed. To produce heat the infants increase their metabolic rate by breaking down brown fat cells. The stress of heat production places the baby at greater risk for hypoxemia, acidosis, bradycardia, and hypoglycemia.

TABLE 14.1 Causes of Hypoxemia in the Newborn

Conditions During Labor and Delivery	Conditions Present or Developing After Birth
Compression of the umbilical cord during delivery	Airway obstruction from secretions or meconium
Stress from a difficult labor and delivery	Hypothermia and cold stress
Maternal hemorrhage from placenta previa or placenta abruptio	Large blood loss
	Immature lungs in a premature infant

**TABLE 14.2   Mechanisms of Heat Loss in Newborns
and Appropriate Management**

Mechanisms of Heat Loss	Temperature Control Management
Evaporation: Heat loss from moisture vaporizing from the skin surface	Dry the skin surface. Cover with dry towel or blanket. Wrap in cellophane or bubble wrap.
Conduction: Heat loss into a cold surface on which the baby is placed.	Use warm blankets or towels. Place on mother's abdomen and cover. Cover head.
Convection: Heat loss to the cooler air circulating and moving over the infant.	Prevent exposure to air currents. Cover the infant's head. Avoid use of cool oxygen.
Radiation: Heat loss to cooler objects not in direct contact with the infant.	Heat the ambulance interior prior to transport. Place heat packs around the baby, not in direct contact with the skin.

Imminent Delivery

When called to care for an obstetrical emergency, you have both the mother and at least one newborn as patients. One person should have primary responsibility to care for the mother while the other prehospital provider cares for the newborn. In this way, neither patient will be forgotten in the excitement of the birth.

If you arrive on the scene prior to delivery, it is necessary to determine if time exists to transport the mother to the nearest hospital. It is of course preferable that the delivery occur at the hospital under controlled circumstances, with all needed equipment and personnel to care for both the mother and infant.

History

To determine how much time you have for transport before delivery may occur, ask the following questions:

- What is the mother's due date? How many months pregnant is she?
- When did labor begin? How many minutes are there between contractions? Has her water broken? Does she have an urge to move her bowels?
- Has there been any vaginal bleeding?
- How many children has she previously had?
- Were there complications with prior pregnancies?
- Did she have a prior C-section?

Assessment

Delivery is imminent when the mother's contractions are 2 minutes or less apart, her water has broken, and she has an urge to move her bowels. If crowning is evident after inspecting the mother's perineal area, prepare for delivery prior to transport. Decisions to transport for less imminent delivery should be based upon transport time to the nearest hospital and local protocols. Vaginal bleeding is a sign of early separation of the placenta from the uterus, an emergency that places the mother and newborn in danger. Immediate transport is required.

Management

BLS care for the mother with impending delivery includes the following:

- Designate one provider to care for the mother while the other provider cares for the infant.
- Collect all needed supplies to care for the infant.
- Heat the ambulance to protect the newborn from hypothermia.
- Follow guidelines for care of the newborn beginning on page 211.
- If the mother is transported to the hospital prior to delivery, place her on her left side. Monitor her ABC's and progress in labor. Administer oxygen by face mask.
- For ALS care and the management of labor and delivery complications, refer to appropriate EMT textbooks.

Care of the Newly Born Infant

Newborns often need only supportive care to make the transition from fetus to independent life. Those newborns needing more extensive resuscitation are born to mothers with complications such as premature labor, improper presentation of the newborn, hemorrhage, substance abuse, and chronic illnesses such as diabetes.

History

When delivery will be managed by you, or the child has been born prior to your arrival, you should question the mother about the status of her pregnancy, in addition to the questions about the progress of her labor (see page 209).

- Has she seen a doctor regularly for prenatal care?
- Did she have any illnesses or need special care for a chronic disease during her pregnancy?
- Has the mother used street drugs during the pregnancy? When was the last dose taken?
- If the infant has already been born, ask the mother or birth assistant how long ago the birth occurred, and whether the baby breathed immediately.

Assessment

Most full-term newborns present to the world head first, covered with blood and amniotic fluid. The baby appears long and skinny, and the skin is generally dry, flaky, and wrinkled. The baby makes spontaneous movements of the extremities but maintains the arms and legs in a flexed, fetal position. Cyanosis of the hands and feet is common when the newborn is trying to conserve heat. Cyanosis of the mucous membranes indicates hypoxemia or a congenital heart defect.

Assessment and management of the newborn are usually performed together. As with any primary survey, airway is the initial concern, followed by the initiation of breathing, and maintenance of the heart rate. Prevention of hypothermia should be done simultaneously with the primary survey. See Table 14.3 for normal birth weights and vital signs of the full-term newborn infant. The APGAR score is commonly taken at 1 and 5 minutes after birth to evaluate the baby's respiratory, circulatory, and neurologic systems and the need for supportive care. The five categories evaluated include color, pulse, grimace, muscle tone, and respiratory effort. See Table 14.4 for the APGAR scoring criteria.

Management

If time permits, the prehospital provider should put on a gown, gloves, and goggles to reduce exposure to the mother's blood during the birth. BLS management of the newborn includes the following:

Airway Control
- As the head is delivered, inspect for the presence of the umbilical cord around the neck of the newborn and attempt to loosen and unwrap it if present. If it cannot be unwrapped, place two clamps on the cord and cut it between the clamps. Permitting the delivery to proceed without loosening the cord will asphyxiate the infant.

- Suction the mouth first, and then the nose, with a bulb syringe after the head has been delivered. Suctioning the nose first will often trigger spontaneous breathing, and potential aspiration of the contents of the mouth. Remember to depress the bulb syringe before placing it at the baby's nose (see Figure 14.1, page 213).

- Note the presence of green- or black-colored substance, which is indicative of meconium (see Caution box for management, page 214).

- Hold the baby with the head in neutral position as delivery progresses, taking care not to drop the slippery infant.

Temperature Control
- Dry the infant with a warmed towel. Discard the wet towel and wrap the baby in another warmed, dry towel or blanket. This stimulation frequently causes the baby to breathe spontaneously.

- Place the infant on a warmed towel in Trendelenburg position at the same level as the mother, and cut the umbilical cord (see Figure 14.2, page 213).

TABLE 14.3 Normal Vital Signs for Full-term Newborns

Birth weight (37–40 week gestation)	5–10 lb (2.2–4.5 kg), average is 7.5 lb (3.5 kg)
Heart rate	120–160/min
Respiratory rate	30–60/min
Systolic blood pressure	55–75 mm Hg
Temperature	96.8°–98.6°F

TABLE 14.4 APGAR Scoring Criteria

Characteristic Evaluated	Score		
	0	1	2
Appearance (color)	Blue or pale	Body pink, extremities blue	Completely pink
Pulse rate	Absent	<100/min	>100/min
Grimace (reflex irritability)	No response	Grimace	Cough or sneeze
Activity (muscle tone)	Limp	Some flexion of extremities	Active move- ment
Respiratory effort	Absent	Slow or irreg- ular	Good crying

KEY: *Directions for Administration of the APGAR*

Appearance (color) reflects peripheral tissue oxygenation. For nonwhite newborns, it is important to inspect the color of the mucous membranes of the mouth and conjunctiva, as well as the color of the lips, palms of the hands, and soles of the feet.

Pulse rate should be counted for at least 30 seconds for accuracy.

Grimace (reflex irritability) is judged by the infant's response to passing a catheter into the tip of the nose after suctioning. It can also be evaluated by slapping the sole of the foot with the palm of your hand. The usual response from a healthy newborn is a loud, angry cry.

Activity (muscle tone) refers to the degree of flexion and resistance offered by the infant when you attempt to extend the extremities. Any attempt to alter the normal flexed position of the extremities should be met by resistance.

Respiratory effort evaluates the adequacy of ventilation. Look for slow, shallow, irregular, or gasping respirations, which would be scored as 1.

CALCULATING THE APGAR SCORE

Individual scores are summed to give a total ranging from 0 to 10, indicating the type of resuscitation needed. Make every effort to give an accurate score to the emergency room personnel.

- 7 to 10, no resuscitation is needed;
- 4 to 6, stimulate, suction, and give oxygen;
- 0 to 3, begin ventilation and CPR.

Source: V. A. Apgar, "A Proposal for a New Method of Evaluation of the Newborn Infant," *Current Research in Anesthesia and Analgesia,*" vol. 32 (1953), pp. 260–67.

Ventilations

- If breathing has not yet started, further stimulate the baby by flicking or slapping the feet and rubbing the back (see Figure 14.3, page 214).

- If no spontaneous breathing occurs after stimulation, artificial ventilation with a bag-valve mask must be initiated. Ventilate with high-concentration oxygen (warmed and humidified if available) at a rate of 40 breaths/min. (See guidelines for use of oxygen, page 215.) The initial breath should be made with the pop-off valve of the bag-valve mask disabled. This provides enough pressure to open the lung tissue for oxygen exchange to occur. Subsequent breaths should be provided with less pressure, only enough to make the chest rise.

- Infants are obligate nose breathers; they do not breathe through their mouth unless they are crying or an oral airway is in place. Make sure the nasal passages remain clear of mucous.

Bradycardia

- Monitor the heart rate. Palpate the umbilical stump or the brachial pulse. If the heart rate is less than 100/min, continue bag-mask ven-

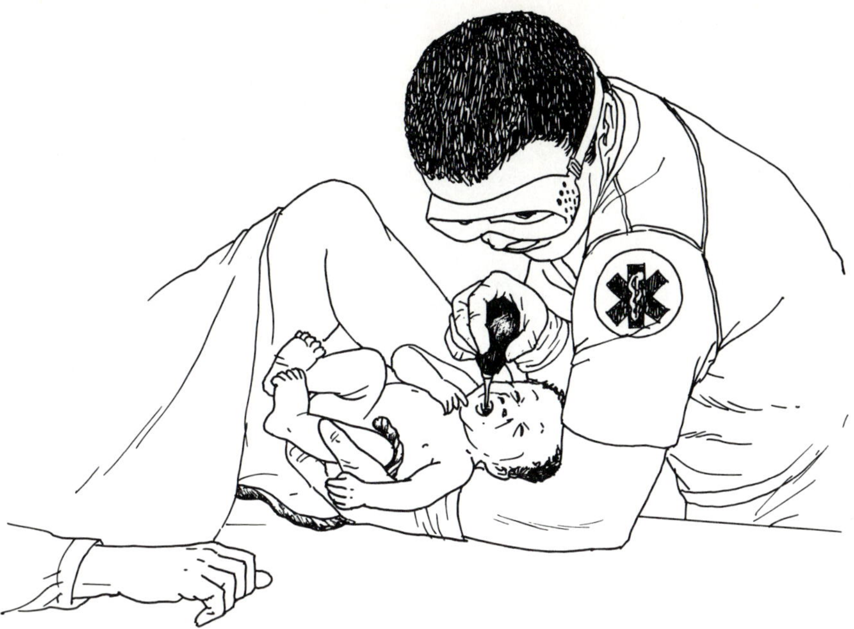

FIGURE 14.1 Suctioning the newborn's airway with the bulb syringe. Suction the mouth first and then the nose. Stimulating the nose may trigger spontaneous breathing before the airway is clear of mucous or meconium.

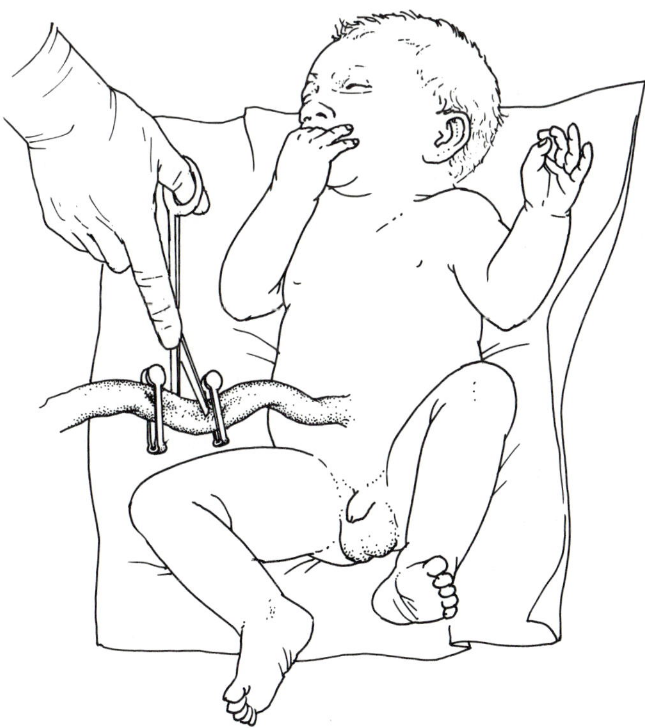

FIGURE 14.2 After the infant has been dried, place in a clean, warmed towel in Trendelenburg position prior to cutting the umbilical cord.

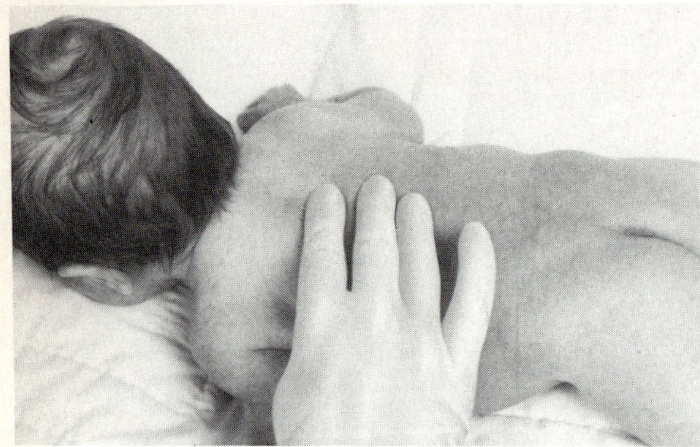
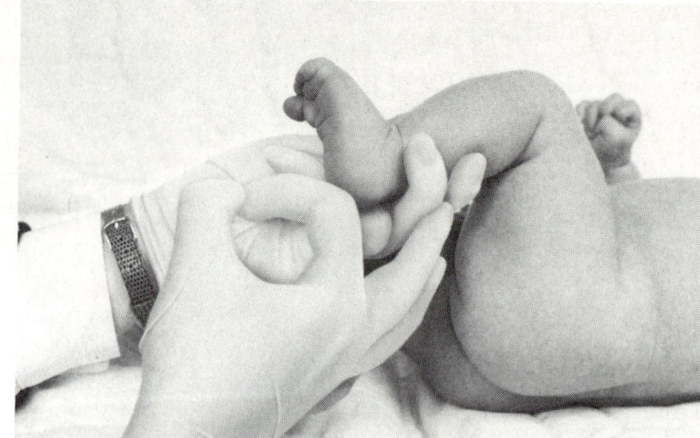

A   B

FIGURE 14.3 Stimulate breathing by (A) rubbing the infant's back or (B) flicking the feet.

tilation at a rate of 40–60/min with high-concentration oxygen. The heart rate should increase within 15–30 seconds.

- If the heart rate is less than 60/min or between 60–80/min and not responding after 30 seconds of bag-mask ventilation, begin chest compressions (see Chapter 5).
- Rapidly transport the distressed infant to the hospital. A less urgent transport is needed for the stable mother and newborn. Position the baby on its side to prevent aspiration of secretions.
- Discontinue artificial ventilation when the infant breathes spontaneously and perfuses adequately and maintains a heart rate above 100/min.

ALS providers should perform the following additional care to a distressed infant:

- Assess the approximate weight of the newborn.
- Intubate when there is no response to bag-mask ventilation and oxygen. Monitor the heart rate for further decrease in heart rate.

CAUTION! 

Meconium Staining and Aspiration
When an infant's skin has a dark greenish stain, the baby was distressed during labor or delivery. Meconium is a dark green-black, thick, sticky bowel movement. You may see the green-black staining as the baby's head emerges. Get prepared to suction the baby's mouth and nose while the head is being delivered. If meconium is in the mouth and airway, and the infant breathes spontaneously prior to suctioning, aspiration of meconium will occur. These infants have a high mortality rate. The infant must be aggressively suctioned prior to stimulation of spontaneous breathing, even at the risk of causing bradycardia. BLS providers should use a DeLee suction trap to get adequate suction to remove the meconium.

The ALS provider should examine the trachea with the laryngoscope and intubate the infant, followed by suctioning if meconium is seen. Bag-mask ventilation should be initiated as soon as most of the meconium is removed.

Newborn Management

Reoxygenate for 20 seconds with bag-mask ventilation if intubation takes longer than 30 seconds.

- Give epinephrine, 0.1 ml/kg of 1:10,000 solution, by endotracheal tube or IV if bradycardia does not respond to ventilation, oxygenation, and chest compressions.
- Depending upon local protocol, an IV can be started either with a peripheral line, umbilical cannulation, or intraosseous line.
- Naloxone, 0.01 mg/kg IV, may be used in a nonresponsive newborn if the mother has recently taken or suspected to have taken a narcotic.

Guidelines for the Use of Oxygen in Newborns

The newborn's brain cells are very sensitive to hypoxia, and permanent brain damage will result if hypoxemia is prolonged. For this reason, oxygen should never be withheld from a newborn suspected to have hypoxia.

Give oxygen by blow-by when bag-mask ventilation is not needed at 5–10 l/min. Use a bag-valve mask with reservoir when high-concentration oxygen is needed for resuscitation.

Cold oxygen blown directly on the baby's face around the nose, in the distribution of the trigeminal nerve, will cause apnea. Apnea is triggered by the mammalian diving reflex. Warmed oxygen does not cause apnea. If cold blow-by oxygen is being administered, direct the oxygen to the nose from one side of the baby's face (see Figure 14.4). This will reduce the chances of triggering the diving reflex.

Premature Infants

Premature infants are generally those born prior to 37 weeks of gestation. Their weight may range from 1.5 to 5 pounds (0.6–2.2 kg). Size of the newborn should not be the criteria you use to initiate resuscitation. Some fetuses are malnourished and very small, but they may be near full-term. It is also not possible to determine which small premature infants will survive. The lower limit of survival for premature infants is now 24–26 weeks when cared for in an intensive care nursery.

Assessment

The premature infant's degree of immaturity determines the physical characteristics seen on examination. The infant generally has a large trunk and shorter-appearing extremities, which maintain a frog-like position. Their skin is generally transparent and less wrinkled than are full-term infants.

Management

- In the case of a very small infant, initiate resuscitation if the infant has any signs of life, such as breathing, movement, or a heart rate.

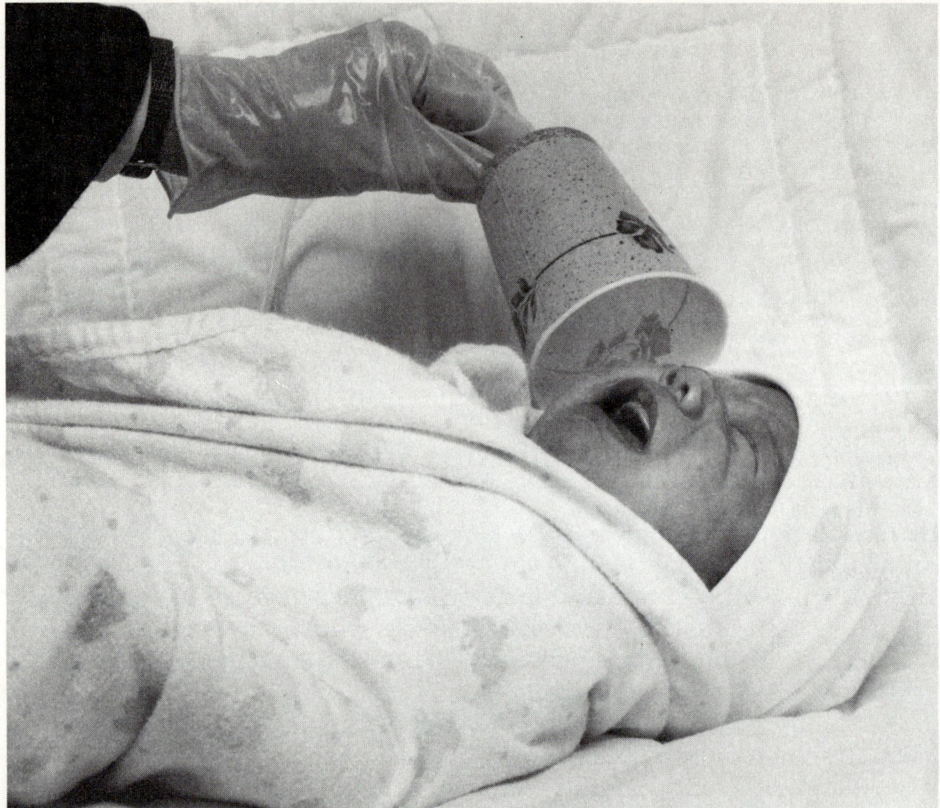

FIGURE 14.4 When oxygen cannot be warmed, direct the flow of oxygen to the nose from one side of the newborn's face rather than directly on the face around the nose. This will reduce the chance of triggering the mammalian diving reflex, which causes apnea.

- Follow guidelines for management of the newborn on pages 211–215.
- Keep the infant well oxygenated and warm. Use insulated blankets, caps, or plastic wrap to help the infant retain body heat (see Figure 14.5).
- Transport the infant to a hospital with specialized services for low birth-weight infants, if available.

CAUTION! 

Oxygen Use in Low Birth-Weight Infants

Low birth-weight infants are at risk for retrolental fibroplasia. Concentration of oxygen is one factor associated with the development of this disorder. However, the amount of oxygen used during routine prehospital transport is not believed to cause the condition. It is more important to ensure that the infant is *well oxygenated to prevent brain damage.* Administer enough oxygen to keep the infant pink and well perfused. Remember to keep the infant warm, which will also reduce oxygen demands.

ALS providers should have equipment that measures oxygen saturation levels for longer transport times. The concentration of oxygen to be administered to the low birth-weight infant can then be more precisely calculated.

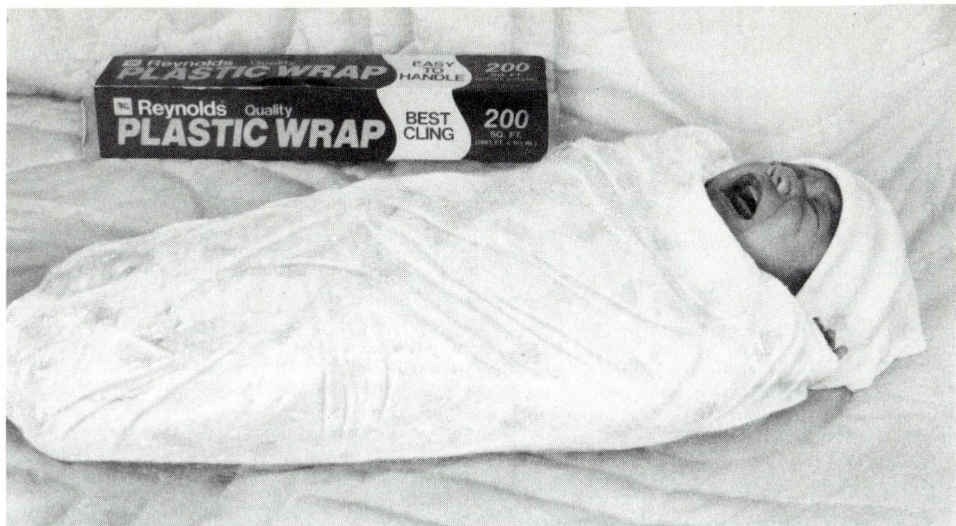

FIGURE 14.5   Keep small newborns warm during transport by wrapping them in insulated blankets or plastic wrap.

Respiratory Distress in Newborns

Newborn respiratory distress is caused by a number of disorders, including the following:

- Obstruction of the nasal passages either by mucous or a congenital blockage (choanal atresia);
- Meconium aspiration;
- Amniotic fluid aspiration; and
- Lung immaturity.

Each of these problems could progress to cardiac arrest if appropriate intervention is not provided early for hypoxemia.

Assessment

Signs of respiratory distress in the newborn include the following:

- See-saw or paradoxical breathing (the chest and abdomen do not rise and fall together with each breath; the chest rises as the abdomen falls and vice versa);
- Intercostal retractions;
- Nasal flaring; and
- Expiratory grunting that can be heard without a stethoscope.

Management

Prehospital care of the newborn in respiratory distress is the same as that provided to the normal newborn. Airway management and ventilation with high-concentration oxygen must be well controlled. This infant needs

Newborn Management References

BANTA, S. A., "Transition to extrauterine life," *Neonatal Network*, (June 1985), pp. 35–39.

CHAMEIDES, L., ed., *Textbook of Pediatric Advanced Life Support.* Dallas: American Heart Association and American Academy of Pediatrics, 1988.

DIERKING, B. H., "Neonatal resuscitation," *Emergency*, 21, no. 8 (August 1989), pp. 19–22.

DODMAN, N., "Newborn temperature control," *Neonatal Network*, (June 1987), pp. 19–23.

EDWARDS, M. C., "Delivery room resuscitation of the neonate," *Pediatric Annals*, 17, no. 7 (July 1988), pp. 458–466.

FRIGOLETTO, F. D., and LITTLE, G. A., eds., *Guidelines for Perinatal Care*, 2nd. ed. Chicago: American Academy of Pediatrics and American College of Obstetricians and Gynecologists, 1988.

SILVERMAN, B. J., ed., *Advanced Pediatric Life Support.* Dallas: American College of Emergency Physicians, 1989.

15

Apnea and Sudden Infant Death Syndrome

OBJECTIVES

When you have completed this chapter you should be able to

* Differentiate between sleep apnea and sudden infant death syndrome (SIDS).
* Describe the physical findings noted on the SIDS victim.
* List the current research findings associated with SIDS.
* Describe the parents' or caretaker's reactions to the SIDS emergency.
* Describe the responsibilities of the EMS field providers in caring for the family experiencing a SIDS emergency.

Apnea and Apparent Life-Threatening Events

Apnea is a temporary break in breathing, and when it is severe it places an infant at risk for recurrent hypoxia and hypoventilation. Newborns and infants commonly have short episodes of respiratory pause with spontaneous respiration interrupting the apnea. These episodes of *periodic breathing* last less than 20 seconds and are not considered to be abnormal.

Infantile apnea is a condition in which the infant develops irregular and sporadic breathing patterns, generally lasting longer than 20 seconds. A shorter duration of apnea accompanied by signs of bradycardia, pallor, or cyanosis is also defined as infantile apnea. These episodes generally occur during sleep and are referred to as *sleep apnea.* These infants are believed to be at increased risk for sudden infant death syndrome (SIDS). Premature infants have a higher incidence of apnea, probably associated with their immaturity. Its occurrence is thought to peak between 1 month and 4 months of age.

Apnea is also defined by mechanism of breathing pause. In *central apnea* there is neither chest movement, muscle movement, nor air passing through the nose or mouth, because the infant is making no breathing effort. In cases of *obstructive apnea* there is chest movement and the infant is trying to breathe, but an obstruction is blocking air movement. Often there is *mixed apnea,* a combination of the two types.

An *apparent life-threatening event* (ALTE) is an episode in infants, usually infants less than 6 months of age, characterized by some combination of apnea (usually central, but occasionally obstructive), color change, marked decrease in muscle tone, and choking or gagging. These episodes have previously been called "near miss SIDS." While research has identified only a small overlap between infants with ALTE and those who subsequently die from SIDS, there is an increased risk of SIDS in infants with ALTE. Infants at greatest risk are those requiring vigorous stimulation or resuscitation to terminate the apnea.

ALTE is approximately twice as common as SIDS, occurring in 2–3% of the population. No cause is found in half of these cases. ALTE has been associated with specific conditions such as infection, airway obstruction, heart defects, choking, seizures, and breath-holding spells.

History

Important information to obtain from the parent or care provider includes the following:

- Did someone observe the episode or was the baby found with symptoms? If the episode was observed, ask the care provider what happened.
- Was resuscitation started prior to arrival of EMS?
- Has the infant had any other episodes like this? Is the parent using an apnea monitor?
- Does the infant have any known medical problems or an acute illness?

Assessment

During the primary survey the infant with an ALTE may appear lifeless with marked limpness, pallor or cyanosis, no respiratory effort, and no response to mild stimulation. Either bradycardia or no pulse will be detected. Alternately, the infant may have an irregular respiratory pattern with apnea spells longer than 20 seconds, choking, or gagging. The infant with some respirations will be pale, cyanotic or reddish, bradycardic, limp, but responsive to mild stimulation.

Management

BLS care for the infant with an ALTE includes the following:

- Assess and monitor ABC's.
- Administer high-flow, high-concentration oxygen and bag-mask ventilate at 40 breaths/min.
- Initiate CPR if no heart rate is detected.
- Transport patient rapidly to nearest emergency department.
- If infant responds to stimulation or resuscitation with spontaneous regular respirations, continue high-flow, high-concentration oxygen while enroute.
- Provide reassurance to the parents that you are doing everything you can for the infant.

ALS providers may want to add the following management:

- Begin intubation.
- Attach a cardiac monitor.
- Start an IV of Ringer's Lactate at a keep-open rate.
- Initiate the ACLS (Advanced Cardiac Life Support) drug protocol if the heart rate does not increase with oxygen or no pulse and/or no respiratory effort are present.

Sudden Infant Death Syndrome

Sudden infant death syndrome (SIDS), also known as "crib death" or "cot death," is the unexpected death of a presumably healthy infant. It is a distinct medical diagnosis made after the exclusion of all other causes of death from history, examination of the death scene, and autopsy. It is the leading cause of death of infants between 1 and 12 months of age; approximately 6500 infants die from SIDS each year in the United States. At the present time SIDS is unpredictable and unpreventable. The onset and death are believed to be rapid, with no suffering.

Research has revealed common characteristics of SIDS infants and its occurrence. SIDS occurs more often in the fall and winter months. The peak age for SIDS is between 2 and 4 months, and the majority of cases occur before 7 months of age. Death usually occurs during sleep. Infants believed to be at higher risk for SIDS include the following:

- Male (60% of cases);
- Black infants;
- Twin or triplet (2.5 times more frequently a victim);
- Low birth-weight infants (4 times more frequent);
- Infants of young unmarried mothers of low socioeconomic status, even though it occurs in families of all socioeconomic levels;
- Infants of mothers who did not receive prenatal care, who used cocaine, methadone, or heroin during pregnancy.

History

Questions should be phrased so blame is not implied. Questions should not include "you," such as "When did you . . . ?" The parents will already feel guilty, and such questions will make them take on additional blame. If open-ended questions are used, such as "What happened?" most of the necessary information will be provided.

- Who discovered the infant; when and where?
- What action was taken by that person?
- When was the baby put to bed, or when did the baby fall asleep?
- What is the age and weight of the infant?
- What has the baby's general health been like? Have there been any recent illnesses? When was the child last seen by the doctor?
- Were there any health problems identified in the baby at birth?

Assessment

EMS will be activated when the parent or care provider finds the infant lifeless with no pulse or respiratory effort. The baby will be cool or cold if adequate time has elapsed since death. The infant may be limp, or stiff if rigor mortis is present. Lividity or purple marks may be noted on the dependent parts of the body where blood has settled.

By the time the EMTs arrive, the parents may have picked up the infant and/or initiated CPR. If the infant is still lying in the crib, the following signs are usually present:

- No evidence of having been disturbed during sleep, or the infant may have changed position at the time of death. It is not uncommon for infants to be found wedged in the corner of the crib.
- Blood-tinged fluid around the mouth and nose, or on bed covers. This discharge is associated with muscle relaxation after death rather than vomitus, which could have caused an airway obstruction.
- The infant's head may be covered with a blanket; however, suffocation has been ruled out as a cause of death in these infants because oxygen levels were adequate to sustain life.

Parents may demonstrate a wide range of behavior to emergency personnel. Most are anxious for help in saving their infant. When the parent suspects the infant is dead or has it confirmed, a number of grief reactions are possible, including the following:

- Shock, disbelief, denial (they do not recognize the reality of the situation);
- Hysteria;
- Inability to make decisions; disorganization and difficulty functioning;
- Guilt and self-blame;
- Withdrawal and depression.

Management

Emergency care in the case of an apparently dead infant, assumed to be the victim of SIDS, is to be supportive of the parents and assist them in the grieving process. Often BLS and ALS providers will follow the same protocols, especially when death occurred hours earlier. Parents will be helped the most if they feel that everything possible was done to save their infant.

- Assess and monitor ABC's.
- Initiate CPR, usually with BLS maneuvers only. (This action is not taken in some jurisdictions when signs indicate death occurred hours earlier.)
- Even when you have limited or no hope of successful resuscitation, support the parents and demonstrate your concern by explaining what is being done. Do not offer false hope that the infant will recover. Parents will have selective memory of the entire resuscitation episode. Your gestures to help the child and offer them some assistance will be remembered, even if the details are forgotten.
- Transport the infant and parent(s) to the hospital. If the parent cannot be transported in the ambulance, arrange for other transport. Parents are too distraught to drive themselves.
- If possible when at the hospital, try to offer some comfort to the parents by sitting with them; while the infant is cared for by hospital personnel, listen to the parents if they want to talk, offer to make phone calls for them, etc.
- If local protocol does not permit transport of the dead infant to the hospital, such as when the coroner is called to the scene, do not leave the parents alone in the home with the dead infant. If the rescue squad must leave, arrange for a neighbor, family member, or the clergy to stay with the parents until the coroner arrives.

Sudden Infant Death Syndrome and Child Abuse

In the recent past, infants initially thought to be victims of child abuse have later been determined to be SIDS victims. Parents were subjected to accusations and criminal investigations, which obstructed their grieving process. Overdiagnosis of SIDS in infants who could possibly be victims of child abuse is still a controversial subject. Concrete evidence from the autopsy and the scene to diagnose child abuse has not been present in these cases, but circumstantial evidence has made many people suspect it. (See Table 15.1 to distinguish between signs of SIDS and child abuse.) Child abuse is another major cause of death in infants, and it is important to be alert to the possibility. However, do not make judgments about the infant's cause of death or indirectly blame the parents for the child's death.

Assessment

Make a brief assessment of the death scene, noting any discrepancies among the history, the environment, the behavior of the parents, and your assessment of the infant. Observations to make when you are suspicious of child abuse include the following:

- Physical appearance of the baby, especially before CPR is initiated. If the parents initiated first aid, this may account for some of the marks on the body.
- The position of the baby in the crib may account for marks noted on the child's head and body—i.e., lividity in dependent body parts, or pressure marks from lying against side rails.
- Physical appearance of the crib and objects in the crib.

TABLE 15.1 How to Distinguish Between SIDS and Child Abuse and Neglect

Sudden Infant Death Syndrome	Child Abuse and Neglect
Incidence: Deaths: 6500–7500/year Highest: 2 to 4 months of age When: Winter months	*Incidence:* Deaths: 1000–4000/year Deaths in infants: 300/year When: No seasonal difference
Physical Appearance: Exhibits no external signs of injury Exhibits "natural" appearance of dead baby: • Lividity—settling of blood; frothy drainage from nose/mouth • Small marks, e.g., diaper rash looks more severe • Cooling/rigor mortis—takes place quickly in infants (about 3 hours) Appears to be well-developed baby, though may be small for age	*Physical Appearance:* Distinguishable and visible signs of injury • Broken bone(s) • Bruises • Burns • Cuts • Head trauma (black eye) • Scars • Welts • Wounds May be obviously wasted away (malnutrition) Other siblings may show patterns of injuries commonly seen in child abuse
May Initially Suspect SIDS: All of the above characteristics PLUS Parents say that infant was well and healthy when put to sleep (last time seen alive).	*May Initially Suspect Child Abuse or Neglect:* All of the above characteristics PLUS Parents' story does not "sound right" or cannot account for all of injuries on infant.

Source: Bureau of Community Health Services (HSA/PHS). *Training Emergency Responders: Sudden Infant Death Syndrome. An Instructor's Manual.* 1979, p. C–3. Used with permission, National SIDS Clearinghouse.

- Unusual or dangerous items in the room (sharp objects, plastic bags).
- Behaviors of people present.
- Medications or drugs that are present; intended for the infant or adult (you may choose to take medications to the hospital).
- Appearance of the room and house.

Management

All prehospital providers should perform the following care:

- Do NOT delay treatment or transport to make the scene investigation.
- Report your findings objectively, not your assumptions about the case based upon evidence seen. All information should be objectively and factually documented in your report. Your suspicions and objective information should be reported confidentially to the emergency department staff at the receiving hospital.
- Let the police do the investigation; your job is to care for the family.

Apnea and SIDS References

ANDREWS, M. M., and others, "Home apnea monitoring in the Intermountain West," *Journal of Pediatric Health Care*, 1, no. 5 (September/October 1987), pp. 255–260.

ARIAGNO, R. L., "Evaluation and management of infantile apnea," *Pediatric Annals*, 13, no. 3 (March 1984), pp. 210–217.

BARKIN, R. M., and ROSEN, P., eds., "Apnea." In *Emergency Pediatrics*, 3rd. ed. St. Louis: The C.V. Mosby Co., 1990.

BASS, M., KRAVATH, R. E., and GLASS, L., "Death scene investigation in sudden infant death," *New England Journal of Medicine*, 315, no. 2 (1986), pp. 100–105.

DOUGHERTY, J. E., "SIDS: The silent killer," *Emergency*, 19, no. 10 (October 1987), p. 38.

Fact Sheet: SIDS Information for the EMT. Rosslyn, Va: National SIDS Clearinghouse, 1983.

Fact Sheet: Current Research in Sudden Infant Death Syndrome. Rosslyn, Va: National SIDS Clearinghouse, 1984.

LAWRENCE, D., "SIDS: Handle with care," *JEMS* 13, no. 12 (December 1988), pp. 51–53.

WEDDINGTON, W. W., "Immobilization as a reaction to sudden death," *Resident and Staff Physician* (September 1982), pp. 69–71.

ZEBEL, B. H., and WOOLSEY, S. F., "SIDS and the family: The pediatrician's role," *Pediatric Annals*, 13, no 3 (March 1984), p. 237.

16

Suicide in Children and Adolescents

OBJECTIVES

When you have completed this chapter you should be able to

✱ Recognize the potential of a suicide attempt or gesture in the child or adolescent.

✱ Describe appropriate ways to communicate with the suicidal child or adolescent.

Suicide and Suicide Attempts

Suicide and suicide attempts are difficult situations to handle when the patient is an adult. However, it becomes an incomprehensible and highly charged emotional event when the person is a child or adolescent. You must be able to recognize potential suicidal behavior in the child. Recognition, evaluation, and documentation of this behavior are vital to receiving hospital personnel. Rapid decisions and referrals for psychosocial intervention must be made early to assure the child's protection from further harmful acts.

Suicide is a self-inflicted injury that results in death. A *suicide attempt or gesture* refers to an attention-seeking behavior that threatens suicide often without any real effort to die. All suicide attempts or gestures must be taken seriously and the child should be considered at high risk for further suicidal behavior.

Epidemiology

Incidence

- Suicide has been identified in preschoolers as young as $2\frac{1}{2}$ years of age.

- Each year in the United States over 12,000 children ages 5 to 14 are admitted to psychiatric hospitals because of suicidal ideations or behavior.

- Suicide is five times as frequent in the 5–14-year age group as is meningitis.

- The suicide rate for youths 15 to 19 years of age has tripled over the last three decades and is now thought to be the second leading cause of death for this age group.

- Males commit suicide three times more frequently than females in all age groups. However, more males 12 years and under will attempt suicide than will females; the sex distribution reverses itself after 12 years of age.

- The suicide rate, though equally distributed among all socioeconomic groups, is more common in white teenagers than in blacks, and the risk is considerably higher for teens who are unemployed or married.

The actual number of suicides in children is unknown for a variety of reasons. Many suicides are masked as accidents, such as single-car crashes with the driver as the only passenger. Ingestions of poisons in children 5 years and older are highly suspicious. Parents may actually try to conceal suicide attempts because of strong feelings of failure and guilt, denial, and a tendency to minimize the suicidal ideations of their children.

Physicians and medical examiners are often unwilling to record suicide as a cause of death owing to a lack of clear-cut evidence or to keep from stigmatizing the parents. Sometimes the parents themselves will request that suicide not be recorded on the death certificate.

Mechanism of Injury

The methods that children will use to commit or attempt suicide vary by age group. Children 10 years or under will, typically, stab themselves or set themselves on fire. Older children and adolescents commonly use firearms (especially males), hanging, self-poisoning, and single-car crashes as the method. According to a recent study, 70% of adolescents who are successful or failed suicide victims chose firearms as the method. Further evidence shows that suicide by firearms is directly related to their availability.

Psychosocial Risk Factors

Disruption within the family unit, *intrafamilial*, is often the primary factor that contributes to the suicidal ideations of the younger child. Disruptions outside the family unit, *extrafamilial*, often increase in significance as the child gets older (see Table 16.1).

Developmental Concepts of Death and Related Suicidal Ideations

Under 3 Years of Age

Infants and toddlers, up to about 3 years of age, view death as separation.

3 to 7 Years of Age

Children from 3 to 7 years of age are unable to grasp death as permanent and will personify death; for example, death is a wicked witch or a monster in the closet. During a crisis, death may be viewed as desirable and a temporary means of escape. Children may even fantasize about their own death. For example, they fantasize themselves lying in a coffin while family members are crying and wishing them back to life, making statements such as, "I should never have yelled at her, and if she comes back I'll give her everything she wants." This age group is incapable, developmentally, of skills of strategy and foresight. This is particularly dangerous because it leads to impulsive behavior.

7 to 12 Years of Age

Children initially begin to grasp the permanency of death between the ages of 7 and 12; however, 50% of 12-year-olds still believe death is not permanent, but reversible. This age group does not differentiate between thoughts and actions; therefore, they view suicidal thoughts and actions as the same thing. They are developmentally capable of strategy and foresight and will premeditate, or plan, when and how to commit suicide.

TABLE 16.1 Psychosocial Risk Factors of Suicide Behavior in Children and Adolescents

Family Influences	Other Societal Influences
Divorce	Peer pressure
Death of parent or other family member (sibling, grandparent)	Fear of being different
	Low self-esteem
Separation—actual or threatened	Graduation from high school
Rejection—real or imagined	Loss of love relationship
Child abuse or neglect	Drug abuse
	Uncertainty about future
	Imitation-contagion theory
	Depression
	Legal problems

12 Years through Adolescence

Adolescents generally begin to recognize that death is permanent. It is important to remember that this age group is exposed to high family stress as well as increasing peer group and societal stress, which puts them at higher risk for suicide than any other age group (refer to Table 16.1).

Children may vary from the development ages listed above owing to a variety of environmental factors and life experiences. The sex of the child can also determine his/her emotional and developmental level at any particular age. Therefore, the individual child should be considered when doing your assessment using the above information only as a guide.

Common Misconceptions About Suicide

There are many misconceptions about suicide that apply to all age groups. Becoming aware of these is key to the complete management of the suicidal child. Some of the most common misconceptions are listed below.

Those Who Talk About Suicide Never Do It

Many children will make an attempt, usually verbally, to let someone know. They may not come right out and say "I'm going to kill myself"; rather, they may say, "I want to die" or "Nobody cares about me anyway." *Take these statements seriously! They are a cry for help.*

Suicide Happens Without Warning

Numerous hints or warnings are often given either verbally or in the form of gestures, such as becoming accident prone or taking only a few pills. The child may give away cherished belongings to a friend or sibling. These are nonverbal clues to suicide ideations.

Once Suicidal, Always Suicidal

There is a 24–72-hour peak danger period following a crisis. Children tend to believe that the pain they are feeling will continue forever. They do not have the life experiences to recall and remember that the pain they are feeling is temporary and will eventually subside, probably within a few days.

Once an Attempt Is Survived, There Will Never Be Another Attempt

There is a high risk for future attempts if prior attempts are not followed by psychosocial intervention. Future attempts become more lethal and usually occur within a year of the first attempt. You can reduce the chance of future attempts by relaying pertinent information to the appropriate medical personnel so that psychosocial intervention can begin early in the child's medical care.

Suicide Victims Always Leave Notes

Only a small number of individuals leave notes. This is one of the reasons why many suicides are classified as accidents.

*Never Use the Word "Suicide" When Talking
with Children: It May Give Them the Idea*

The word *suicide* won't put the idea into the mind of a child who is not suicidal. Using the word can actually invite the suicidal child to verbalize feelings of despair. It can help establish rapport and trust by showing the child that you are taking his or her feelings seriously.

Suicide Is Hereditary

Though the tendency may be increased in a family with a prior suicide, it is not genetically inherited. A child may view the suicide of a family member as an appropriate way to solve a problem. Typically, children have not yet learned how to cope effectively, reduce stress, and work toward a more promising future.

History and Assessment

A complete history should be obtained from the child and any available family members. Note and document all pertinent information heard and seen at the scene.

- Is there a note, pill bottles, a firearm, rope, etc.?
- Listen and communicate directly with the child, whenever possible.

The "High Risk–Low Rescue Factors" outlined below should be used to *evaluate the child's degree of suicidal risk* at this time. Talking with the child will promote building trust and rapport with the child. There will be times when the family or a family member hinders your efforts to obtain this information. You may have to separate the child from this person or persons. Do this in a calm and compassionate manner. It may be as simple as letting the family member ride in the front of the ambulance so that you can talk privately to the child in the back. It is important for information about the child, the family situation, and the environment to be documented and passed on to the personnel at the medical facility.

High Risk–Low Rescue Factors

- Did the attempt take place in isolation and at a time when discovery was unlikely?
- Did the child not seek help before, during, or after the attempt?
- Was a final act performed; for example, did the child give away cherished possessions?
- Was the expected outcome death?
- Was premeditation present?
- Was a suicide note written?

An answer of yes to any or all of the above questions shows that the child is at high risk. The child's rescue was accidental and unintended by the child. Document the information gathered. This child needs immediate psychosocial intervention.

Management

ALS and BLS providers must provide prompt care treating the self-inflicted injury as well as offering psychological support during transport.

- Assess and monitor ABC's.
- Manage all life-threatening injuries.
- Use caution to preserve evidence for potential police investigation. You may need to request police backup.
- Transport the child with the parents whenever possible.
- Remember to document and pass on both medical reports and discussions with the child to the receiving hospital personnel.

Psychological Support During Management and Transport

Provide psychological support to the child using the following guidelines of appropriate interventions.

- Ensure a safe environment.
- Isolate the child from further tension and provocation.
- Move the child to a private area whenever possible.
- Take the child's threats seriously. This will help gain the child's trust and assist you in establishing rapport with the child. It is possible that you may be the first person that has not negated the patient's feelings.
- Listen with interest and sensitivity. Only one responder should work directly with the child. Others should remain present but silent.
- Offer support, understanding, and compassion for what the child is telling you. Let them know that you are there to help them.
- Validate the child's feelings. This does not mean that you agree with their actions but you can relate, to some degree, to their feelings of hopelessness and despair.
- Avoid making statements such as "I know how you feel" as this may bring out a negative response. Instead, say something to the effect of, "I understand why you feel so lonely" or "That must have made you very sad."
- Question the child about the attempt. Ask what happened to make life so difficult, and where did the pills, gun, etc., come from. Ask children who attempt suicide why they did what they did and what they thought would happen. Find out when they first thought about doing this and if they ever attempted suicide in the past. If they tell you they have attempted suicide in the past, find out when. Find out if there is anyone to stop them. They may be alone most of the time.

Avoid the following inappropriate behaviors or actions when caring for the suicidal child.

- *DO NOT* act judgmental, either verbally or nonverbally. Examples of this are saying something to the effect of: "Why would you do such a silly thing?" or "You're such a pretty girl and you have so much to live for." Rolling your eyes at a response is an example of nonverbal judgmental behavior.
- *DO NOT* make moral judgments. While the situation that caused the child's suicidal behavior may seem silly to you, it is very real and painful to them. Children cannot rationalize situations like

adults can because they lack experience in coping with difficult situations.

- *DO NOT* make light of the situation.

- *DO NOT* argue with the child about his or her feelings. Examples of this are saying something to the effect that "You don't really feel that way." Obviously they do or they would not attempt to commit suicide.

- *DO NOT* discount the child's desire to die. For example, you can say "It's OK to feel like you want to die, but to try to kill yourself is not acceptable." This is the difference between feelings and actions, which is a difficult concept for children to understand.

Reactions of the EMS Provider

It is common for the prehospital care provider to have a very strong emotional reaction associated with a suicide or attempted suicide, especially when it involves a child. You may feel anger, both toward the child and the parents, as well as depression or anxiety. Helplessness is a common emotion EMTs and other people feel when someone contemplates suicide or actually commits the act.

Finally, it is of utmost importance to your emotional well-being to remember that it is not within your power to keep someone from committing suicide if that person really wants to die. Do not accept responsibility for someone's actions beyond providing that individual with the best medical care you are able to provide. Consult Chapter 17, "Crisis and Stress Management," for assistance with your own response to this type of rescue.

Suicide References

BASSAK, E. L., and others, *Behavioral Emergencies: A Field Guide for EMT's and Paramedics.* Boston: Little, Brown, 1983.

BRENT, D. A., PERPER, J. A., and ALLMAN, C. J., "Alcohol, firearms, and suicide among youth," *Journal of the American Medical Association,* 257, no. 24 (June 26, 1987), pp. 3369–3372.

CAPUZZI, D., "Adolescent suicide: Preventions and intervention," *Counseling and Human Development,* 19, no. 2 (1986), pp. 1–9.

CHRISTOFFEL, K. K., and others, "Adolescent suicide and suicide attempts: A population study," *Pediatric Emergency Care,* 4, no. 1 (March 1988), pp. 32–40.

CUMMING, P., "This is our child, this is your patient," *Caring,* (November 1986), p. 30.

EISENBERG, L., "Does bad news about suicide beget bad news?" *New England Journal of Medicine,* 315, no. 11 (Sept. 11, 1986), pp. 705–707.

FINIGAN, J., "Assessment of childhood and adolescent depression and suicide potential," *Journal of Emergency Nursing,* 12, no. 1 (January 1986), pp. 35–38.

MESSIER, L. D., "Suicide." In Mitchell, J. T., and Resnik, H. P., eds., *Emergency Response to Crisis.* Bowie, Md.: Robert J. Brady Co., 1981.

ROSENTHAL, R. A., and ROSENTHAL, S., "Suicide behavior by preschool children," *American Journal of Psychiatry,* 141, no. 4 (April 1984), pp. 520–525.

SHAW, K. R., SHEEHAN, K. H., and FERNANDEZ, R. C., "Suicide in children and adolescents," *Advances in Pediatrics,* 34 (1987), pp. 313–334.

VALENTE, S. M., "Assessing suicide risk in the school-age child," *Journal of Pediatric Health Care,* 1, no. 1 (January/February 1987), pp. 14–20.

WEISMAN, A. D., and others, "Risk-rescue rating in suicide assessment," *Archives of General Psychiatry,* 26 (June 1972), pp. 553–560.

17

Crisis and Stress Management

OBJECTIVES

When you have completed this chapter you should be able to

* Identify the psychological hazards of the EMS profession.
* Describe the differences among acute, delayed, and cumulative stress reactions.
* Describe the coping strategies that help reduce stress before, during, and after an event.
* Describe a debriefing session.

Work and Stress

EMS providers care very much about their work and about others. They dedicate enormous numbers of hours, in addition to their regular jobs, as professional volunteers on a rescue squad. Often, paid EMS professionals volunteer after hours on a unit in their community. These are people who place themselves at risk for a high degree of stress in their lives. This stress should not automatically be considered harmful stress, unless the providers do not recognize and accept its existence, or that their reactions to it are normal. Learned coping mechanisms and techniques for stress management make the difference between surviving stress or being harmed by it.

Characteristics of the EMS Profession

Personalities

EMS professionals are action oriented, like to be needed, and have a high level of energy. They are willing to take risks, make sacrifices, and do not give up easily, even when faced with overwhelming odds. They like to maintain control and are sensitive, yet many have learned to suppress their emotions to events that those outside of the profession cannot.

Job Qualities

Many aspects of the EMS profession can be considered exhilarating. It is a profession that attracts specially trained personnel and tests them beyond the breaking point, causing them to feel elite when they are successful. However, these are the very qualities that can create high levels of stress and stressful environments. For example, consider the following scenario: The scene is such that your abilities are tested to their limit; the patient is seriously ill or in a seriously injured state, and the management of the scene is at its most difficult. There is a long extrication, and bystanders are difficult to handle, *yet the patient survives.* You can be left feeling elite and good about yourself, your co-workers, and the work you do. You feel great personal reward for your efforts.

But how often does the scenario, described above, occur? How often were you told, early on in your career, that a "save" is the exception rather than the rule? More often than not the scenario goes more like this: The scene is a difficult one, with bystanders pulling and yelling at you. The weather is miserable; it's cold or hot, it's pouring rain or else snowing. Then the rescue takes longer than usual. The last crew shift did not have time to restock the ambulance, and you are missing necessary supplies. You need and use every skill you've ever learned, but the patient is going downhill fast. You've been pushed to the limit of your endurance and you've met the challenge, but the patient doesn't survive.

Both scenarios create stress; the difference is that the first resulted in a positive response to that stress; the second, a negative response leaving you feeling angry, frustrated, unsure of yourself and your abilities.

Occupational Hazards

As was mentioned in the chapters on child abuse and suicide, dealing with children can intensify your stress reactions, especially if the event results in death or injury from abuse, neglect, or suicide. However, children in general rank high on the list of occupational hazards that create a high degree of stress attributable to a variety of emotional and societal factors.

Children bring out the protective side of adults, whether they are parents or not. Children are cute, small, and vulnerable, evoking our sense of responsibility and desire to take care of them. They are young and we envision them growing up, not dying. Our society places a higher value on children; they are our future. Our feelings tend to come closer to the surface when confronted with a child, and these feelings are intensified when a child's life is at risk. Many EMS professionals have reported that becoming a parent themselves increased their level of stress reaction to ill and injured children. These are some of the underlying emotional and societal factors that create an environment that sets us up for stronger-than-normal stress reactions. Additionally, the injury or death of someone you know, the injury or death of one of your own colleagues, or any event that draws extraordinary media coverage also rank high on the list of events that can create high stress.

 **CAUTION!**

Stress must be recognized as a real potential for disrupting your mental health and well-being. It must be accepted as a real part of EMS, and when combined with stressful events related to family, friends, and/or additional jobs, the reaction to the stress of a particular event, or chain of events, increases. 

Types of Stress

Acute

Acute stress happens at the time the personnel is engaged in rescue efforts. It can cause mental and emotional breakdown, sometimes resulting in cardiac arrest. Symptoms can include physical, cognitive, and emotional reactions. See Table 17.1 for the range of signs and symptoms commonly identified.

Delayed Posttraumatic Stress

Delayed stress reactions can occur minutes to weeks, months, or sometimes years after a stressful event. Signs and symptoms of a delayed stress reaction include the following:

- Increased feelings of anxiety, depression, and irritability;
- Sleep disturbances;
- Changes in eating habits;
- Loss of emotional control;

- Feelings of isolation;
- Decreased sexual drive and menstrual cycle changes;
- Decreased interest in loved ones;
- Increased marital disharmony;
- Changes in personality and behavior;
- Flashbacks;
- Marked differences in job performance.

There are three primary characteristics of delayed posttraumatic stress. These include the following:

- Intrusive mental images. These can be in the form of dreams, nightmares, or flashbacks.
- Fear of repetition of the event, either real or imagined. The event remains so powerful that one begins to avoid activities associated with the event.
- Physical and emotional symptoms include sleep disturbances, fatigue, depression, and irritability.

Cumulative Stress

Cumulative stress is a state of chronic fatigue and frustration resulting from many disappointments and unrelieved stress. It is sometimes referred to as "burnout" and is difficult to differentiate from clinical depression. Signs and symptoms of cumulative stress include the following:

- Depression;
- Fatigue;
- Irritability;
- Apathy and disillusionment;
- Excessive defensiveness and withdrawal;
- Increased use of alcohol and drug abuse;
- Loss of energy;
- Increased illness.

TABLE 17.1 Signs and Symptoms of Acute Stress Reaction

Physical	Cognitive	Emotional
Nausea and upset stomach	Impaired thinking and decision making	Anxiety
Profuse sweating and tremors	Poor concentration and confusion	Fear
Dizziness and disorientation	Difficulty performing calculations	Grief and depression
Lack of coordination	Loss of memory	Feeling lost and abandoned
Increased heart rate	Concentration problems	Withdrawal
Increased blood pressure	Flashbacks	Anger
Headaches, muscle soreness	Poor attention span	Feeling shocked, numb, and overwhelmed
Difficulty sleeping		

Source: Adapted from Mitchell, J. T., Maryland Crisis Intervention and Preparedness Team, Baltimore, Maryland Institute for Emergency Medical Services System, 1985.

Crisis and Stress Management

Management and Coping Skills

The following recommendations should be used as guidelines to help you manage and cope with the stress associated with the emotionally charged work you perform daily.

- Obtain extensive EMS training; being well prepared can help prevent additional stress.
- Be part of a team; it can help reduce feelings of isolation.
- Learn communication skills and stress-management techniques.
- Establish social and psychological support groups.
- Learn deep-breathing skills; this helps to diffuse tension and increase attention.
- Use physical exercise, brisk walking, jogging, or calisthenics as a method to reduce a stress reaction. This should be done within a few hours after an event.
- Eat healthy meals, high in vitamins and protein.
- Try to maintain a normal schedule and avoid boredom.
- Express your feelings.
- Attend a Critical Incident Stress Debriefing when available.

The following actions may interfere with your ability to cope with stress.

- *DO NOT* use excessive humor to break tension. It may hurt the feelings of bystanders and colleagues.
- *DO NOT* exaggerate efforts to control your emotions. Expressing emotions is healthier than suppressing them.
- *DO NOT* consume alcohol and/or drugs; they will only temporarily mask a stress response.
- *DO NOT* consume large doses of caffeine or sugar; they can heighten your stress reaction.
- *DO NOT* fight too hard against dreams and flashbacks; they are a normal response to a stressful event and will diminish over time.

Critical Incident Stress Debriefings (CISD's)

CISD's are group sessions for everyone involved in the stressful event. They are conducted by one or two mental health professionals and peer-support personnel who have been trained to assist the group to express their feelings and work through stressful events in EMS. CISD's are held within 24 to 72 hours after the event and attendance is voluntary.

If a Critical Incident Stress Debriefing is not offered after a highly stressful event, request one. If you are experiencing signs and symptoms of stress it is likely that others involved in the incident are also experiencing them. If your symptoms persist beyond 6 weeks, seek additional help from a mental health professional experienced in crisis intervention and/or EMS providers and the problems they encounter in the field. Remember, without appropriate intervention a stress reaction can become damaging to your mental health and well-being.

Crisis and Stress References

BASSUK, E. L., and others, *Behavioral Emergencies: A Field Guide for EMT's and Paramedics.* Boston: Little, Brown, 1983.

MITCHELL, J. T., and DONOHOE, M. A., "Critical incident stress: A videotape for emergency personnel." Catonsville: University of Maryland, Baltimore County, 1985.

MITCHELL, J. T., and RESNIK, H. P., *Emergency Response to Crisis.* Bowie, Md.: Robert J. Brady Co., 1981.

Index

EMS profession (*cont.*)
  job qualities, 236
  occupational hazards, 237
  personalities, 236
Epidural hemorrhage, 164
Epiglottic folds, 29
Epiglottitis:
  assessment, 109–10
  history, 109
  management, 110–12
Epinephrine, 90, 91, 94, 98, 105, 215
Epiphyseal fractures, 179
Epiphyseal plate, 178
Exposure, 155–56
  assessment, 155–56
  management, 156
External jugular placement, 68
Extremities, 32, 42
  management, 158–59
  palpitation of, 42
  secondary trauma survey, 158–59
Extremity injuries, 177–81
  fractures, 177–79
    types of, 178–79
Eyes, chemical burns to, 191

F

Face mask, 51
Facial contusions, 164
Fear, 2–3
  and blood pressure readings, 41
  in infants, 5–6
  in parents, 16–17
  in toddlers, 7
Febrile seizures, 114
Fever, *See* Hyperthermia
Fireworks injuries, 185
First-degree burns, 187
Flail chest, 150, 176
Flame burns, 184–85
Flushing:
  of eye to remove poisons, 145
  localized, 37
Fontanelles, 27
Forehead contusions, 164
Fractures, 32, 177–79
  compartment syndrome, 180
  open fracture, 180
  potential for disability, 179
  splinting management, 180–81
  types of, 22

G

Gastrointestinal system, effect of drugs/poison
    on, 140–41
Glasgow Coma Scale (GCS), 155, 166
  modifications for infants, 43
Green-stick fracture, 179
Grunting, 38
Gurgling, 38

H

Hallucinogens, effect on body systems, 141
Head, 27–28
Head injury, 156–57, 162–70
  assessment, 166
    increase intracranial pressure, 167–68
    secondary survey, 166
  characteristics of, 168
  history, 164–65
  incidence of, 162
  intubation risks, 169
  management, 168–69
  mechanism of, 162
  patient care, 164–69
  physiology, 162–63
  and shock, 166
  types of, 163–64
Hearing, sense of, 4
Heart and circulation, 31–32
Heart rate, 40
Heated oxygen, 50
Heat stroke, 115
Hemophilus influenzae, 109, 120
Hemorrhage, 158, 164
Hemothrorax, 174
High-pitched cry, 38
High-technology equipment, children dependent
    on, 133–34
High-voltage electrical burns, management of,
    192
Hoarseness, 38, 107
Honesty, 4, 19, 35
Hospice care, and terminal illness, 134
Humidified oxygen, 50
Hydrocarbons, effect on body systems, 141
Hyperactive children, and child abuse, 196–97
Hyperthermia (fever), 107, 114–16
  assessment, 114–15
  history, 114
  management, 115–16
  sponging, 116
Hypoglycemia, 118, 130–31
  assessment, 130
  history, 130
  management, 130–31
Hypotension, 31
Hypothermia, 27, 40, 95, 116–18, 155
  assessment, 117
  history, 117
  management, 117–18
  in newborns, 208
    prevention of, 211
  severe, drowning with, 96
  signs/symptoms, 117
Hypovolemic shock, 153–54, 168–69
  signs of, 166
Hypoxemia, 31, 134, 154, 168
  causes that result in cardiac arrest, 78
  in newborns, 208
Hypoxia, 220
Hysterical behavior, toward EMT, 22